Early Detection and Management of Mental Disorders

Early Detection and Management of Mental Disorders

Edited by

Mario Maj
University of Naples, Italy

Juan José López-Ibor
Complutense University of Madrid, Spain

Norman Sartorius
University of Geneva, Switzerland

Mitsumoto Sato
Tohuko University School of Medicine, Sendai, Japan

Ahmed Okasha
Ain Shams University, Cairo, Egypt

WILEY

Telephone (+44) 1243 779777

Email (for orders and customer service enquiries): cs-books@wiley.co.uk
Visit our Home Page on www.wileyeurope.com or www.wiley.com

Other Wiley Editorial Offices

John Wiley & Sons Inc., 111 River Street, Hoboken, NJ 07030, USA

Jossey-Bass, 989 Market Street, San Francisco, CA 94103-1741, USA

Wiley-VCH Verlag GmbH, Boschstr. 12, D-69469 Weinheim, Germany

John Wiley & Sons Australia Ltd, 33 Park Road, Milton, Queensland 4064, Australia

John Wiley & Sons (Asia) Pte Ltd, 2 Clementi Loop #02-01, Jin Xing Distripark, Singapore 129809

John Wiley & Sons Canada Ltd, 22 Worcester Road, Etobicoke, Ontario, Canada M9W 1L1

Wiley also publishes its books in a variety of electronic formats. Some content that appears in print may not be available in electronic books.

Library of Congress Cataloging-in-Publication Data

Early detection and management of mental disorders / edited by Mario Maj ... [et al.].
p. ; cm.
Includes bibliographical references and index.
ISBN 0-470-01083-5 (alk. paper)
1. Mental illness – Diagnosis. 2. Mental illness – Treatment. 3. Psychiatry. I. Maj, Mario, 1953–
[DNLM: 1. Mental Disorders – diagnosis. 2. Early Diagnosis. WM 141 E12 2005]
RC469.E217 2005
616.89–dc22

2004055349

British Library Cataloguing in Publication Data

A catalogue record for this book is available from the British Library

ISBN 0-470-01083-5

Typeset in 10/12pt Palatino by Dobbie Typesetting Ltd, Tavistock, Devon
Printed and bound in Great Britain by TJ International Ltd, Padstow, Cornwall
This book is printed on acid-free paper responsibly manufactured from sustainable forestry in which at least two trees are planted for each one used for paper production.

Contents

List of Contributors

Hagop S. Akiskal International Mood Center, Department of Psychiatry, University of California at San Diego, 9500 Gilman Drive, La Jolla, CA 92093-0603, USA

Kareen Akiskal International Mood Center, Department of Psychiatry, University of California at San Diego, 9500 Gilman Drive, La Jolla, CA 92093-0603, USA

Paul Carey Medical Research Council Unit on Anxiety Disorders, Department of Psychiatry, University of Stellenbosch, PO Box 19063, Tygerberg 7505, Cape Town, South Africa

Regina C. Casper Department of Psychiatry and Behavioral Sciences, Stanford University Medical School, 401 Quarry Road, Stanford, CA 94305-5723, USA

Jane Edwards Early Psychosis Prevention and Intervention Centre, Department of Psychiatry, University of Melbourne, Locked Bag 10, Parkville, 3052 Victoria, Australia

Adrienne K. Elliott National Institute of Mental Health, Section on Clinical and Experimental Neuropsychology, Suite 203-B, 5415 West Cedar Lane, MSC 2615, Bethesda, MD 20892-2615, USA

Heinz Häfner Schizophrenia Research Unit, Central Institute of Mental Health, J5, D-68159 Mannheim, Germany

Brian Harvey School of Pharmacy, Division of Pharmacology, North West University, Private Bag X6001, Potchefstroom 2520, South Africa

Joon Kang Department of Child and Adolescent Psychiatry, Children's Hospital of Philadelphia, 34th & Civic Center Blvd, Philadelphia, PA 19104, USA

Iris Manor Geha Psychiatric Hospital, PO Box 102, 49100 Petach-Tikvah, Israel

Gabriele Masi IRCCS Stella Maris, Scientific Institute of Child Neurology and Psychiatry, University of Pisa, Via Dei Giacinti 2, 56018 Calambrone (Pisa), Italy

Kurt Maurer Schizophrenia Research Unit, Central Institute of Mental Health, J5, D-68159 Mannheim, Germany

Patrick McGorry Early Psychosis Prevention and Intervention Centre, Department of Psychiatry, University of Melbourne, Locked Bag 10, Parkville, 3052 Victoria, Australia

Allan F. Mirsky National Institute of Mental Health, Section on Clinical and Experimental Neuropsychology, Suite 203-B, 5415 West Cedar Lane, MSC 2615, Bethesda, MD 20892-2615, USA

Soraya Seedat Medical Research Council Unit on Anxiety Disorders, Department of Psychiatry, University of Stellenbosch, PO Box 19063, Tygerberg 7505, Cape Town, South Africa

Roomana Sheikh Department of Child and Adolescent Psychiatry, Drexel University College of Medicine, Eppi, 3200 Henry Avenue, Philadelphia, PA 19129, USA

Dan J. Stein Medical Research Council Unit on Anxiety Disorders, Department of Psychiatry, University of Stellenbosch, PO Box 19063, Tygerberg 7505, Cape Town, South Africa

Sam Tyano Geha Psychiatric Hospital, PO Box 102, 49100 Petach-Tikvah, Israel

Andre Tylee Health Services Research Department, Section of Primary Care Mental Health, Institute of Psychiatry, King's College, De Crespigny Park, London SE5 8AF, UK

Paul Walters Health Services Research Department, Section of Primary Care Mental Health, Institute of Psychiatry, King's College, De Crespigny Park, London SE5 8AF, UK

Elizabeth Weller Department of Child and Adolescent Psychiatry, Children's Hospital of Philadelphia, 34th & Civic Center Blvd, Philadelphia, PA 19104, USA

Ronald Weller Department of Psychiatry, University of Pennsylvania, 3535 Market Street, 2nd Floor, Philadelphia, PA 19104, USA

Alison Yung Early Psychosis Prevention and Intervention Centre, Department of Psychiatry, University of Melbourne, Locked Bag 10, Parkville, 3052 Victoria, Australia

Michael Zaudig Windach Hospital and Institute for Neurobehavioral Research and Therapy, Schützenstraße 16, 86949 Windach, Germany

Preface

A common theme in the recent literature on most mental disorders is that they often remain undetected and untreated for quite a long time, not rarely for several years, after the occurrence of their first manifestations. For some disorders – namely bipolar disorder, schizophrenia and some anxiety disorders – clinical research has directly documented the average interval between their onset and the time of their diagnosis and the start of appropriate treatment. For depressive disorders, a different way to document the same phenomenon has been the finding that a high proportion of cases are missed by general practitioners, although part of them are recognized in subsequent consultations. For other conditions – especially eating disorders and some anxiety disorders – the main focus has been on the multiple barriers to help seeking, which often delay recognition and treatment. In the case of Alzheimer's disease, neuropsychological and biological research has been decisive in documenting the latency between the first manifestations of the disease and the clinical diagnosis.

The argument underlying this vast and diverse body of literature has been that an early diagnosis and management of the various disorders may be essential in improving their course and outcome and in reducing or even preventing their social consequences. This hypothesis has received up to now only a partial empirical support for most of the above-mentioned disorders, but represents a major focus of research for virtually all of them. Moreover, it has been repeatedly pointed out that the reconstruction of the early phases of development of mental disorders may contribute significantly to the elucidation of their etiopathogenesis and, in the case of some of them, may allow devising prevention programmes.

Early detection and management of a mental disorder implies the availability of a thorough description of the prodromal manifestations of the disorder, the existence of assessment and screening instruments with a satisfactory sensitivity and specificity, the feasibility of screening programmes in the general population or in vulnerable groups, the successful engagement of a significant proportion of the subjects found to be at high risk, and the availability of validated programmes of intervention focused on the early phases of the disorder. All these elements are currently being developed for most of the above-mentioned mental disorders, and are already part of clinical practice in several contexts for some of them (notably schizophrenia).

This volume aims to provide an update on this complex and dynamic area of research and clinical practice, with a description of the precursors and prodromes of the various mental disorders (more or less extensive and detailed, depending on the current state of knowledge and on the complexity of the individual disorders); an outline of the available instruments for the assessment of the prodromal symptoms of the disorders and, when available, for their screening in the general population or in vulnerable groups; and a critical review of the screening, management and preventive interventions which have been tested up to now by empirical research. Emphasis is laid on the importance of sensitizing general practitioners to the early manifestations of the various disorders, and on the complexity of the ethical issues which arise in relation to the recognition and management of early psychosis.

Two chapters focus on research conducted in the offspring of patients with schizophrenia and bipolar disorder, because of the essential contribution that such research can provide to the elucidation of clinical, personological and biological precursors, of possible resilience factors, and of the prodromal symptoms and signs of these disorders. One chapter deals with the differential diagnosis of mental disorders in children, emphasizing the risk of overdiagnosis as well as of underdiagnosis of these disorders, the problems raised by psychiatric comorbidity and diagnostic instability in this age group, and the role of the environment in shaping the clinical picture of the disorders.

We hope that this volume will contribute to call the attention of psychiatrists and other mental health professionals to this rapidly growing and fascinating area of modern psychiatry, and to encourage some of them to approach it with the appropriate dose of optimism and pragmatism.

Mario Maj
Juan José López-Ibor
Norman Sartorius
Mitsumoto Sato
Ahmed Okasha

This volume includes several chapters developed from presentations delivered at the 12th World Congress of Psychiatry (Yokohama, Japan, 24–29 August, 2002).

CHAPTER

1

Prodromal Symptoms and Early Detection of Schizophrenia

Heinz Häfner and Kurt Maurer

Schizophrenia Research Unit, Central Institute of Mental Health, Mannheim, Germany

INTRODUCTION

Prodromal symptoms occurring before the first-ever onset or relapse of schizophrenia were observed a long time ago. In 1861 the pioneer of modern, scientifically oriented psychiatry, the Berlin-based psychiatrist Wilhelm Griesinger [1], described a melancholic prodromal stage that tends to precede psychosis. Kraepelin [2] described a series of "minor changes in mood, which may be recurrent or persist for weeks, months or even for years as the only premonitory signs of an imminent mental disorder". The main symptoms of this "stage of the prodrome" were "increased irritability and moodiness, restlessness, unmotivated spells of high or frequently low spirits... Further prodromal signs that can be observed frequently are absent-mindedness, lack of interest or markedly increased activity".

Bleuler [3] called this premonitory stage latent schizophrenia and described it as characterized by irritability, introversion and eccentric behaviour. He put forward the hypothesis, later revived by Häfner [4] and Maier *et al.* [5], that the underlying disease process may come to a halt at any stage of its early development. Such a process ending prematurely may bring forth mild, nonpsychotic symptoms such as schizoid or schizotypal personality disorders.

In the period during and following World War I research on the topic lacked in vigour, but was soon resumed by Sullivan [6] in a hope of finding reliable early prognostic indicators of psychosis as a basis for early treatment. Proceeding from a psychoanalytical–psychodynamic theory, Sullivan based his explicatory models on neurotic reaction patterns, such as hysteria, neurasthenia and obsessive–compulsive reactions. The sequence of these reaction patterns at the prodromal stage of psychosis

Early Detection and Management of Mental Disorders.
Edited by Mario Maj, Juan José López-Ibor, Norman Sartorius, Mitsumoto Sato and Ahmed Okasha.
 ISBN 0-470-01083-5.

was seen by Sullivan as a hierarchical sequence of neurotic defence mechanisms adopted to fend off more severe psychopathology as the disorder progresses.

After Sullivan's unsuccessful endeavours to find reliable prognostic indicators of incipient psychosis, Cameron [7,8] set out to study the prodromal stage of schizophrenia in greater detail by clinical methods. Cameron [7] was also the first to assess the duration of untreated psychosis (DUP): 32.4% of the patients he studied had suffered from more or less rapidly accumulating psychotic symptoms for up to six months from their onset until first admission, 17.5% for six months to two years and 48.1% for more than two years. He found [8] that 83% of these patients first admitted because of schizophrenia had suffered a prepsychotic prodromal stage marked by deteriorating functioning, affective blunting, social withdrawal and bizarre thoughts and convictions. In most cases the prepsychotic prodromal stage showed a smooth transition to paranoid delusions and other positive symptoms of full-blown psychosis.

Cameron defined the DUP by two timepoints that can be determined fairly reliably, i.e. by onset of psychotic symptoms and first admission. For this reason his estimates can be compared with results based on similar definitions from more recent studies, as reflected in the similarity of the results [9,10] presented in Table 1.1.

STAGE MODELS OF THE EARLY COURSE OF SCHIZOPHRENIA

Conrad's Model

The first stage model of the early course of schizophrenia was proposed by the Marburg-based psychiatrist Conrad [21], who studied 107 German soldiers admitted to a military hospital because of a mostly acute schizophrenic psychosis during World War II. On the basis of the symptoms and complaints reported by the patients, Conrad developed four – and a rarer fifth – stages of evolving and two stages of remitting schizophrenia.

Stage 1, called *trema*, could last for several years. Conrad described it as characterized by uncertainty, depression, anxiety, suspiciousness, first signs of attenuated delusions and social withdrawal. He likened what patients at this stage feel to the anxiety that takes possession of actors before entering the stage.

The next stage, *apophany*, brings forth strange experiences that the patients cannot explain, fully elaborated psychotic symptoms – hallucinations,

TABLE 1.1 Duration of the prephase of schizophrenia from onset (first sign, first psychotic symptom) until first contact or first admission (modified from Häfner *et al.* [10])

Study	*n*	Duration from first sign (in years)	Duration from first psychotic symptom (in years)
Gross [11]	290	3.5	
Lindelius [12]	237		4.4
Huber *et al.* [13]	502	3.3	
Loebel *et al.* [14]	70	2.9	1.0
Beiser *et al.* [15]	70	2.1	1.0
McGorry *et al.* [16]	200	2.1	1.4
Lewine [17]	97		1.9
Häfner *et al.* [18]	232	4.8	1.1
Johannessen *et al.* [19]	43		2.2
Ho *et al.* [20]	156	2.7	1.4

delusions, thought disorders etc. – and derealization. Insight and reality control are lost.

The third stage was called by Conrad *anastrophae*. It is characterized by formal thought disorder and a delusional-projective attribution of inexplicable experiences to external causes, which Conrad interpreted as secondary delusions in the manner of Bleuler. The fourth stage that the previous stage of increasing psychotic symptoms may lead to was called by Conrad *apokalypse*. It is identical to full-blown, severe psychosis associated with disorganization, severe anxiety, restlessness and catatonic symptoms.

Sometimes a fifth stage, *catastrophae*, follows, which shows increasingly severe psychotic symptoms, agitation, disorganization and concomitant physical phenomena. According to Conrad, *catastrophae* results in *terminale*, which usually ends in death. This final stage corresponds to the so-called pernicious or febrile catatonia. In those days, when antipsychotic treatment was lacking, it occurred fairly frequently as a consequence of desiccation, electrolyte imbalance, increased body temperature and protein catabolism in the muscles due to sustained and severe psychotic tension.

Docherty *et al.*'s Model

Another stage model designed with the aim of enabling early recognition was published by Docherty *et al.* in 1978 and has been entered especially in the Anglo-American canon of knowledge [22]. The introduction to this work reads like a statement from current research efforts to improve our understanding of the early course of schizophrenia:

> There are many reasons for wanting to know more about the period of onset of schizophrenic psychosis. The dearest benefit is in the area of preventive psychiatry. The establishment of regular premonitory signs might permit a reliable early recognition of impending psychosis and also the staging of the degree of psychological and biological decompensation. That is an assessment of how close a patient is to a psychotic episode. Further this knowledge raises the possibility of developing a clearer rationale for stage-appropriate treatment.
>
> We think that the available data strongly suggest that schizophrenic psychosis is one stage in a process of psychological and biological breakdown that has a specific structure and a characteristic unfolding.... The structure consists of the sequential appearance of hierarchical or distinguishable and recognizable psychological states.

Reflected in these sentences are a few theoretical premises. Docherty *et al.*'s model of the onset of schizophrenic psychosis consists of four – or six – stages. Stages 5 and 6, psychotic resolution and remission, are regarded as phases of remitting psychosis and increasing mental stability. The "empirical basis" of the model were three case histories and a survey of the extremely heterogeneous pertinent literature, including Conrad's stage model.

Stage 1, which Docherty *et al.* called *overextension,* is characterized by experiences of passivity, overstimulation, irritability, persistent anxiety and first signs of cognitive impairment (distractability). This stage tends to show a lengthy, insidious course. Predominant at stage 2, called *restricted consciousness,* are such symptoms as apathy, social withdrawal, hopelessness and somatization, but also deterioration of personal appearance and – here the authors follow Sullivan – obsessional and phobic symptoms. The third stage, *disinhibition,* brings forth symptoms that give the impression of patients losing their inhibitory abilities: hypomania, elevation of mood and occasional ideas of reference. This stage, still part of the prepsychotic prodromal period, is followed by a fourth called *psychotic disorganization,* characterized by disorganization of cognition and perception, hallucinations, ideas of reference, disorders of self and sometimes by catatonic symptoms. In the stages that follow, i.e. psychotic resolution and remission, as stability of the mental state increases, affective and psychotic symptoms remit completely or in part.

Empirical Testing of Conrad's and Docherty *et al.*'s Models

We applied the structural equation modelling technique (SEM) to test the internal validity of Conrad's and Docherty *et al.*'s stage models. As latent variables we chose the symptoms and symptom patterns subsumed under the stages and the stages as such [23]. We also tested external validity, i.e. to what extent the two models tallied with each other and with empirical data on the early course of schizophrenia collected retrospectively using the Interview for the Retrospective Assessment of the Onset of Schizophrenia (IRAOS) [24–28] in a representative sample of first illness episodes of schizophrenia ($n = 232$) from the Age, Beginning, Course (ABC) Schizophrenia Study. Our analysis is based on a subsample of 170 patients who had experienced a clear-cut prepsychotic prodromal stage (73% of 232).

Neither of the two models was significantly supported or even converged in the analysis of internal and external validity or in the comparisons with the empirical data. Conrad's model explained 74% (goodness of fit: 0.79, adjusted 0.74) and Docherty *et al.*'s model 71% (goodness of fit: 0.75, adjusted 0.71) of the empirical data, thus failing to attain the conventional level of goodness of fit of $\geq$90% [23].

This result is no surprise. The reasons lie not only in the construction weaknesses of these models, but also in the partly imprecise description of the symptoms and their occurrence at the stages.

Because of the difficulties posed by a comprehensive validation, we had earlier compared the sequence of symptom onset over time as an indicator of the sequence of stages in Conrad's model with a slightly different set of the IRAOS data from the ABC study [29]. The results confirmed Conrad's model only with respect to prepsychotic "trema" as the first stage of illness (this was the case in 76% of the first-admission sample, of whom 84% were first illness episodes and of these first-episode cases 73% had experienced a prepsychotic prodromal stage). But the comparison failed to provide any evidence for the sequence of the other stages. To conclude, Conrad's model provides a correct representation only of the distinction between a prepsychotic prodromal stage, which he called "trema", and the subsequent stage of psychosis.

Foulds' Model

A third stage model, not limited to schizophrenia, of how mental disorders develop and remit, was proposed by Foulds [30]. The model proceeds from the premise that there is a natural sequence of stages from minor to increasingly severe psychopathology and a symmetrically reversed sequence in remitting illness. The stages of evolving illness consist of dysphoric symptoms, neurotic symptoms, psychotic symptoms, integrated delusions and disintegrated delusions combined with psychotic disorganization on top.

Construed as applicable to all types of mental illness, this model can hardly be expected to be of sufficient specificity in terms of diagnostic power. Because of that, it is no surprise that de Jong *et al.* [31], studying a sample of first-episode cases of schizophrenia assessed by the Present State Examination (PSE) in Groningen, and Biehl *et al.* [32], who studied a first-episode sample of 70 patients with schizophrenia from Mannheim, found a sufficient goodness of fit for the sequence of Foulds' stages in about 85% of their samples. This result means that Foulds' stage model is applicable to the early course of schizophrenia without any substantial benefit in terms of the information it provides, but probably also to many other illnesses with progressive types of courses culminating in psychosis.

RECONSTRUCTING ILLNESS ONSET AND EARLY COURSE

The ABC Schizophrenia Study

Using the IRAOS interview, the ABC Schizophrenia Study examined a population-based sample of 232 first illness episodes, representing 84% of 276 first treatment episodes, and a representative subsample of 130 subjects, who were compared with two age- and gender-matched control samples – one from the "healthy" population ($n = 130$), the other first hospitalized with a diagnosis of depressive episode ($n = 130$).

Survival analysis of the duration of early illness course from onset to first admission as target event revealed a distribution of durations of the early illness course that was markedly skewed to the left. One third (33%) of the broadly defined cases of schizophrenia took less than one year from prodromal onset to develop psychotic symptoms. Only 18% had an acute type of onset of four weeks or less, 15% a subacute type of 4 weeks to one year and 68% a chronic type of onset of one year or more. Only 6.5% started with positive symptoms; 20% presented both positive and negative symptoms within the same month. A prepsychotic prodromal stage with negative or nonspecific symptoms prior to the emergence of the first positive symptom was experienced by 73%.

Nonspecific and negative symptoms started to increase early, positive symptoms quite late, the first of them appearing one year and one month before the climax of the first episode and one year and three months before first admission. In the psychotic episode all three symptom categories accumulated rapidly and reached a maximum followed by almost parallel decreases.

Defining and Operationalizing the Prodromal Stage and the Milestones of the Early Course of Schizophrenia

The "clinical" end of the early illness stage (first treatment contact or first admission) is easy to define. But this event is determined not only by the increase in serious symptoms and impairment, but also by patients' help-seeking behaviour and the availability of adequate care. A suitable illness-related event to mark the end of the early illness stage is the climax of the first psychotic episode, operationalized as the maximum of positive symptoms [18]. Figure 1.1, based on data from the ABC Schizophrenia Study, depicts the mean durations (and medians) of the intervals between the milestones or stages of evolving schizophrenia.

In practice, but also in many epidemiological and clinical studies, the onset of schizophrenia and of many other disorders is defined by the first contact with mental health services. This fact, namely, that the prodromal and the psychotic phase preceding first contact may last a few years, has implications for the interpretation of research results based on first admission as the definition of illness onset. This holds, for example, for reports of a significant excess of first admissions for schizophrenia from the lowest social class and from poor disintegrated neighbourhoods of big cities [33,34] as well as their possible interpretation as social causation versus social selection [35,36]. The same is also true for studies that do not distinguish the prodromal stage from "premorbid" development

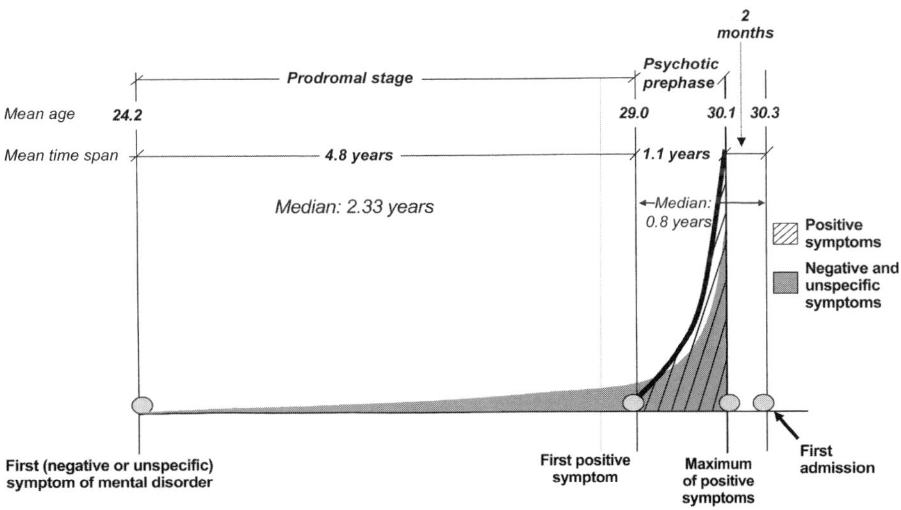

Figure 1.1 The prephases of schizophrenia from first sign of mental disorder to first admission. Modified from Häfner *et al.* [10] by permission of Springer-Verlag

(adjustment): when poor global functioning represents an early consequence of the prodromal stage of the disorder, it is no wonder that "premorbid" functioning possesses such high prognostic power for the social course of the disorder [37]. Prognoses of this type merely tell us that fairly stable features of the disorder continue to persist in the further illness course.

Psychosis onset as the end of the prodromal stage can be determined fairly reliably by the timepoint at which the first psychotic symptom appears. Considering the fairly common occurrence of single psychotic symptoms in the nonpsychotic general population [38–40], with lifetime rates ranging from 5% to 15%, it is advisable to operationalize psychosis onset by persistence of psychotic symptoms for at least one week. By this criterion the fairly rare brief limited intermittent positive symptoms (BLIPS) [41], defined by persistence for up to one week, are subsumed under the prodromal stage or classified as not yet progressing risk indicators.

The onset of the prodromal stage is marked primarily by symptoms not specific to schizophrenia, and for this reason it is far more difficult to define. An operational definition must distinguish between stable, persistent single symptoms on the one hand and early or premonitory signs of other mental disorders on the other hand. An optimal solution to this problem has not yet been found either at the psychopathological or the biological level. For this reason in the ABC Study we used an operational definition based on the different specificities of the three symptom categories: nonspecific symptoms qualified as first signs of the disorder only if they persisted continuously until first admission, negative symptoms, if they were continuous or recurrent, and positive symptoms in any case, even if they had occurred only once for at least two weeks. But it might well be that in the future a neurobiological indicator will be found that marks the onset of the most active neurodegenerative phase in the course of schizophrenia.

DURATION OF UNTREATED ILLNESS AND UNTREATED PSYCHOSIS AS INDICATORS OF AN UNFAVOURABLE FURTHER ILLNESS COURSE

In current clinical practice, the first treatment contact of persons falling ill with schizophrenia is preceded by incipient psychosis with a mean duration of about a year or more (DUP) and a prepsychotic prodromal phase with a mean of several years (duration of untreated illness, DUI = duration of the prodrome+DUP) (see Table 1.1).

DUP and, in rare studies, also DUI have been described as prognostic indicators of unfavourable aspects of course and outcome in schizophrenia. The following short-term effects of a lengthy untreated first psychotic episode have been reported: delayed and incomplete remission of the first episode versus better therapy response and more rapid remission [14,16,42–46], longer active illness or longer presence of psychotic and negative symptoms [47,48], reduced level of global functioning [49] and a longer duration of hospitalization and higher treatment costs [45,46,50].

The results on the association between DUP or DUI and medium- or long-term outcome are less clear-cut. McGorry *et al.* [16], in their investigation of 200 patients (about 50% with schizophrenia), demonstrated a positive association between DUP and positive and negative symptoms, global functioning and quality of life 12 months after first assessment. Johnstone *et al.* [42], Larsen *et al.* [51] and McGorry *et al.* [16] observed an increased frequency and severity of relapses. Helgason [52] found a higher risk of relapse and a longer duration of hospitalization and less compliance. A greater burden on the family and a higher expressed emotions level have also been reported [53,54]. Other effects observed are a less supportive social network [51], higher risk of depression and suicide [55–58], more stress in work- and education-related situations [59,60] and more substance abuse and delinquent behaviour [61]. In sum, almost all the characteristics that make up an unfavourable course of schizophrenia have been reported.

Analyses based on a representative follow-up sample of first illness episodes of schizophrenia in the ABC study [62] showed that DUP was a significant predictor only of psychotic and nonspecific symptoms at five-year follow-up. In contrast, DUI predicted negative and nonspecific symptoms and social outcome. Neither DUI nor DUP significantly predicted the frequency and duration of, and intervals between, psychotic relapses. This result sounds quite plausible because, apart from the nonspecific component, the powerful predictions were limited to the symptom categories prominent in these two phases. A prolonged DUI is characterized mainly by negative symptoms, a short DUP primarily by positive symptoms.

In contrast, three studies found no such association: Craig *et al.* [63] could not demonstrate any association between DUP, illness course and clinical outcome 24 months after first assessment, nor could Robinson *et al.* [64,65] or Ho *et al.* [66] in a well-designed and systematic study (Table 1.2).

The inconsistency of the results from the studies on the topic is very likely explained by great differences in the study samples. It is reasonable to presume that a prolonged prodromal stage – whatever its underlying cause may be – involving a great number and severity of negative symptoms and presumably also associated with a lengthy psychotic stage is an unfavourable prognostic indicator of the further illness course. Edwards and

Table 1.2 Selected studies on short- and long-term prediction of course and outcome by duration of untreated psychosis (DUP) or duration of untreated illness (DUI)

Study	Subjects	Observation period	Shorter DUP or DUI predicts better outcome or shorter first episode	Longer-perspective course and outcome
Altamura *et al.* [67]	67 DSM-III-R schizophrenia spectrum	4 years	Yes	Short DUP → less psychotic relapses
Malla *et al.* [68]	106 non-affective psychoses	1 year	Yes	Short DUP → positive outcome; long DUI → higher negative and disorganization factor scores
Malla *et al.* [68]	53 non-affective psychoses	13 months	Yes	Little evidence of any association between DUP or DUI and course of schizophrenia; long DUI more likely unemployed, alone or homeless
Ho *et al.* [20]	156 DSM-IV schizophrenia spectrum disorder	First episode and retrospective until onset	No	No significant correlations between DUP and neurocognitive functioning
Joyce *et al.* [69]	136 schizophrenia, 81 controls	1 year	Yes	Long DUP → neuropsychological deficits and clinical deterioration
McGorry *et al.* [70]	203 schizophrenia	1 year	Yes	Long DUP → strong and consistent prediction of severity of symptoms and functional outcome
Hoff *et al.* [71]	50 schizophrenia	1 year	Yes	Long DUP → no association after recovery from first episode
Craig *et al.* [63]	155 schizophrenia, 115 bipolar disorder, 75 unipolar depression	2 years	No	No association
Barnes *et al.* [72]	53 schizophrenia (first episode)	First episode and retrospective until onset	No	No association
Harrigan *et al.* [73]	354 schizophrenia	1 year	Yes	Long DUP → deterioration of functioning
Häfner *et al.* [62]	115 schizophrenia (first episode)	5 years	Yes	Long DUP → more psychotic and unspecific symptoms; long DUI → more negative symptoms and poorer social outcome

McGorry [74] have published a fairly comprehensive, but unsystematic list of the potential risks of delayed treatment:

1. slower and less complete recovery;
2. poorer prognosis (subsumed under this heading are numerous results or hypotheses on the further course of the disorder, measures of symptoms and impairment, relapse rates and duration of symptom-free intervals in particular);
3. increased risk of depression and suicide;
4. interference with psychological and social development;
5. strain on relationships;
6. loss of family and social support;
7. disruption of patient's parenting skills (for those with children);
8. distress and increased psychological problems within the patient's family;
9. disruption of study and employment;
10. substance misuse;
11. violence/criminal activity;
12. unnecessary hospitalization;
13. loss of self-esteem and self-confidence;
14. increased costs of management.

The Hypothesis of the Neurotoxicity of Psychotic Episodes

In his early writings, Kraepelin [2] had presumed that the "florid bouts of illness" – psychotic episodes – lead to a certain amount of irreversible consequences he called "defects". This model, implying that schizophrenia shows a deteriorating course in the form of steps, as depicted in the trajectory proposed by Breier *et al.* [75], has been revived by Wyatt [76,77], Loebel *et al.* [14] and Lieberman *et al.* [78,79]: "The illness gets gradually worse during that period indicating that untreated psychosis may constitute an active morbid process, 'toxic' to the brain. If this disease process is not treated and suppressed early enough, it may become chronic" [14,76,79]. McGlashan and Johannessen [80] presume that the plasticity of the brain can be preserved and prevented from deteriorating if the persons affected receive both antipsychotic medication and simultaneously social stimulation at a sensitive stage of the illness.

The neurodegenerative effect of the first psychotic episode – if it really exists – should become visible as pronounced deterioration following the psychotic "bout" in first-episode cohorts. But this does not seem to be the case when judged by mean symptom scores and measures of social impairment in methodologically sound, prospective first-episode studies.

Nor can the effect be demonstrated on mean scores from neuropsychological tests in the majority of studies [81]. In fact, global impairment and its social consequences emerge as early as the prodromal stage without clear signs of gaining momentum in the psychotic episode.

If the duration or severity of psychotic episodes were causally associated with indicators of a poor further illness course, evidence for such an association would be provided by findings that psychotic symptoms predict subsequent negative symptoms. For this purpose we operationalized the symptom dimensions of schizophrenia on the basis of Liddle's three-factor model [82–84] to obtain comparable measurements [85]. We prospectively assessed the representative ABC follow-up sample of 115 first-illness episodes at six cross-sections over five years after first admission. The negative factor remained independent of the two other factors, throughout the cross-sections, but highly significantly correlated with itself from cross-section to cross-section. In conformity with results from numerous follow-up studies, the negative factor turned out to be the most stable component independent of the course of the psychotic symptom dimensions in schizophrenia. The two other factors (reality distortion and disintegration) showed a few autocorrelations and significant intercorrelations at several cross-sections as well as courses independent of the negative factor. Similar results have been reported by Arndt *et al.* [86], who showed that Liddle's three factors varied independently over two years, and Salokangas [87], who showed the same over five years.

The analysis discussed above of how DUP and DUI influence five-year outcome can also be regarded as a test of the hypothesis about the neurotoxicity of psychosis. The result that significant effects could be shown to exist only at the level of the quantitatively predominant symptoms corresponds to the results on the stability of the factors.

To test the neurotoxicity hypothesis, Ho *et al.* [20] recently conducted a cross-sectional study of 156 first episodes of schizophrenia at the levels of symptoms, neuropsychological test results and brain morphology. The authors were unable to find significant correlations of DUP either with changes in grey matter volumes, symptoms or neuropsychological test results.

The reasons for the inconclusiveness of the findings concerning the effects of DUP and DUI probably lie in the great methodological differences of these studies (Table 1.2). Exact comparisons of the two periods concerned, DUP and DUI, are hardly possible due to differences in the definitions used and/or non-use of appropriate assessment instruments. With a few exceptions, the samples studied were not representative. Because of the extremely heterogeneous course of schizophrenia, the proportions of unfavourable courses in the study samples probably varied a great deal. The difficulties encountered in studying associations between

DUP and illness course are by no means minor in studies based on magnetic resonance imaging (MRI) and computed tomography (CT) scans. Some studies have shown that morphological brain changes occur early in the illness, before the psychotic stage. Other studies have demonstrated that compared with age-matched controls brain volume reduction increases over time (five years) in some cases [88]. However, it is not yet possible to tell the exact proportion of these cases in the total of people with schizophrenia (Table 1.3).

Does a Shortened DUP Lead to a More Favourable Illness Course and Better Outcome?

This important question stems from a hope of reducing the adverse consequences of the disorder by shortening the untreated early illness period. But objections have been raised against the implied causal association: "is the link due to a common underlying factor, such as a more severe form of the illness with functional impairment after an insidious onset, more negative symptoms, more paranoid ideation?" [74]. At any rate, it has been known since Kraepelin's days that an insidious onset with a long prodromal phase featuring negative symptoms and impairments is a clinical indicator of a poor illness course. In contrast, a highly acute onset without a prodromal stage seems to be associated with a favourable illness course as an intrinsic factor of the disease process. Verdoux *et al.* [95] have shown that demographic and clinical factors that predict a poor prognosis may also be associated with delayed presentation to psychiatric services.

Evidence for the assumption that shortening the early illness stages (DUP, DUI) ameliorates the further illness course could only be obtained in randomized controlled intervention studies among patients at early stages of their illness. Because of the unresolved problems posed by early recognition and reliably predicting psychosis risk, the studies were based on conventional definitions of high psychosis risk. The study conducted by McGorry *et al.* [70], which was based on 59 ultra-high-risk (UHR) probands, showed that, after one year of targeted cognitive behavioural therapy and low doses (on average 1.3 mg pro die) of risperidone, 7.1% of the fully compliant patients transited to psychosis, compared with 29.4% of the not fully compliant index cases and 35.7% of the controls, who had received unspecific therapy. Lewis *et al.* [96], in a study in which high-risk probands at the prodromal stage received cognitive behavioural therapy and social support, also found significant differences in outcome between the index cases and controls.

Table 1.3 Changes in brain morphology at the prodromal stage of schizophrenia according to selected studies

Study	Subjects	Brain imaging	Before or at first psychotic episode	At follow-up
Johnstone *et al.* [89] Lawrie *et al.* [90]	162 psychotic risk; 18.1% psychotic (11.6% schizophrenia), 33% partly psychotic Risk period: 6 years	MRI	High-risk subjects: reduced hippocampal and thalamic volumes, changes occur before psychosis	High-risk subjects show reductions in temporal lobe volumes; with approaching psychosis anomalies increase
Hoff *et al.* [71]	50 first episode schizophrenics 25 controls	MRI volumetry	First episode: structural anomalies	No significant correlation of DUP with severity of either cognitive or structural brain deficits
Fannon *et al.* [91]	37 first-episode schizophrenics Risk period: 1 year	MRI	First episode: smaller brain volumes and cortical grey matter volumes and larger lateral and third ventricle	No association between DUP and any changes
Ho *et al.* [20]	156 DSM-IV schizophrenia Risk period: 2 years (1 episode)	MRI grey and white volumetric and surface anatomy measurement	First episode: no association between DUP and volumetric measures of the brain	No association between DUP and MRI anomalies
Pantelis *et al.* [92]	75 ultra-high-risk (UHR) cases; 31% psychotic Risk period: 1 year	MRI volumetry	High-risk cases: brain changes appear before psychosis and further changes occur	Psychotic cases: reduction in grey matter volume and left caudate and hippocampus
Copolov *et al.* [93]	32 first episodes with schizophrenia; 39 UHR cases Risk period: 1 year	MRI volumetry hippocampus	High-risk subjects: hippocampus ~10% volume reduction	15 of 39 psychotic: no progression of hippocampus reduction
Malla *et al.* [94]	114 first episodes (schizophrenia or schizophreniform)	CT	First episode: modest enlargement of sylvian fissure and ventricle; no association with DUP	Chronic cases: sylvian fissure significantly larger

CT, computed tomography; DUP, duration of untreated psychosis; UHR, ultra high risk.

Hence, appropriate early intervention administered to high-risk individuals from the late prepsychotic stage onwards can succeed in delaying the onset of a psychotic episode. This effect is analogous to that in relapse prevention in schizophrenia. But will early intervention also help to reduce negative symptoms and functional impairment enduringly?

In view of the independent courses of the negative-impairment dimension and the positive-symptom dimension over time, shortening the prodromal stage characterized by negative symptoms or DUI as a whole seems more promising than reducing the purely positive symptoms. In this context it should be kept in mind, as mentioned above, that in the first psychotic episode unspecific and negative symptoms also increase simultaneously with positive symptoms [18]. The aim of early intervention is not only to reduce the most enduring component of the illness, but also to try to reduce or even prevent the early social consequences, which decisively co-determine the social course of the disorder and the kind of life patients will be able to lead. This is why diagnostic recognition and prediction of schizophrenia as early as the prodromal stage are so important.

ASSESSING PRODROMAL SYMPTOMS AND IMPAIRMENT IN THE EARLY COURSE OF SCHIZOPHRENIA

Residual Symptoms as Prodromal Signs

Because of the great difficulty in obtaining information on the onset and early course of schizophrenia prospectively, due to the low incidence rate and a frequent onset with uncharacteristic symptoms, prodromal signs usually go unheeded when they appear. In traditional clinical settings, first contact with mental health services in most cases takes place during the first psychotic episode. Help-seeking is usually precipitated by a loss of working ability and the distress caused by psychosis to the sick person and his/her environment. In the ABC Schizophrenia Study the time span between onset of the first psychotic episode and first contact varied around a mean of 1.3 years (median 0.8 years).

Due to their obscurity, the prodromal symptoms of the first episode were also lacking or listed incompletely in the international classification systems and at first reconstructed on the basis of symptoms occurring in the further illness course [97].

Different attempts have been made to assess prepsychotic prodromal symptoms that do not usually come to clinical observation. Janzarik [98] and Gross [11], proceeding from clinical observation of residual symptoms in the psychosis-free interval in patients with long histories of illness, found above all negative symptoms and signs of functional impairment, at that time called a "defect". Presuming that prodromal and residual symptoms are identical, Janzarik concluded that there must be an "anteceding defect state" observable before the first psychotic episode, whereas Gross [11] and Huber *et al.* [13] spoke of "basic symptoms" which, unlike psychotic symptoms, are direct expressions of degenerative brain changes. Such prodromal symptoms also to be found among the residual symptoms include, for example, affective flattening, avolition, and difficulties of thinking and concentration [13].

This approach is in part well founded, because negative symptoms and functional impairment constitute the most stable symptom dimension in schizophrenia. As retrospective analyses have shown [18], they tend to emerge long before psychosis onset (see Table 1.1). Negative symptoms manifest themselves before and simultaneously with positive symptoms and reach a maximum at the climax of the psychotic episode. As the psychosis remits, they too remit fully or in part [18]. In the further illness course, their prevalence shows a plateau [99]. But prodromal symptoms are not limited to the negative symptoms and functional impairment observable at the residual stage. Affective, especially depressive, dysphoric and other "unspecific" symptoms and behavioural anomalies play an important role at the prepsychotic stage.

Assessing Prodromal Symptoms Before Psychotic Relapses

The first attempts at systematically assessing prodromal signs retrospectively were made in the context of targeted antipsychotic therapy of relapses. The advantages of this procedure are that the prodromal symptoms of relapses are not as remote in time as those of the first episode and that their prognostic efficiency can be prospectively validated [100–105]. The results obtained were valuable, but of insufficient predictive power, presumably due to differences in the type of prodromal signs included in the assessments and insufficient monitoring of their development over time.

In addition it is unclear whether the first psychotic episode is preceded by an interindividually identical pattern of prodromal symptoms and whether the prodromal symptoms in each individual case undergo changes in type and sequence. Meanwhile, intraindividual stability is presumed in clinical practice, and on that basis educational interventions are being offered particularly in relapse-oriented, targeted and crisis-intervention therapy [74,106–109].

TABLE 1.4 The ten most frequent earliest signs of schizophrenia (independent of the course) reported by the patients

	Total ($n = 232$) %	Men ($n = 108$) %	Women ($n = 124$) %
Restlessness	19	15	22
Depression	19	15	22
Anxiety	18	17	19
Trouble with thinking and concentration	16	19	14
Worrying	15	9	20
Lack of self-confidence	13	10	15
Lack of energy, slowness	12	8	15
Poor work performance	11	12	10
Social withdrawal, distrust	10	8	12
Social withdrawal, communication	10	8	12

All items were tested for gender differences. Only "worrying" showed a significant difference ($p < 0.05$).
Source: modified from Häfner *et al.* [10] by permission of Springer-Verlag.

Various items from scales for the identification of early signs and symptoms of psychotic relapses [102,110] have been integrated in subsequently generated instruments for the assessment of onset and early course in schizophrenia [24–26,111,112].

Systematic studies of the onset and prodromal symptoms of schizophrenia have relied on retrospective assessments of representative samples of first-episode cases of schizophrenia. Table 1.4, taken from the ABC Schizophrenia Study, shows the ten most frequent initial symptoms. These symptoms are equally frequent in men and women, except worrying, an item which is also more frequent in women in population studies. The majority of these items belong to two symptom dimensions, the affective–depressive and the negative one. The early occurrence of indicators of functional impairment, such as trouble with thinking and concentration or loss of energy, pointed to a risk of early consequences of the disorder in terms of global dysfunction and social decline.

The Earliest Psychotic Symptoms

In the ABC Schizophrenia Study [18], the earliest positive symptom, delusions, appeared on average 14.3 months, the first hallucination 8.7 months and the first formal thought disorder 8.2 months before first admission. This result provides no evidence for the hypothesis that delusions are an expression of cognitive coping with the distressing experience of hallucinations. The cumulative prevalence of delusions in the early course was 96%, that of auditory hallucinations 69% and that of thought disorder 62%. The fact that their prevalence approaches 100% reflects the role of positive symptoms as the leading diagnostic criteria for schizophrenia and, hence, also the type of patients included in or excluded from study samples of schizophrenia.

The Sequence of First-ever Onset of Symptoms

Arranging the early symptoms by their time of emergence in a time matrix of up to 60 months before first admission, we found that four depressive symptoms (depressed mood, suicide attempt, loss of self-confidence and feelings of guilt) tended to occur five to three years before first admission. In the second time window, four to two years before first admission, with a clear overlap with the depressive syndrome, all the negative symptoms appeared. After a short interval characterized by the emergence of dysphoric symptoms, positive symptoms appeared in the last year before first admission. This sequential pattern of emergence of various types of symptoms gives the impression of a regular sequence of stages reminiscent of Conrad's [21] and Docherty *et al.*'s [22] models. However, these stages of the early course of schizophrenia reconstructed on the basis of group means do not necessarily apply to individual cases.

Depressive Symptoms as Prodromal Signs of Schizophrenia

Several first-episode studies have consistently reported an extremely high frequency of depressive symptoms in the first psychotic episode: depressive mood or at least two depressive symptoms were found in 70–75% of cases [56,57,113–115].

As shown above, depressive symptoms frequently appear long before the first positive symptom [16,114,116]. In the ABC study cohort, the lifetime prevalence of depressive mood of a duration of two or more weeks – assessed until first admission – was 81%. In 39% of cases the symptom was continuously present, in 34% recurrent, and in 8% it occurred only once. Only 19% of the first-episode cases of schizophrenia reported not to have suffered from an episode of depressed mood [114].

A comparison of 57 first-episode patients with schizophrenia with 57 population controls matched by age, sex and place of residence showed that three out of four depressive symptoms were significantly more frequent in patients than in controls [114]. For depressive mood, the lifetime prevalence at first admission was 70.2% in patients versus 19.3% in controls, for feelings of guilt 33.3% versus 10.5%, and for poor self-confidence 59.4% versus 12.3%. The relative risks of these symptoms ranged from 3 to 5. The frequency of attempted suicide at the early illness stage showed a nonsignificant excess of some 40%. This result will probably attain significance in larger samples, thus indicating that early clinical intervention is needed here.

The depressive syndrome emerging at the early prodromal stage of schizophrenia is presumably for the most part a pattern of response of the brain to fairly mild degrees of dysfunction. It seems to be produced by the same neurobiological processes that bring forth psychotic symptoms at a later stage. In contrast, at the beginning of the prodromal stage, the distressing factors associated with the disorder – e.g. traumatic experiences of the psychosis, hallucinations in particular, and social consequences of schizophrenia – do not yet play a role.

Comparison of Prodromal Symptoms in Schizophrenia and Depression

We compared a representative subsample of 130 first admissions for schizophrenia from the ABC study with 130 age- and sex-matched "healthy" controls from the general population and 130 first admissions because of a depressive episode. Of the latter group, 70% suffered from a severe depressive episode. All these samples went through IRAOS interviews. Preliminary results show that DUI was significantly longer in depression (7.2 years) than in schizophrenia (5.3 years) ($p<0.05$). Equal proportions of both samples had received psychotropic medication before first admission: 19% of the patients with schizophrenia and 20% of the depressed patients.

As shown in Table 1.5, the two disorders share eight of their ten most frequent initial symptoms. These shared symptoms are primarily core depressive symptoms and indicators of functional impairment. In the further course of the prodromal stage, cognitive and social functioning deteriorate in depressive illness, too, but less markedly than in schizophrenia. This result is also reflected in a comparison of the cumulative prevalence rates of the ten most frequent symptoms in the early course of schizophrenia and depression (Table 1.6). Towards the end of the prodromal stage, the two disorders become clearly distinguishable, as psychotic symptoms appear and functional impairment clearly increases in schizophrenia and the depressive symptom dimension becomes predominant in depression.

Table 1.5 The ten most frequent initial symptoms (IRAOS items) in schizophrenia and in depression

	Schizophrenic patients		Depressive patients		
Symptom	%	Rank	%	Rank	p
Worrying	19.2	4	14.1	5	n.s.
Headaches, other aches and pains	10.3	–	13.2	8	n.s.
Nervousness, restlessness	21.9	2	6.2	–	<0.001
Anxiety	23.2	1	15.4	4	n.s
Difficulties of thinking, concentration	17.1	5	16.5	3	n.s.
Depressed mood	20.6	3	34.9	1	<0.05
Loss of self-confidence	11.9	8	14.0	6	n.s.
Social withdrawal	11.6	9	13.3	7	n.s.
Disturbed sleep and/or appetite	15.0	6	21.9	2	n.s.
Loss of energy, slowness	13.5	7	8.5	10	n.s.
Loss of libido	4.1	–	8.5	10	n.s.
Oversensitivity	3.3	–	9.3	9	n.s.
Other changes in affect (blunted etc.)	11.1	10	0.8	–	<0.001

Table 1.6 The ten most frequent symptoms (IRAOS items) in the early course of schizophrenia and depression (period prevalence)

	Period prevalence from symptom onset until first hospital admission				
	Schizophrenic patients		Depressive patients		
Symptom	%	Rank	%	Rank	p
Worrying	74.6	9	94.6	4	<0.001
Nervousness, restlessness	88.3	3	81.5	10	n.s.
Anxiety	88.1	4	81.5	10	n.s.
Difficulties of thinking, concentration	93.8	1	96.9	3	n.s.
Depressed mood	84.9	5	100.0	1	<0.001
Loss of self-confidence	68.3	10	89.2	7	<0.001
Social withdrawal	79.8	8	90.8	6	<0.05
Disturbed sleep and/or appetite	93.8	1	98.5	2	n.s.
Loss of energy, slowness	82.5	6	93.8	5	<0.05
Delusional mood	68.3	10	4.6	–	<0.001
Delusional misinterpretations; delusions of reference	80.3	7	6.2	–	<0.001
Reduced spare time activities	63.5	–	89.1	8	<0.001
Reduced interests, citizen role	33.9	–	87.7	9	<0.001

Depression in the Early Illness Course as a Prognostic Indicator of the Later Course

We studied the further illness course and the predictive efficiency of prodromal symptoms in 115 first illness episodes from the representative subsample of 130 first admissions at six cross-sections over five years after first admission [114]. Patients with schizophrenia who suffered from depressive mood ($\geq$14 days) in the early illness course were compared with age- and gender-matched patients without depressive episodes. The group with depression in the early course of schizophrenia showed significantly higher scores of depressive, but also of positive, negative and nonspecific symptoms in the first episode than did nondepressed patients. With remission of the episode, the mean score for depressive symptoms fell with psychotic symptoms without any indication of a "wave" of postpsychotic depression and remained more or less stable until five years after first admission. The presence of depressive symptoms in the early illness course predicted the occurrence of neither positive nor depressive or nonspecific symptoms after remission of the psychotic episode. In contrast, the absence of depressive symptoms in the early course was significantly correlated with affective flattening in the five years following first admission. The implication of this finding is that prodromal depression predicts a severe first psychotic episode, whereas a low score of prodromal depressive symptoms predicts more affective flattening after the remission of the episode.

Early Functional Impairment and Social Consequences

Because of the early emergence of negative symptoms and functional impairment, most patients with schizophrenia started to suffer from social disability (Disability Assessment Schedule, DAS score $\geq$2) 51 to 24 months before first admission, long before they received appropriate treatment. Two years before first admission, 57% of the patients were considerably impaired, when judged by the overall DAS score ($\geq$2), in the domains of work performance, household activities, communication and leisure activitites. This result raises the question at which point do the social consequences actually emerge.

The effect of early social disability on the further illness course can only be judged against a baseline, i.e. the social status or level of social development at illness onset. In the ABC first-episode sample, no significant differences were observable in the fulfilment of six main social roles between patients and controls at the age of illness onset. By the time of first admission, patients with schizophrenia had fallen significantly behind the controls in several roles, most markedly in marriage or stable partnership. In sum, before illness onset, patients with schizophrenia were probably slightly, but not yet markedly and significantly, socially disadvantaged [62].

Age and Gender as Risk Factors

Age and level of social development are highly significantly correlated. Men fall ill with schizophrenia 3 to 4 years earlier and, in our population of origin, married 2.5 years later than women. Their level of social development at illness onset, in the social role of marriage in particular, was therefore considerably lower than that of women. In addition, young men with schizophrenia showed a significant excess of socially adverse behaviour at first admission, e.g. self-neglect, lack of interest in finding a job, deficits in hygiene, aggressive behaviour and an elevated lifetime prevalence of alcohol and drug abuse until first admission. Female patients in contrast showed a significant excess of "social conformity", which presumably reflects a different type of adaptive behaviour. The socially adverse behaviour of young males has been confirmed in many population studies by elevated rates of conduct disorders, aggressiveness, antisocial personality, and alcohol and drug abuse [117,118]. In schizophrenia it must therefore be classified as gender-specific illness behaviour and not as a direct expression of the disorder [18].

The more favourable social course of the disorder observed in premenopausal women has to do with their higher level of social development in our culture as a result of a later illness onset and socially more adaptive illness behaviour. It does not appear to be related to women having a milder form of the disorder.

In a stepwise logistic regression [119], the level of social development at the first psychotic symptom and the socially adverse behaviour at the end of the prephase turned out to be the only factors significantly predicting five-year social outcome. The traditional prognostic indicators – age, gender, symptomatology and type of illness onset – merely had indirect effects via the level of social development at illness onset and illness behaviour. The symptom-related illness course showed no sex difference. It seems that the social course of schizophrenia is largely determined by social status or development at illness onset as well as the functional impairment and social disability that emerge in the early illness course. In early-onset illness, the consequence is social stagnation at a low level of social development; in late-onset illness, when a comparatively high level of social development has been attained, the consequence is social decline [62].

The earlier onset of schizophrenia in men has been widely reported (for review, see 120–122). The difference is not an artefact due to gender differences in diagnostic definitions and procedures, help-seeking behaviour or in the length of the early illness course [123–126]. An analysis of pooled data from 10 centres of the World Health Organization (WHO) Determinants of Outcome of Severe Mental Disorders (DOSMED) study [127] showed a mean difference of 3.4 years and some consistency across countries and cultures.

No such gender difference in age at onset is shown by siblings and twins [128,129], and this is almost exclusively because of women's reduced age of onset. Studying the ABC first-episode sample, Könnecke *et al.* [130] found that two risk factors for schizophrenia (at least one first-degree relative with schizophrenia and pre- and perinatal complications) significantly reduced the gender difference in age at onset by significantly lowering the age of onset in women, but not in men. When neither risk factor was present, the mean age of onset in women was 4.9 years later than in men. Underlying the protective effect of oestrogen that delays illness onset, there seems to be an antagonistic balance between the sex hormone and strength of predisposition to illness. The delaying effect of oestrogen on illness onset is the strongest in cases who have the weakest predisposition to illness or lack the two risk factors.

The duration of the prodromal stage does not differ significantly between the sexes or in five-year age groups over an age range of 12 to 59 years, apart from a slightly shorter duration in early-onset illness. Male onsets peak at 15 to 24 years, female onsets at age 15 to 29 years. Because of decreasing oestrogen secretion with age, women aged 45 to 50 years show a second peak of onsets lower than the first one. The second peak has also been demonstrated on pooled data from the WHO DOSMED study [127] and in the Camberwell case-register population [126]. The explanation of these sex differences by a protective effect of oestrogen [125,131] was supported in animal experiments by the attenuating effect that a four-week oestrogen treatment had on apomorphine-stimulated dopaminergic behaviour as a result of sensitivity reduction in central D2 receptors [132,133].

Further Syndromes of the Prodromal Phase

Less frequent than depressive symptoms in the early course of schizophrenia are manic and hypomanic symptoms. In studies their frequencies range from 3% to 10% of cases depending on the symptoms defined. They are in part associated with other bipolar symptoms and primarily have episodic or intermittent courses [99].

The catatonic syndrome, which was fairly frequent before the advent of neuroleptics and still is in some developing countries, has become rare in Western Europe and the USA. Only recently have catatonic features started to attract renewed interest [134]. They seem to be most prevalent at a young age. But these fairly rare catatonic subtypes do not seem to be very stable over time [135].

Lists of Prodromal Features of Schizophrenia

Yung and McGorry [41] and Edwards and McGorry [74] have listed the prodromal features in first-episode psychosis most commonly described in the literature. All these symptoms have also been included in the IRAOS and were assessed in the ABC Schizophrenia Study:

1. reduced concentration and attention;
2. reduced drive and motivation, anergia;
3. depressed mood;
4. sleep disturbances;
5. anxiety;
6. social withdrawal;
7. suspiciousness;
8. deterioration in role-functioning;
9. irritability.

Edwards and McGorry [74] also list the four symptom categories experienced prior to a first or current psychotic episode. They, too, are based on the literature and the authors' own data:

1. Changes in affect: suspiciousness, depression, anxiety, mood swings, feelings of tension, irritability, anger.
2. Changes in cognition: odd ideas, vagueness, difficulties with concentration or recall.
3. Changes in perception of self, of other people, of the world at large.
4. Physical and perceptual changes: sleep disturbances, appetite change, somatic complaints, loss of energy or motivation, perceptual disturbances.

These indicators of the prodromal stage can be informative but, as they are described in a quasi-cross-sectional manner and no information is provided on their frequencies or sequence of emergence, they are not helpful in reconstructing the early illness course.

It was also the McGorry group which brought to our attention the existence of two further types of symptoms in incipient psychosis, i.e. attenuated psychotic symptoms and the rarer BLIPS [41].

Can Substance Misuse Trigger a Premature Onset of the Prepsychotic Prodromal Stage?

In the ABC Schizophrenia Study, the lifetime prevalence of alcohol abuse until age at first admission was 24% for the first-episode sample and 12% for matched controls from the same population [119,136,137], and that of drug abuse 14% for patients and 7% for controls. Studies on the topic almost invariably show a preponderance of men in substance abuse. We found a cumulative prevalence (until first admission) of any type of substance abuse of 39% for men and 22% for women. Cannabis was the most frequently abused substance (88%), followed by alcohol (58%).

In this study, 35% of the patients with drug abuse and 18% of those with alcohol abuse started with the abuse behaviour in the same month as the onset of schizophrenia occurred. In this small group, precipitation of illness onset by substance abuse cannot be excluded, especially since these patients were significantly younger (8 years) at illness onset than non-abusing patients. In contrast, we could not support in our study the dopamine-receptor hypothesis of a drug-related precipitation of the psychotic episode. However, presence of alcohol and drug abuse in the early illness course predicted an elevated score for positive symptoms in both the psychotic episode and at five cross-sections over five years following first admission. In contrast, substance abuse significantly reduced affective flattening with a latency of several years, probably in the context of a dysfunctional self-therapy of apathy. At the same time, substance and drug abuse may have contributed to poorer compliance with antipsychotic therapy, which again could have contributed to an increased level of positive symptoms [137].

Premorbid Personality Traits

Indicators more closely related with the disorder that have been reported from the recent prospective epidemiological cohort studies seem to offer prospects of identifying at-risk persons. The Swedish conscript study [138] of 50 084 young men aged 18 to 20 years showed that four items (having fewer than two friends, preference for socializing in small groups, feeling more sensitive than others, and not having a steady girlfriend) were associated with a high relative risk (odds ratio: 30.7) of being admitted to inpatient treatment with a diagnosis of schizophrenia in a period of risk of 13 years. But in the total sample a positive response to all four items predicted psychosis only in 3%, because of the high prevalence of these features in the conscript population.

Davidson *et al.* [139] and Rabinowitz *et al.* [37] studied 16- to 17-year-old Israeli male conscripts. The authors identified 692 individuals who had been hospitalized with a diagnosis of schizophrenia for the first time in a mean period of nine years following initial testing. When these individuals were compared with the entire conscript population and with matched controls, the results pointed in the same direction as in the Swedish study. The main indicator of risk was poor social functioning, with an effect size difference of 1.25. With effect sizes ranging from 0.44 to 0.58, the young males later hospitalized with a diagnosis of schizophrenia also fared worse than controls in all tests of cognitive functioning.

As poor communicability and lack of social drive have also been found in population cohort studies of persons later falling ill with schizophrenia, this stable behavioural dimension probably represents the most pronounced psychological indicator of vulnerability to schizophrenia.

In prospective assessments of schizophrenia onset the distinction must be drawn between prodromal symptoms and premorbid antecedents or indicators of other causes. Since schizophrenia onset is marked by unspecific symptoms in 73% of cases, it is a very difficult event to recognize in prospective studies of whatever design. The same is true for the diagnostic classification of the first unspecific symptoms. For this reason, as long as sufficiently powerful discriminatory and predictive early indicators of schizophrenia are lacking, schizophrenia onset and prodromal stage can only be assessed retrospectively in cases clearly diagnosable as schizophrenia, ideally in recent-onset, representative first-episode samples.

Three aspects of transition from a premorbid risk status to a prodromal stage of the disorder can be distinguished: (a) new symptoms appear and those already persisting deteriorate, frequently involving increased subjective distress; (b) symptoms accumulate, probably following a typical pattern (stage model); and (c) progressive deterioration occurs in social and cognitive functioning or in deficits measured by neuropsychological tests. A characteristic of the prodromal stage of key importance is the gradient of change or deterioration.

The early illness stage usually involves increasing communicative and social impairment and behavioural changes detrimental to the person's functioning in the social, school, work and family environment.

INSTRUMENTS FOR ASSESSING THE ONSET AND EARLY COURSE OF SCHIZOPHRENIA

The success of early intervention programmes depends on the degree to which help-seeking can be mobilized among at-risk persons in the population, for example by carrying out awareness programmes that provide basic information on schizophrenia and its treatment [74,140]. Antistigma and information campaigns play an important role, as successfully demonstrated by the WPA Global Programme Against Stigma and Discrimination Because of Schizophrenia [141]. Another precondition is a well-functioning network of low threshold pathways to care [142], that is, easily accessible and as far as possible stigma-free early intervention centres or other suitable mental health services [16,143].

Indicators of Prognostic Accuracy

Early recognition inventories should allow a correct identification of "at-risk mental states". This objective is attained when as large a proportion of at-risk persons as possible is classified as such (i.e. the test for diagnostic ascertainment is highly sensitive) and at the same time as large a proportion of risk-free persons as possible is identified as not being at risk (specificity). But there is no single symptom or single risk factor of sufficient diagnostic efficiency that early recognition could be based on. Usually a selection of several prodromal symptoms is used as a basis for a total score that indicates psychosis risk. Besides symptom scales, other risk factors can be taken into account, e.g. biological indicators such as smooth pursuit eye movement or MRI parameters, in order to create the best possible criteria. A technique for generating combinations of indicators is the Receiver Operating Characteristic Analysis (ROC Analysis), which helps to find out an optimum cut-off based on a combination of single items [112]. Further indicators of the predictive power of early recognition inventories are the positive and the negative predictive power (PPP and NPP). These measures are suited to assessing individual psychosis risk in actual test situations when the persons examined present or do not present a particular symptom (more generally: receive a positive or a negative test result, which usually represents a cut-off based on a selection of several features).

Contemporary early recognition instruments of high sensitivity for identifying large proportions of at-risk persons in the general population all have insufficient specificities. But even if sensitivity and specificity were satisfactory (e.g. 0.95), the number of false positive cases would be rather high, because of the low base rate of schizophrenia in the general population. Let us presume that 1% of the population at large is at risk for schizophrenia. By screening 1000 individuals only 10 at-risk persons would be identified. The problem is the high number of 50 false positives among the 990 persons not being at risk.

Strategies to Improve the Predictive Accuracy of Diagnostic Tests

An attempt to solve this problem is a multi-level procedure of case identification (sequential screening) [144]. If case identification is based, instead of on the general population, on a group of people who have already contacted a general practitioner, psychologist or a counselling service because of mental problems, the rates for false positive cases will drop considerably.

The Early Recognition Inventory (ERIraos), which we developed in the German Research Network on Schizophrenia, pursues a two-step strategy for the identification of at-risk persons. In the first step a screening procedure of a high sensitivity and slightly increased risk threshold is applied in general practices, counselling services or schools. In these populations at an increased risk, the ratio of risk persons to non-risk persons is far better in balance and the number of false positives much lower. The risk persons thus identified are referred to a specialist service or an early intervention centre where they will be examined by more differentiated instruments of the highest possible diagnostic and predictive power. In the efforts to validate such early recognition inventories, which have to be practical and economic to use and produce favourable results, biological tests may follow at a third level of risk identification. Designs of that type are being pursued in the Edinburgh high-risk study [89] and in a multicentre study in Germany [145].

An early recognition inventory successfully validated and fulfilling all the requirements mentioned is not yet available. To achieve an acceptable number needed to treat (NNT) and, hence, to meet the main economic and ethical requirements, risk predictions in early recognition instruments (state criteria) will be supplemented by "longstanding biobehavioural markers" [146]. The ones most frequently used are age of risk (e.g. up to 30 years), family history (at least one first-degree relative with schizophrenia), schizotypal personality and history of obstetric complications. An example of a set of risk criteria, which has been prospectively validated, was developed by Yung *et al.* [147,148] and Edwards and McGorry [74] with their operationalized concept of ultra-high risk (UHR) for psychosis. Included are the following trait factors [147]: age of risk 16 to 30 years, schizotypal personality or a first-degree relative with a history of psychotic disorder. As state indicators they chose attenuated psychotic symptoms or BLIPS and a change in mental state and functioning which results in a loss of 30 points or more in the Global Assessment of Functioning (GAF) scale for at least one month. Such a definition of an increased risk has considerable advantages in terms of diagnostic and prognostic power. Its weaknesses are the selective nature of risk assessment and that it does not include a rule for quantitative risk estimation.

The Chapman Scales

Chapman and colleagues [149–154] produced a list of early symptoms by studying first-episode cases of schizophrenia retrospectively. They focused on the cognitive character of the changes preceding the psychotic symptom pattern – disturbances of attention, perception and memory – supplemented by indicators of psychomotor functioning. They were the first to develop experimental procedures for assessing disordered perception on this observational basis. Proceeding from the construct of "psychosis proneness", they developed several scales for the assessment of psychotic and psychotic-like experiences [153]: the 35-item Perceptual Aberration Scale, the 30-item Magical Ideation Scale, the Impulsive Nonconformity Scale (51 items) and the Social Anhedonia Scale (40 items). The scales were tested for internal consistency and retest reliability. The authors concluded that their scales are suited to identifying persons with schizophrenia proneness, but not to reliably predicting schizophrenia risk, nor do the scales permit one to distinguish between risk for schizophrenia and other types of psychotic disorder or affective illness with psychotic symptoms. If we enter the numbers of psychotic transitions as based on psychosis proneness in the four-cell matrix for calculating the usual indices of diagnostic efficiency, the probands identified by the two subscales tested as valid and the control group yield a high sensitivity of 0.92, an extremely low rate of false negatives (0.003%) and a negative predictive power of 99%. In contrast, the values for specificity (0.43), false positives (55%) and positive prognostic power (5.6%) are less favourable. The conclusion that the number of people with psychosis proneness by far exceeds the number of persons ever falling ill with schizophrenia may be correct, but it also means that the concept is hardly suitable for identifying persons at risk for psychosis if the aim is to refer them to treatment. Nevertheless the concept can be used for screening purposes, because it is fairly easy to use and helps to identify all at-risk persons at an early stage (10 to 15 years before the onset of psychotic symptoms).

The Bonn Scale (BSABS)

On the basis of the results of a follow-up study of 502 first admissions to the University Hospital in Bonn [11,13], Gross and colleagues constructed the Bonn Scale for the Assessment of Basic Symptoms (BSABS) [155], which includes subscales on "dynamic deficiency", cognitive disturbances of thought, perception and motor action, "coenaesthesias" and disturbances of the central autonomic nervous system and sleep disturbances. Each single item is rated by its closeness to positive symptoms in three degrees: (1) characteristic, which means the phenomenon observed is sufficiently similar to certain full-blown psychotic symptoms, (2) accompanied by a sense of strangeness, splitting or restlessness, and (3) associated with a delusional explanation. The instrument does not include a time matrix that would help to determine the gradient of change or timepoint and/or order of appearance, persistence and remission of symptoms.

The prodromal symptoms listed in the BSABS have attained the highest predictive power so far in predicting transition to psychosis, without taking the three degrees of intensity into account. Klosterkötter *et al.* [156] demonstrated transition from attenuated positive symptoms to full-blown psychosis in a descriptive design and predicted onset of schizophrenia in a prospective study over a mean follow-up period of 9.6 years [157]. Of a total of 338 patients who had been referred to any of the five German university hospitals participating in the study under various diagnoses because of suspected incipient schizophrenia, 160 patients who did not present psychotic symptoms at the initial assessment according to clinical records were followed up over a mean period of 9.6 years after first assessment. By the time of follow-up, 79 of these patients had fallen ill with DSM-IV schizophrenia – women on average after 4.3 years, men after 6.7 years [112]. Only two of these cases had not shown any basic symptoms at initial assessment, which yields a high sensitivity of 0.98 and a very low rate of false negatives of only 1.3%. Of the 81 patients who did not develop a DSM-IV schizophrenia during the study period, 33 had presented at least one basic symptom and 48 no basic symptoms. This corresponds to a rather high proportion of false negatives (20.6%) and a clearly lower specificity of 0.59. On the whole, however, a remarkably high proportion of the predicted outcomes were classified correctly (78%).

Klosterkötter *et al.* [112] also analysed the prognostic accuracy of the BSABS subsyndromes and found that "information processing disturbances" yielded the best result (PPP = positive predictive power: 0.77).

Information on the probands' diagnoses and other characteristics of this highly selected group at entry into the study is lacking. Therefore, it is unclear to what type of at-risk population the results are applicable. Nevertheless, several of the basic symptoms have been included in other early recognition instruments and are being subjected to further tests of validity.

Instruments Developed by the McGorry Group

McGorry and colleagues in Melbourne started their analyses with the Royal Park Multidiagnostic Instrument for Psychosis (RP-MIP) [158,159]. This covers a large number of symptoms and diagnostic categories, using repeated interviews and multiple information sources. It is designed for the assessment of patients during the inital period of a psychotic episode and based on established international diagnostic instruments and classifications.

The Comprehensive Assessment of At-Risk Mental States (CAARMS), developed by the McGorry group [160], is an instrument designed for the prospective assessment of sub-threshold psychotic symptoms in high-risk groups. It consists of eight subsections (TC = disorders of thought content; PA = perceptual abnormalities; CD = conceptual disorganization; MD = motor disturbances; CA = disorders of concentration, attention, and memory; EA = disorders of emotion and affect; E = impaired energy and S = impaired tolerance to normal stress). Included in the TC scale, which measures attenuated and sub-threshold delusions, are five dimensions: content, conviction, action, frequency and duration. In the other domains three main aspects are distinguished and assessed for each symptom: intensity, frequency and duration, and degree of severity is determined by a combination of these aspects. A further subsection includes eight of Huber's basic symptoms, the last section three dissociative symptoms (amnesia, depersonalization, derealization). The interview is semistructured, sample questions (probes) are given for each symptom, and each section closes with additional questions on duration, frequency and pattern of symptoms.

Instruments Developed by the McGlashan Group

Researchers at the Prevention through Risk Identification, Management, and Education (PRIME) Research Clinic of Yale University developed the Structured Interview for Prodromal Syndromes (SIPS) [161] and, to assess the severity of prodromal symptoms, the Scale of Prodromal Symptoms (SOPS) [162]. The SIPS is a diagnostic interview, the SOPS an associated severity scale. The aim of these instruments is to help to exclude current or previous psychosis, to diagnose one of three types of prodromal states and to assess the severity of prodromal symptoms. The following three prodromal states are distinguished: (a) recent psychotic symptoms of short duration (in particular BLIPS), (b) attenuated psychotic symptoms and (c) a combination of genetic risk and recent deterioration of functioning. The symptoms are rated on a six-point severity scale. The five psychotic symptoms (unusual thought content/delusional ideas; suspiciousness/persecutory ideas; grandiosity; perceptual abnormalities/hallucinations; conceptual disorganization) denote a clear-cut psychotic state only at the highest severity, and stages 1 to 5 denote different degrees of prepsychotic severity. The six negative symptoms (social isolation or withdrawal; avolition; decreased expression of emotion; decreased experience of emotions and self; decreased ideational richness; deterioration in role functioning) as well as the four disorganization symptoms (odd behaviour or appearance; bizarre thinking; trouble with focus and attention; impairment in personal hygiene/social attentiveness) and the four general symptoms (sleep disturbance; dysphoric mood; motor disturbances; impaired tolerance to normal stress) are also rated on a six-point scale.

Results from a reliability and validity study are presented by Miller *et al.* [163]: inter-rater reliability as based on 18 patients (prodromal versus non-prodromal) was 93% (kappa: 0.81). As evidence for the prognostic power of the instruments the authors found that 6 out of 13 prodromal patients transited to psychosis within 6 months (46.2%) and seven (53.8%) within a year.

Instruments Developed by the Häfner Group

The Interview for the Retrospective Assessment of the Onset of Schizophrenia (IRAOS)

The IRAOS [24–26] is the most differentiated of the currently available retrospective early-recognition instruments. It is now available in an enlarged version [27], applicable to all types of psychotic illness and fully compatible with the first version [24–26]. It comprises the assessment of individual biography and social development in the most important social roles, of premorbid adjustment, emergence and accumulation of prodromal signs, of symptoms, abnormal behaviour, functional impairment and social disability. On the basis of IRAOS data it is possible to assess symptom onset, prodromal and psychotic onset, accumulation of symptoms and impairments, and social course. The IRAOS is used by psychiatrists or psychologists.

The development of the IRAOS started with the compilation of a list of prodromal signs and symptoms on an empirical basis. First the literature was skimmed through for symptoms of incipient schizophrenia. A total of 240 symptoms were identified and were included in a questionnaire submitted to experts. Psychiatrists with at least two years work experience at four psychiatric hospitals were asked to rate the relevance of the prodromal and psychotic symptoms listed in incipient schizophrenia.

The list of symptoms generated in this way was integrated in the IRAOS in the form of closed questions and supplemented by open questions that the patient or his/her key informant are asked on the symptoms marking the onset of the disorder and on the timepoint of their emergence. During the revision of the IRAOS the symptom list was expanded to include 128 items, in order to be able to determine at which point in time the person assessed first fulfilled the criteria for an ICD-10 diagnosis of schizophrenia, affective disorder or other psychosis.

Biographical data on social development and illness course are collected on the basis of six roles relevant in the professional and family context and to the individual's objective social status. In this way individual social development, baseline at illness onset and possible interruptions or delays in social ascent can be determined. Besides the general sociodemographic data the IRAOS provides information on the patient's physical health, family situation and history of mental illness. Major life events are assessed on the basis of a layered time matrix divided into units which increase in length with growing distance to the interview (weeks, months, years). Individual anchor events, such as birthdays, holidays and family celebrations are recorded, which help the interviewee to remember the time of symptom emergence in relation to these events. Symptom emergence and remission are recorded in a calendar of episodes.

In a test–retest design two independent interviewers evaluated the IRAOS symptoms in a period varying from 7 to 15 months (mean: 10.4 months). As kappa values were low due to skewed symptom distributions, we report pairwise agreement rates (PAR): for 47% of the IRAOS symptoms PAR was between 0.60 and 0.79, and for another 27.3% it was between 0.80 and 1.00. Only in 4.5% of the symptoms was PAR below 0.40.

To control for recall deficits or memory biases, data were collected from three sources: patient, his/her closest relative and documents (e.g. medical records). The comparison of prodromal signs and symptoms as perceived by the patients and their significant others and registered by a family doctor, in school records etc. offered an important chance for testing the reliability of the information given by the patients. Hambrecht and Häfner [164] compared individual IRAOS data obtained from the patients in the ABC first-episode sample with the data provided by their family members who were in sufficiently close contact with the patients during the period of onset and early illness. Self-perceived symptoms such as subjective thought disorders, which usually cannot be observed by others, had relatively low kappa and percentual agreement rates. High agreement rates of 0.8 and 0.9 were achieved on observable behaviour such as attempted suicide or disturbances of concentration and thinking. Concerning the time of symptom emergence, single psychotic phenomena such as delusions and hallucinations were frequently observed by the relatives with an average of only one month's delay. Nonspecific and negative symptoms, such as mild depression or loss of energy, were frequently noticed by the family members with a mean delay of six months. Still somewhat later (up to 12 months), these symptoms were noted in the documents such as medical case records etc., demonstrating that the patients communicated the onset of their first symptoms with a shorter delay to their relatives than to their doctors. The authors found a surprisingly high degree of agreement in overall estimates of the time of illness onset and of the milestones of the early course between the patients and their family members. As a result, the retrospectively collected IRAOS data yields a valid representation of the early course of schizophrenia at least as far as mean values are concerned.

Meanwhile, the IRAOS has been applied not only in the ABC study, but also by a great number of research teams working on the early and later course of psychosis in many countries (e.g. 165,166).

The Early Recognition Inventory (ERIraos)

The ERIraos is a two-step procedure. First, potential at-risk persons are identified using a checklist. Then the persons thus identified are examined at an early intervention centre using the complete symptom list of the inventory as well as the modules and associated instruments designed for the assessment of risk factors.

The 17-item screening instrument of the ERIraos, the checklist, is designed to make persons at an increased risk of psychosis aware of this risk in order to enable them to get in touch with an early intervention centre. The checklist should sharpen the awareness of general practitioners, counselling services, psychologists, teachers etc. and facilitate the recognition of psychosis risk as early as the prodromal phase. If a defined cut-off is reached, the person in question should be referred to an early intervention centre for a more detailed risk assessment. The checklist is designed to avoid a hastened exclusion of at-risk persons (so-called false negatives) thus providing a low threshold in order to make sure that as few false decisions as possible are made at this stage of diagnosis.

The checklist is available as an interview and as a questionnaire. The checklist interview is administed by a general practitioner or some other professional contact person, whereas the questionnaire version is done by the respondent without assistance.

The core element of the ERIraos is the symptom list, which includes 110 symptoms of beginning schizophrenia. It mainly contains prodromal symptoms of schizophrenia (unspecific symptoms, depressive symptoms, basic symptoms), but in addition it also includes psychotic symptoms, because in some at-risk persons obvious psychotic symptoms of short duration are already present in the prodromal phase. The inclusion of psychotic symptoms makes it possible to identify transition to psychosis, a prerequisite for recognizing psychotic episodes earlier than under the current conditions of treatment. It also allows one to study the course of schizophrenia from onset to full blown psychosis and the long-term course of the disorder.

The ERIraos symptom list is divided into 12 sections:

S01 Introductory questions
S02 Changes in mood, interest and drive
S03 Disturbance of sleep and appetite
S04 Changes in personality
S05 Dysfunctional behaviour
S06 Anxiety and obsessive–compulsive symptoms
S07 Thought disorder
S08 Disorders of self and delusions
S09 Impaired bodily sensations (coenaesthesia)
S10 Abnormal perceptions
S11 Motor disorder
S12 Observed behaviour

For risk persons, both the present state and previous course of illness before the first interview are recorded. To monitor the success of intervention, the ERIraos symptom list is carried out prospectively at different timepoints. The months in between the follow-ups are rated retrospectively. Of main interest at the first interview are the questions of how far the illness, e.g. the prodromal phase, has already progressed, and the sequence of symptom occurrence. Included in the ERIraos are roughly two thirds of the IRAOS symptoms, but its aim is to assess not only symptom onset, but also the increase in symptom severity (distress) and functional impairment. The symptom list of the ERIraos should help us to decide whether the persons assessed require intervention or not because of a risk for schizophrenia.

In order to improve predictions of illness risk by considering further risk factors, four modules were additionally integrated in the ERIraos and supplemented by two associated instruments. These are family (genetic) risk, complications during pregnancy and childbirth, developmental retardation during infancy, comorbidity (especially if linked to alcohol and drugs), delinquency and schizotypal personality. The diagnostic criteria for schizotypy can be evaluated on the basis of the symptom list. A fourth module is presented as a questionnaire and given after the interview to assess ordinary life situations, serving as a further assessment of schizotypal features. The module on medication includes questions on the type and dosage of already prescribed medications, either current or earlier [172].

To determine the reliability of the ERIraos symptom list, videotaped interviews were presented to 9 or 10 interviewers at three rating sessions. The symptom ratings of the interviewers were compared with the standard ratings of the trainer team. Kappas for "symptom present in the year before interview" range between 0.56 and 0.77; for the rating of "subjective stress associated with the symptom" between 0.54 and 0.77. The reliabilities increased from the first to the third assessment.

An analysis based on 83 checklist interviews was also carried out. Prodromal symptoms assessed by the checklist have been present at least in 24.1% (ideas of reference) at-risk persons and in a maximum of 84.3% (tension, nervousness, restlessness). Checklist symptoms are more frequent in the late prodrome compared to the early prodrome ($p<0.05$ for ten symptoms). The most frequent prodromal symptoms are nonspecific (negative symptoms: loss of energy, loss of concentration, social withdrawal; depressive symptoms: depressive mood, loss of self-confidence, increased fatigability).

ERIraos data of 75 patients, interviewed at the early intervention centres in Bonn, Cologne, Dusseldorf and Munich, have been collected. Symptom onset dates back between 4.7 and 9.1 years. The earliest symptom is "preoccupation with mysterious things", but this item probably indicates a persistent schizotypal personality trait. The most frequent early symptoms are nonspecific (worries about mental functions, depressed mood, tension and restlessness) and are negative symptoms/social disabilities and depressive symptoms. In all, 73% of the patients fulfilled the checklist criteria already one year before inclusion in the early intervention programme.

In addition to the prodromal symptoms, 85% of the sample report further risk factors: 60% report difficulties in everyday situations, indicating schizotypal personality traits, 58% report alcohol or drug use, 21% obstetric or birth complications, 21% delinquency and 11% familial load with psychosis. In the subgroup with additional risk factors, the percentage of patients fulfilling the checklist criteria one year before inclusion in the early intervention study is increased from 73% to 87%.

EVALUATING (VALIDATING) PRODROMAL SIGNS AND CRITERIA

Validating the DSM-IIIR Prodromal Symptoms

Listed in the DSM-IIIR were nine prodromal symptoms of schizophrenia, generated by consensus and not empirically [167]: social isolation or withdrawal; marked impairment in role functioning; markedly peculiar behaviour; marked impairment in personal hygiene; blunted, flat or inappropriate affect; dissociative or metaphoric speech; odd or bizarre ideation; unusal perceptional experiences; marked lack of initiative, interests or energy.

The first attempt at cross-sectionally validating these prodromal signs was made by Jackson *et al.* [168] in a sample of 313 first episodes of various functional psychoses. Where the standard DSM-IIIR assessment is utilized, inter-rater reliability is poor, as is test–retest reliability [97]. Analysing the comparative frequencies and diagnostic efficiencies of the prodromal signs in a retrospective design, the authors found relatively poor distinguishing efficacies between diagnoses. In a second study, McGorry *et al.* [169] followed up the prevalence of these nine prodromal symptoms prospectively in a large representative sample ($n = 2525$) of Australian school children at mean ages of 12, 14 and 16 years. The result supported the low discriminatory efficacy of these prodromal symptoms found in comparisons of diagnosed functional mental disorders: the prevalences ranged from 8% to 51% indicating a high frequency in the healthy population and a low specificity for schizophrenia.

A third study to improve the diagnostic efficiency and predictive power of these prodromal symptoms was conducted by McGorry *et al.* [170]. Of 200 individuals experiencing a first-onset psychosis and aged 14 to 46 years (mean: 25.23), 61 (30.5%) suffered from schizophrenia, 49 (24.5%) from schizophreniform disorder. Two sources were interviewed, patients and relatives, to obtain detailed information on the prodromal period. This information was registered in the RP-MIP. The result was that three items and more had a higher predictive power than single items. When the duration of the prodromal phase and especially prepsychotic deterioration in functioning were taken into account, the predictive power rose considerably. This means that the gradient of change – in clinical terms the observed deterioration – plays an important role in prognosis. Hence, the key finding was that prodromal deterioration which is relatively prolonged – a feature of course in combination with a symptom cluster – predicts schizophrenia within a first episode of psychosis sample as quite likely, but not with sufficient certainty. Meanwhile, the prodromal symptoms of schizophrenia listed in the DSM-IIIR were dropped from the DSM-IV.

First Results from Prospective Validation Studies of Early Recognition Inventories and Risk Criteria

Meanwhile, first studies on the risk of transition to psychosis in UHR individuals have been published. Yung *et al.* [147] identified 20 UHR individuals aged 16 to 30, referred for treatment and followed up at monthly intervals over 6 months. Eight (40%) of these patients developed a frank psychosis. Five of the patients became psychotic as early as the first month. Later studies conducted in larger samples have yielded very similar results for risk periods of one to two years, with the proportion of patients transiting to psychosis ranging from 25% to 41% [74]. A further independent validation of the UHR criteria was done in a control group of UHR cases in a randomized early-intervention study [70]. At one year of follow-up, the rate of transition to psychosis was 35.7% for the controls.

CONCLUSIONS

On all dimensions of the disorder we call schizophrenia – symptoms, neuropsychological changes and functional impairment – the prodromal stage and the early psychotic stage preceding the climax of the first episode constitute the most active, most rapidly progressing and hence the most decisive period in terms of the social consequences of the disorder. It may even be of far greater importance for further illness course and social outcome than any of the later stages of illness. The prodromal period usually interferes with educational and occupational career at a stage most vulnerable to influence. In accordance with results from the ABC Schizophrenia Study, Eaton and Harrison [171] describe the onset of schizophrenia as follows: "The type of symptoms that show up first are affective, negative and cognitive and social dysfunction: depressed mood, trouble with concentration, poor work performance, subtle social deficits".

The durations of the prodromal stages and of the psychotic episode until the climax of psychosis vary a great deal. According to studies on the topic, the mean duration of the prepsychotic prodromal stage ranges from two to five years (ABC Study: 4.8 years), and the psychotic stage until first admission currently still lasts slightly more than a year. In two thirds of cases more than a year elapses from illness onset until first admission, whereas only some 15% experience an acute type of onset of four weeks or less. Especially in patients with a chronic early course, early intervention appears promising and, since first successful results have appeared, also meaningful. The precondition is that individuals at incipient risk seek help, diagnosis can be given early and the time of onset of the psychotic episode and the future illness course are predicted with sufficient accuracy. Three quarters of all cases of schizophrenia experience a prodromal stage without specific psychotic symptoms. We must find ways of detecting and recognizing the illness and of predicting its further course earlier than is currently the case, by using appropriate instruments and designs at early-intervention centres and by increasing awareness and knowledge in the population at risk.

When prodromal signs have appeared and symptoms and/or functional impairments increase (a positive gradient), it is very likely that it will come to a full-blown psychosis. When psychotic symptoms have emerged and persisted for at least one week, a schizophrenia spectrum disorder can be diagnosed and antipsychotic therapy initiated. The validation of early recognition inventories as a basis for early intervention will be a focal point of future research.

ACKNOWLEDGEMENTS

The ABC study was supported by the Deutsche Forschungsgemeinschaft (DFG, German Research Association) as part of the Special Research Branch (Sonderforschungsbereich) 258 at the Central Institute of Mental Health until December 1998. From January 1999 to September 2002 it was continued to be funded by the DFG as an independent project. This chapter was written within the framework of the German Research Network on Schizophrenia and was funded by the German Federal Ministry for Education and Research BMBF (grant 01 GI 0236).

REFERENCES

1. Griesinger W. (1861). *Pathologie und Therapie psychischer Krankheiten*, 2nd edn. Krabbe, Stuttgart.
2. Kraepelin E. (1893). *Psychiatrie. Ein Lehrbuch für Studierende und Aerzte*, 4th edn. Barth, Leipzig.
3. Bleuler E. (1911). Dementia praecox oder Gruppe der Schizophrenien. In: Aschaffenburg G. (ed.) *Handbuch der Psychiatrie*. Deuticke, Leipzig, pp. 1–420.
4. Häfner H. (1995). Was ist Schizophrenie. In: Häfner H. (ed.) *Was ist Schizophrenie?* Fischer, Stuttgart, pp. 1–44.
5. Maier W., Rietschel M., Linz M., Falkai P. (2002). Genetics of schizophrenia and related disorders. In: Häfner H. (ed.) *Risk and Protective Factors in Schizophrenia*. Springer-Verlag, Berlin, pp. 9–28.
6. Sullivan S.H. (1927). The onset of schizophrenia. *Am. J. Psychiatry*, **6**, 105–134.
7. Cameron D.E. (1938). Early diagnosis of schizophrenia by the general practitioner. *N. Engl. J. Med.*, **218**, 221–224.
8. Cameron D.E. (1938). Early schizophrenia. *Am. J. Psychiatry*, **95**, 567–578.

9. Häfner H., Maurer K., Löffler W., Riecher-Rössler A. (1993). The influence of age and sex on the onset and early course of schizophrenia. *Br. J. Psychiatry*, **162**, 80–86.
10. Häfner H., an der Heiden W., Löffler W., Maurer K., Hambrecht M. (1998). Beginn und Frühverlauf schizophrener Erkrankungen. In: Klosterkötter J. (ed.) *Frühdiagnostik und Frühbehandlung psychischer Störungen*. Bayer-ZNS-Symposium XIII. Springer-Verlag, Berlin, pp. 1–28.
11. Gross G. (1969). Prodrome und Vorpostensyndrome schizophrener Erkrankungen. In: Huber G. (ed.) *Schizophrenie und Zyklothymie*. Thieme, Stuttgart, pp. 177–187.
12. Lindelius R. (1970). A study of schizophrenia: a clinical, prognostic and family investigation. *Acta Psychiatr. Scand.*, **216** (Suppl.), 1–125.
13. Huber G., Gross G., Schüttler R. (1979). *Schizophrenie. Eine Verlaufs- und sozialpsychiatrische Langzeitstudie*. Springer-Verlag, Berlin.
14. Loebel A.D., Lieberman J.A., Alvir J.M.J., Mayerhoff D.I., Geisler S.H., Szymanski S.R. (1992). Duration of psychosis and outcome in first-episode schizophrenia. *Am. J. Psychiatry*, **149**, 1183–1188.
15. Beiser M., Erickson D., Flemming J.A.E., Iacono W.G. (1993). Establishing the onset of psychotic illness. *Am. J. Psychiatry*, **150**, 1349–1354.
16. McGorry P.D., Edwards J., Mihalopoulos C., Harrigan S.M., Jackson H.J. (1996). EPPIC: an evolving system of early detection and optimal management. *Schizophr. Bull*, **22**, 305–326.
17. Lewine R.J. (1980). Sex differences in age of symptom onset and first hospitalization in schizophrenia. *Am. J. Orthopsychiatry*, **50**, 316–322.
18. Häfner H., Maurer K., Löffler W., Bustamante S., an der Heiden W., Riecher-Rössler A., Nowotny B. (1995). Onset and early course of schizophrenia. In: Häfner H., Gattaz W.F. (eds) *Search for the Causes of Schizophrenia*, vol. III. Springer-Verlag, Berlin, pp. 43–66.
19. Johannessen J.O., Larsen T.K., McGlashan T. (1999). Duration of untreated psychosis: an important target for intervention in schizophrenia? *Nord. J. Psychiatry*, **53**, 275–283.
20. Ho B.C., Alicata D., Ward J., Moser D.J., O'Leary D.S., Arndt S., Andreasen N.C. (2003). Untreated initial psychosis: relation to cognitive deficits and brain morphology in first-episode schizophrenia. *Am. J. Psychiatry*, **160**, 142–148.
21. Conrad K. (1958). *Die beginnende Schizophrenie. Versuch einer Gestaltanalyse des Wahns*. Thieme-Verlag, Stuttgart.
22. Docherty J.P., van Kammen D.P., Siris S.G., Marder S.R. (1978). Stages of onset of schizophrenic psychosis. *Am. J. Psychiatry*, **135**, 420–426.
23. Häfner H., Maurer K., Löffler W., an der Heiden W., Hambrecht M., Schultze-Lutter F. Modeling the early course of schizophrenia. *Schizophr. Bull.*, **29**, 325–340.
24. Häfner H., Riecher A., Maurer K., Meissner S., Schmidtke A., Fätkenheuer B., Löffler W., an der Heiden W. (1990). Ein Instrument zur retrospektiven Einschätzung des Erkrankungsbeginns bei Schizophrenie (Instrument for the Retrospective Assessment of the Onset of Schizophrenia – "IRAOS") Entwicklung und Ergebnisse. *Z. Klin. Psychol.*, **19**, 230–255.
25. Häfner H., Riecher-Rössler A., Hambrecht M., Maurer K., Meissner S., Schmidtke A., Fätkenheuer B., Löffler W., an der Heiden W. (1992). IRAOS: an instrument for the assessment of onset and early course of schizophrenia. *Schizophr. Res.*, **6**, 209–223.

26. Häfner H., Riecher-Rössler A., Fätkenheuer B., Maurer K., Meissner S., Löffler W. (1992). *Interview for the Retrospective Assessment of the Onset of Schizophrenia (IRAOS)* (trans. G. Patton). Published by H. Häfner.
27. Häfner H., Löffler W., Maurer K., Riecher-Rössler A., Stein A. (1999). *IRAOS. Interview für die retrospektive Erfassung des Erkrankungsbeginns und -verlaufs bei Schizophrenie und anderen Psychosen*. Hans Huber Verlag, Bern.
28. Häfner H., Löffler W., Maurer K., Riecher-Rössler A., Stein A. (2003). *IRAOS – Interview for the Retrospective Assessment of the Onset and Course of Schizophrenia and Other Psychoses*. Hogrefe & Huber, Göttingen.
29. Hambrecht M., Häfner H. (1993) "Trema, Apophänie, Apokalypse" – Ist Conrads Phasenmodell empirisch begründbar? *Fortschr. Neurol. Psychiatr.*, **61**, 418–423.
30. Foulds G.A. (1976). *The Hierarchical Nature of Personal Illness*. Academic Press, London.
31. de Jong A., Giel R., Lindeboom E.G., Slooff C.J., Wiersma D. (1984). Foulds' hierarchical model of psychiatric illness in a Dutch cohort: a re-evaluation. *Psychol. Med.*, **14**, 647–654.
32. Biehl H., Maurer K., Jung E., Krumm B., Schubart C. (1987). Zum "natürlichen Verlauf" schizophrener Erkrankungen – Begriff und Beispiele zum beobachteten Verhalten in einer prospektiven Studie. *Nervenheilkunde*, **6**, 153–163.
33. Faris R.E., Dunham W. (1939). *Mental Disorders in Urban Areas. An Ecological Study of Schizophrenia and Other Psychoses*. University of Chicago Press, Chicago, IL.
34. Dauncey K., Giggs J., Baker K., Harrison G. (1993). Schizophrenia in Nottingham: lifelong residential mobility of a cohort. *Br. J. Psychiatry*, **163**, 613–619.
35. Kohn M. (1969). *Class and Conformity: A Study of Values*. Dorsey Press, Homewood, IL.
36. Eaton W.W. (1999). Evidence for universality and uniformity of schizophrenia around the world: assessment and implications. In: Gattaz W.F., Häfner H. (eds) *Search for the Causes of Schizophrenia*, vol. IV: *Balance of the Century*. Steinkopff, Darmstadt; Springer-Verlag, Heidelberg, pp. 21–33.
37. Rabinowitz J., Reichenberg A., Weiser M., Mark M., Kaplan Z., Davidson M. (2000). Cognitive and behavioural functioning in men with schizophrenia both before and shortly after first admission to hospital. *Br. J. Psychiatry*, **177**, 26–32.
38. Van Os J., Verdoux H., Maurice-Tison S., Gay B., Liraud F., Salamon R., Bourgeois M. (1999). Self-reported psychosis-like symptoms and the continuum of psychosis. *Soc. Psychiatry Psychiatr. Epidemiol.*, **34**, 459–463.
39. Hanssen M.S.S., Bak M., Bijl R., Vollebergh W., van Os J. (2002). Is prediction of psychosis in the general population feasible? *Eur. Psychiatry*, **17** (Suppl. 1), 74.
40. Verdoux H., van Os J. (2002). Psychotic symptoms in non-clinical populations and the continuum of psychosis. *Schizophr. Res.*, **54**, 59–65.
41. Yung A.R., McGorry P.D. (1996). The prodromal phase of first-episode psychosis: past and current conceptualisations. *Schizophr. Bull.*, **22**, 353–370.
42. Johnstone E.C., Crow T.J., Johnson A.L., McMillan J.F. (1986). The Northwick Park study of first episodes of schizophrenia: I. Presentation of the illness and problems relating to admission. *Br. J. Psychiatry*, **148**, 115–120.
43. Norman R.M., Malla A.K. (2001). Duration of untreated psychosis: a critical examination of the concept and its importance. *Psychol. Med.*, **31**, 381–400.
44. Birchwood M., McMillan J.F. (1993). Early intervention in schizophrenia. *Aust. N. Zeal. J. Psychiatry*, **27**, 374–378.

45. Linszen D., Lenior M., de Haan L., Dingemans P., Gersons B. (1998). Early intervention, untreated psychosis and the course of early schizophrenia. *Br. J. Psychiatry*, **172** (Suppl. 33), 84–89.
46. McEvoy J.P., Schooler N.R., Wilson W.H. (1991). Predictors of therapeutic response to haloperidol in acute schizophrenia. *Psychopharmacol. Bull.*, **27**, 97–101.
47. Haas G.L., Gattatt L.S., Sweeney J.A. (1998). Delay to first antipsychotic medication in schizophrenia: impact on symptomatology and clinical course of illness. *J. Psychiatr. Res.*, **32**, 151–159.
48. Szymanski S.R., Cannon T.D., Gallacher F., Erwin R.J., Gur R.E. (1996). Course of treatment response in first-episode and chronic schizophrenia. *Am. J. Psychiatry*, **153**, 519–525.
49. Bottlender R., Strauss A., Möller H.-J. (2000). Impact of duration of symptoms prior to first hospitalization on acute outcome in 998 schizophrenic patients. *Schizophr. Res.*, **44**, 145–150.
50. McGorry P.D., Edwards J. (1997). *Early Psychosis Training Pack*. Gardiner-Caldwell Communications, Victoria Mill, Australia.
51. Larsen T.K., Johannessen J.O., Opjordsmoen S. (1998). First-episode schizophrenia with long duration of untreated psychosis. Pathways to care. *Br. J. Psychiatry*, **172**, 45–52.
52. Helgason L. (1990). Twenty years' follow-up of first psychiatric presentation for schizophrenia: what could have been prevented? *Acta Psychiatr. Scand.*, **81**, 231–235.
53. Stirling J., Tantam D., Thomas P., Newby D., Montague L., Ring N., Rowe S. (1991). Expressed emotion and early onset schizophrenia: a one-year follow-up. *Psychol. Med.*, **21**, 675–685.
54. Stirling J., Tantam D., Thomas P., Newby D., Montague L., Ring N., Rowe S. (1993). Expressed emotion and schizophrenia: the ontogeny of EE during an 18-month follow-up. *Psychol. Med.*, **23**, 771–778.
55. Addington J., Addington D. (1998). Effect of substance misuse in early psychosis. *Br. J. Psychiatry*, **172** (Suppl. 33), 134–136.
56. Addington D., Addington J., Patten S. (1998). Depression in people with first-episode schizophrenia. *Br. J. Psychiatry*, **172**, 90–92.
57. Koreen A.R., Siris S.G., Chakos M., Alvir J., Mayerhoff D., Lieberman J. (1993). Depression in first episode schizophrenia. *Am. J. Psychiatry*, **150**, 1643–1648.
58. Strakowski S.M., Keck P.E. Jr, McElroy S.L., Lonczak H.S., West S.A. (1995). Chronology of comorbid and principal syndromes in first-episode psychosis. *Compr. Psychiatry*, **36**, 106–112.
59. Johnstone E.C., McMillan J.F., Frith C.D., Benn D.K., Crow T.J. (1990). Further investigation of the predictors of outcome following first schizophrenic episodes. *Br. J. Psychiatry*, **157**, 182–189.
60. Larsen T.K., McGlashan T.H., Moe L.C. (1996). First-episode schizophrenia: I. Early course parameters. *Schizophr. Bull.*, **22**, 241–256.
61. Humphreys M.S., Johnstone E.C., McMillan J.F., Taylor P.J. (1992). Dangerous behaviour preceding first admissions for schizophrenia. *Br. J. Psychiatry*, **161**, 501–505.
62. Häfner H., Maurer K., Löffler W., an der Heiden W., Könnecke R., Hambrecht M. (2002). The early course of schizophrenia. In: Häfner H. (ed.) *Risk and Protective Factors in Schizophrenia*. Steinkopff, Darmstadt, pp. 207–228.

63. Craig T.J., Bromet E.J., Fennig S., Tanenberg-Karant M., Lavelle J., Galambos N. (2000). Is there an association between duration of untreated psychosis and 24-month clinical outcome in a first-admission series? *Am. J. Psychiatry*, **157**, 60–66.
64. Robinson D.G., Woerner M.G., Alvir J., Ma J., Geisler S., Koreen A., Sheitman B., Chakos M., Mayerhoff D., Bilder R., *et al.* (1999). Predictors of treatment response from a first episode of schizophrenia or schizoaffective disorder. *Am. J. Psychiatry*, **156**, 544–549.
65. Robinson D.G., Woemer M.G., Alvir J., Ma J., Bilder R., Goldman R., Geisler S., Koreen A., Sheitman B., Chakos M., *et al.* (1999). Predictors of relapse following response from a first episode of schizophrenia or schizoaffective disorder. *Arch. Gen. Psychiatry*, **56**, 241–247.
66. Ho B.C., Andreasen N.C., Flaum M., Nopoulos P., Miller D. (2000). Untreated initial psychosis: its relation to quality of life and symptom remission in first-episode schizophrenia. *Am. J. Psychiatry*, **157**, 808–815.
67. Altamura A.C., Bassetti R., Sassella F., Salvadori D., Mundo E. (2001). Duration of untreated psychosis as a predictor of outcome in first-episode schizophrenia: a retrospective study. *Schizophr. Res.*, **52**, 29–36.
68. Malla A.K., Norman R.M., Manchanda R., Ahmed M.R., Scholten D., Harricharan R., Cortese L., Takhar J. (2002). One year outcome in first episode psychosis: influence of DUP and other predictors. *Schizophr. Res.*, **54**, 231–242.
69. Joyce E., Hutton S., Mutsatsa S., Gibbins H., Webb E., Paul S., Robbins T., Barnes T. (2002). Executive dysfunction in first-episode schizophrenia and relationship to duration of untreated psychosis. *Br. J. Psychiatry*, **181** (Suppl. 43), 38–44.
70. McGorry P.D., Yung A.R., Phillips L.J., Yuen H.P., Francey S., Cosgrave E.M., Germano D., Bravin J., Adlard S., McDonald T., *et al.* (2002). Randomized controlled trial of interventions designed to reduce the risk of progression to first episode psychosis in a clinical sample with subthreshold symptoms. *Arch. Gen. Psychiatry*, **59**, 921–928.
71. Hoff A.L., Sakuma M., Razi K., Heydebrand G., Csernansky J.G., DeLisi L.E. (2000). Lack of association between duration of untreated illness and severity of cognitive and structural brain deficits at the first episode of schizophrenia. *Am. J. Psychiatry*, **157**, 1824–1828.
72. Barnes T.R., Hutton S.B., Chapman M.J., Mutsatsa S., Puri B.K., Joyce E.M. (2000). West London first-episode study of schizophrenia: clinical correlates of duration of untreated psychosis. *Br. J. Psychiatry*, **177**, 207–211.
73. Harrigan S.M., McGorry P.D., Krstev H. (2003). Does treatment delay in first-episode psychosis really matter? *Psychol. Med.*, **33**, 97–110.
74. Edwards J., McGorry P.D. (2002). *Implementing Early Intervention in Psychosis*. Dunitz, London.
75. Breier A., Schreiber J.L., Dyer J., Pickar D. (1991). National Institute of Mental Health longitudinal study of chronic schizophrenia: prognosis and predictors of outcome. *Arch. Gen. Psychiatry*, **48**, 239–246.
76. Wyatt R.J. (1991). Neuroleptics and the natural course of schizophrenia. *Schizophr. Bull.*, **17**, 325–351.
77. Wyatt R.J. (1995). Early intervention for schizophrenia: can the course of the illness be altered? *Biol Psychiatry*, **38**, 1–3.
78. Lieberman J.A., Perkins D., Belger A., Chakos M., Jarskog F., Boteva K., Gilmore J. (2001). The early stages of schizophrenia: speculations on pathogenesis, pathophysiology and therapeutic approaches. *Biol. Psychiatry*, **50**, 884–897.

79. Lieberman J.A., Tollefson G., Tohen M., Green A.I., Gur R.E., Kahn R., McEvoy J., Perkins D., Sharma T., Zipursky R., *et al.* (2003). Comparative efficacy and safety of atypical and conventional antipsychotic drugs in first-episode psychosis: a randomized, double-blind trial of olanzapine versus haloperidol. *Am. J. Psychiatry*, **160**, 1396–1404.
80. McGlashan T.H., Johannessen J.O. (1996). Early detection and intervention with schizophrenia: a rationale. *Schizophr. Bull.*, **22**, 201–222.
81. Goldberg T.E., David A., Gold J.M. (2003). Neurocognitive deficits in schizophrenia. In: Hirsch S.R., Weinberger D.R. (eds) *Schizophrenia*, 2nd edn. Blackwell, Oxford, pp. 168–184.
82. Liddle P.F. (1987). Schizophrenic syndromes, cognitive performance and neurological dysfunction. *Psychol. Med.*, **17**, 49–57.
83. Liddle P.F. (1987). The symptoms of chronic schizophrenia: a re-examination of the positive–negative dichotomy. *Br. J. Psychiatry*, **151**, 145–151.
84. Liddle P.F., Barnes T.R.E. (1990). Syndromes of chronic schizophrenia. *Br. J. Psychiatry*, **157**, 558–561.
85. Löffler W., Häfner H. (1999). Dimensionen der schizophrenen Symptomatik. *Nervenarzt*, **70**, 416–429.
86. Arndt S., Andreasen N.C., Flaum M., Miller D., Nopoulos P. (1995). A longitudinal study of symptom dimensions in schizophrenia – prediction and patterns of change. *Arch. Gen. Psychiatry*, **52**, 352–360.
87. Salokangas R.K.R. (1997). Structure of schizophrenic symptomatology and its changes over time: prospective factor-analytical study. *Acta Psychiatr. Scand.*, **95**, 32–39.
88. DeLisi L.E., Sakuma M., Ge S., Kushner M. (1998). Association of brain structural change with the heterogeneous course of schizophrenia. *Psychiatry Res.*, **84**, 75–88.
89. Johnstone E.C., Russell K.D., Harrison L.K., Lawrie S.M. (2003). The Edinburgh High Risk Study: current status and future prospects. *World Psychiatry*, **2**, 45–49.
90. Lawrie S.M., Whalley H.C., Abukmeil S.S., Kestelman J.N., Donnelly L., Miller P., Best J.J.K., Owens D.G.C., Johnstone E.C. (2001). Brain structure, genetic liability, and psychotic symptoms in subjects at high risk of developing schizophrenia. *Biol. Psychiatry*, **49**, 811–823.
91. Fannon D., Chitnis X., Doku V., Tennakoon L., O'Ceallaigh S., Soni W., Sumich A., Lowe J., Santamaria M., Sharma T. (2000). Features of structural brain abnormality detected in first-episode psychosis. *Am. J. Psychiatry*, **157**, 1829–1834.
92. Pantelis C., Velakoulis D., McGorry P.D., Wood S.J., Suckling J., Phillips L.J., Yung A.R., Bullmore E.T., Brewer W., Soulsby B., Desmond P., McGuire P.K. (2003). Neuroanatomical abnormalities before and after onset of psychosis: a cross-sectional and longitudinal MRI comparison. *Lancet*, **361**, 281–288.
93. Copolov D., Velakoulis D., McGorry P., Mallard C., Yung A., Rees S., Jackson G., Rehn A., Brewer W., Pantelis C. (2000). Neurobiological findings in early phase schizophrenia. *Brain Res. Brain Res. Rev.*, **31**, 157–165.
94. Malla A.K., Mittal C., Lee M., Scholten D.J., Assis L., Norman R.M. (2002). Computed tomography of the brain morphology of patients with first-episode schizophrenic psychosis. *J. Psychiatry Neurosci.*, **27**, 350–358.
95. Verdoux H., Maurice-Tison S., Gay B., Van Os J., Salamon R., Bourgeois M.L. (1998). A survey of delusional ideation in primary-care patients. *Psychol. Med.*, **28**, 127–134.

96. Lewis S., Tarrier N., Haddock G., Bentall R., Kinderman P., Kingdon D., Siddle R., Drake R., Everitt J., Leadley K. *et al.* (2002). Randomised, controlled trial of cognitive–behaviour therapy in early schizophrenia: acute phase outcomes. *Br. J. Psychiatry*, **181**, 91–97.
97. Jackson J.H., McGorry P.D., McKenzie D. (1994). The reliability of DSM-III prodromal symptoms in first episode psychotic patients. *Acta Psychiatr. Scand.*, **90**, 375–378.
98. Janzarik W. (1968). *Schizophrene Verläufe*. Springer-Verlag, Berlin.
99. Häfner H., an der Heiden W. (2003). Course and outcome of schizophrenia. In: Hirsch S.R., Weinberger D.R. (eds) *Schizophrenia*, 2nd edn. Blackwell, Oxford, pp. 101–141.
100. Gaebel W., Frick U., Köpcke W., Linden M., Müller P., Müller-Spahn F., Pietzcker A., Tegeler J. (1993). Early neuroleptic intervention in schizophrenia: are prodromal symptoms valid predictors of relapse? *Br. J. Psychiatry*, **163** (Suppl. 21), 8–12.
101. Gaebel W., Frommann N. (2000). Long-term course in schizophrenia: concepts, methods and research strategies. *Acta Psychiatr. Scand.*, **102**, 49–53.
102. Birchwood M., Smith J., Macmillan F., Hogg B., Prasad R., Harvey C., Bering S. (1989). Predicting relapse in schizophrenia: the development and implementation of an early signs monitoring system using patients and families as observers. A preliminary investigation. *Psychol. Med.*, **19**, 649–656.
103. Carpenter W., Heinrichs D. (1983). Early intervention, time limited targeted pharmacotherapy for schizophrenia. *Schizophr. Bull.*, **9**, 533–542.
104. Hirsch S.R., Jolley A.G. (1989). The dysphoric syndrome in schizophrenia and its implications for relapse. *Br. J. Psychiatry*, **155** (Suppl. 5), 46–50.
105. Cutting J., Dunne F. (1989). Subjective experience of schizophrenia. *Schizophr. Bull.*, **15**, 217–231.
106. Jolley A.G., Hirsch S.R., McRink A., Manchanda R. (1989). Trial of brief intermittent neuroleptic prophylaxis for selected schizophrenic outpatients: clinical outcome at one year. *Br. Med. J.*, **298**, 985–990.
107. Marder S.R., Wirshing W.C., Van Putten T., Mintz J., McKenzie J., Johnston-Cronk K., Lebell M., Liberman R.P. (1994). Fluphenazine vs. placebo supplementation for prodromal signs of relapse in schizophrenia. *Arch. Gen. Psychiatry*, **51**, 280–287.
108. Herz M.I., Lamberti J.S., Mintz J., Scott R., O'Dell S.P., McCartan L., Nix G. (2000). A program for relapse prevention in schizophrenia: a controlled study. *Arch. Gen. Psychiatry*, **57**, 277–283.
109. McGorry P.D. (1995). Psycho-education in first-episode psychosis: a therapeutic process. *Psychiatry*, **58**, 329–344.
110. Herz M., Melville C. (1980). Relapse in schizophrenia. *Am. J. Psychiatry*, **137**, 801–805.
111. Maurer K., Häfner H. (1995). Methodological aspects of onset assessment in schizophrenia. *Schizophr. Res.*, **15**, 265–276.
112. Klosterkötter J., Hellmich M., Steinmeyer E.M., Schultze-Lutter F. (2001). Diagnosing schizophrenia in the initial prodromal phase. *Arch. Gen. Psychiatry*, **58**, 158–164.
113. Biehl H., Maurer K., Schubart C., Krumm B., Jung E. (1986). Prediction of outcome and utilization of medical services in a prospective study of first onset schizophrenics – results of a prospective 5-year follow-up study. *Eur. Arch. Psychiatry Neurol. Sci.*, **236**, 139–147.

114. Häfner H., Löffler W., Maurer K., Hambrecht M., an der Heiden W. (1999). Depression, negative symptoms, social stagnation and social decline in the early course of schizophrenia. *Acta Psychiatr. Scand.*, **100**, 105–118.

115. Dobmeier P., Bottlender R., Wittmann J., Groß A., Wegner U., Strauß A., Möller H.-U. (2000). Depressive Symptome bei schizophrenen Erkrankungen – Ergebnisse der Münchner 15-Jahres-Katamnese. In: Maier W., Engel R.R., Möller H.-U. (eds) *Methodik von Verlaufs- und Therapiestudien in Psychiatrie und Psychotherapie*. Hogrefe, Göttingen, pp. 179–188.

116. Davidson L., McGlashan T.H. (1997). The varied outcomes of schizophrenia. *Can. J. Psychiatry*, **42**, 34–43.

117. Döpfner M., Pluck J., Berner W., Fegert J.M., Huss M., Lenz K., Schmeck K., Lehmkuhl U., Poustka F., Lehmkuhl G. (1997). Psychische Auffälligkeiten von Kindern und Jugendlichen in Deutschland – Ergebnisse einer repräsentativen Studie: Methodik, Alters-, Geschlechts- und Beurteilereffekte. *Z. Kinder Jugendpsychiatr. Psychother.*, **25**, 218–233.

118. Choquet M., Ledoux S. (1994). Epidémiologie et adolescence. *Confrontations psychiatriques*, **27**, 287–309.

119. Häfner H., Maurer K., Löffler W., an der Heiden W., Stein A., Könnecke R., Hambrecht M. (1999). Onset and prodromal phase as determinants of the course. In: Gattaz W.F., Häfner H. (eds) *Search for the Causes of Schizophrenia*, vol. IV: *Balance of the Century*. Steinkopff, Darmstandt; Springer-Verlag, Heidelberg, pp. 35–58.

120. Lewine R.R.J. (1988). Gender and schizophrenia. In: Nasrallah H.A. (ed.) *Handbook of Schizophrenia*, vol. 3. Elsevier, Amsterdam, pp. 379–397.

121. Angermeyer M.C., Kühn L. (1988). Gender differences in age at onset of schizophrenia. *Eur. Arch. Psychiatry Neurol. Sci.*, **237**, 351–364.

122. Häfner H., Riecher A., Maurer K., Löffler W., Munk-Jörgensen P., Strömgren E. (1989). How does gender influence age at first hospitalization for schizophrenia? A transnational case register study. *Psychol. Med.*, **19**, 903–918.

123. Häfner H., Behrens S., Vry J. de, Gattaz W.F. (1992). An animal model for the effects of estradiol on dopamine-mediated behavior: implications for sex differences in schizophrenia. *Psychiatry Res.*, **38**, 125–134.

124. Loranger A.W. (1984). Sex difference in age of onset of schizophrenia. *Arch. Gen. Psychiatry*, **41**, 157–161.

125. Seeman M.V., Lang M. (1990). The role of estrogens in schizophrenia gender differences. *Schizophr. Bull.*, **16**, 185–194.

126. Castle D.J., Wessely S., van Os J., Murray R.M. (1998). *Psychosis in the Inner City: The Camberwell First Episode Study*. Psychology Press, Hove, East Sussex.

127. Hambrecht M., Maurer K., Häfner H., Sartorius N. (1992). Transnational stability of gender differences in schizophrenia? *Eur. Arch. Psychiatry Clin. Neurosci.*, **242**, 6–12.

128. DeLisi L.E., Bass N., Boccio A., Shilds G., Morganti C., Vita A. (1994). Age of onset in familial schizophrenia. *Arch. Gen. Psychiatry*, **51**, 334–335.

129. Albus M., Maier W. (1995). Lack of gender differences in age at onset in familial schizophrenia. *Schizophr. Res.*, **18**, 51–59.

130. Könnecke R., Häfner H., Maurer K., Löffler W., an der Heiden W. (2000). Main risk factors for schizophrenia: increased familial loading and pre- and perinatal complications antagonize the protective effect of oestrogen in women. *Schizophr. Res.*, **44**, 81–93.

131. Häfner H. (1987). Epidemiology of schizophrenia. In: Häfner H., Gattaz W.F., Janzarik W. (eds) *Search for the Causes of Schizophrenia*. Springer-Verlag, Berlin, pp. 47–74.
132. Häfner H., Behrens S., Vry J. de, Gattaz W.F. (1991). Oestradiol enhances the vulnerability threshold for schizophrenia in women by an early effect on dopaminergic neurotransmission. *Eur. Arch. Psychiatry Clin. Neurosci.*, **241**, 65–68.
133. Gattaz W.F., Behrens S., Vry J. de, Häfner H. (1992). Östradiol hemmt Dopamin-vermittelte Verhaltensweisen bei Ratten – ein Tiermodell zur Untersuchung der geschlechtsspezifischen Unterschiede bei der Schizophrenie. *Fortschr. Neurol. Psychiatr.*, **60**, 8–16.
134. Stöber G., Ungvari G.S. (eds) (2001). Catatonia: a new focus of research. *Eur. Arch. Psychiatry Clin. Neurosci.*, **251** (Suppl. 1), 1–34.
135. Mimica N. (1996). Schizophrenia and its catatonic subtype instability during long-term follow-up. *Schizophr. Res.*, **18**, 101.
136. Hambrecht M., Häfner H. (1996). Substance abuse and the onset of schizophrenia. *Biol. Psychiatry*, **40**, 1155–1163.
137. Bühler B., Hambrecht M., Löffler W., an der Heiden W., Häfner H. (2002). Precipitation and determination of the onset and course of schizophrenia by substance abuse – a retrospective and prospective study of 232 population-based first illness episodes. *Schizophr. Res.*, **54**, 243–251.
138. Malmberg A., Lewis G., David A., Allebeck P. (1998). Premorbid adjustment and personality in people with schizophrenia. *Br. J. Psychiatry*, **172**, 308–313.
139. Davidson M., Reichenberg A., Rabinowitz J., Weiser M., Kaplan Z., Mark M. (1999). Behavioral and intellectual markers for schizophrenia in apparently healthy male adolescents. *Am. J. Psychiatry*, **156**, 1328–1335.
140. Johannessen J.O., Larsen T.K., Horneland M., Joa I., Mardal S., Kvebaek R., Friis S., Melle I., Opjordsmoen S., Simonsen E., *et al.* (2001). The TIPS Project. A systematized program to reduce duration of untreated psychosis in first episode psychosis. In: Miller T., Mednick S.A., McGlashan T.H., Libiger J., Johannessen J.O. (eds) *Early Intervention in Psychotic Disorders*. Kluwer, Dordrecht, pp. 151–166.
141. Sartorius N. (1998). Stigma: what can psychiatrists do about it? *Lancet*, **352**, 1058–1059.
142. Sainsbury Centre for Mental Health (1998). *Keys to Engagement: Review of Care for People with Severe Mental Illness who are Hard to Engage with Services*. Sainsbury Centre Publications, London.
143. McGorry P.D. (2002). The recognition and optimal management of early psychosis: an evidence-based reform. *World Psychiatry*, **1**, 76–83.
144. Bell R.Q. (1992). Multiple-risk cohorts and segmenting risk as solutions to the problem of false positives in risk for the major psychoses. *Psychiatry*, **55**, 370–381.
145. Wölwer W., Buchkremer G., Häfner H., Klosterkötter J., Maier W., Möller H.-J., Gaebel W. (2003). German Research Network on Schizophrenia – bridging the gap between research and care. *Eur. Arch. Psychiatry Clin. Neurosci.*, **253**, 321–329.
146. Cornblatt B., Obuchowski M., Schnur D., O'Brien J.D. (1998). Hillside study of risk and early detection in schizophrenia. *Br. J. Psychiatry*, **172** (Suppl. 33), 26–32.

147. Yung A.R., Phillips L.J., McGorry P.D., McFarlane C.A., Francey S., Harrigan S., Patton S.G., Jackson H.J. (1998). Prediction of psychosis. A step towards indicated prevention of schizophrenia. *Br. J. Psychiatry*, **172** (Suppl. 33), 14–20.
148. Yung A.R., Phillips L.J., Yuen H.P., Francey S.M., McFarlane C.A., Hallgren M., McGorry P.D. (2003). Psychosis prediction: 12 month follow-up of a high risk ("prodromal") group. *Schizophr. Res.*, **60**, 21–32.
149. Chapman J.P. (1966). The early symptoms of schizophrenia. *Br. J. Psychiatry*, **112**, 225–251.
150. McGhie A., Chapman J. (1961). Disorders of attention and perception in early schizophrenia. *Br. J. Med. Psychol.*, **34**, 103–115.
151. Chapman L.J., Chapman P.J. (1980). Scales for rating psychotic or psychotic-like experiences as continua. *Schizophr. Bull.*, **6**, 476–489.
152. Chapman J.P., Chapman L.J. (1996). The psychometric assessment of schizophrenia proneness. In: Matthysse S., Levy D.L., Kagan J., Benes F.M. (eds) *Psychopathology. The Evolving Science of Mental Disorder*. Cambridge University Press, Cambridge, pp. 313–333.
153. Chapman L.J., Chapman J.P., Raulin M.L. (1976). Scales for physical and social anhedonia. *J. Abnorm. Psychol.*, **85**, 374–382.
154. Chapman L.J., Chapman J.P., Raulin M.L. (1978). Body-image aberration in schizophrenia. *J. Abnorm. Psychol.*, **87**, 399–407.
155. Gross G., Huber G., Klosterkötter J., Linz M. (1987). *Bonner Skala für die Beurteilung von Basissymptomen* (BSABS: Bonn Scale for the Assessment of Basic Symptoms). Springer-Verlag, Berlin.
156. Klosterkötter J., Hellmich M., Schultze-Lutter F. (2000). Ist die Diagnose schizophrener Störungen schon in der initialen Prodromalphase vor der psychotischen Erstmanifestation möglich? *Fortschr. Neurol. Psychiatr.*, **68** (Sonderheft 1), 13–21.
157. Klosterkötter M. (2002). Predicting the onset of schizophrenia. In: Häfner H. (ed.) *Risk and Protective Factors in Schizophrenia*. Steinkopff-Verlag, Darmstadt, pp. 193–206.
158. McGorry P.D., Copolov D.L., Singh B.S. (1990). Royal Park Multidiagnostic Instrument for Psychosis: Part I. Rationale and review. *Schizophr. Bull.*, **16**, 501–515.
159. McGorry P.D., Singh B.S., Copolov D.L., Kaplan I., Dossetor C.R., van Riel R.J. (1990). Royal Park Multidiagnostic Instrument for Psychosis: Part II. Development, reliability, and validity. *Schizophr. Bull.*, **16**, 518–536.
160. Yung A.R. (2000). *The Comprehensive Assessment of At-Risk Mental States (CAARMS)*. University of Melbourne, Australia.
161. McGlashan T.H., Miller T.J., Woods S.W., Rosen J.L., Hoffman R.E., Davidson L. (2001). *Structured Interview for Prodromal Syndromes*. PRIME Research Clinic, Yale School of Medicine, New Haven, CT.
162. Miller T.J., McGlashan T.H., Woods S.W., Stein K., Driesen N., Corcoran C.M., Hoffman R., Davidson L. (1999). Symptom assessment in schizophrenic prodromal states. *Psychiatr. Q.*, **70**, 273–287.
163. Miller T.J., McGlashan T.H., Rosen J.L., Somjee L., Marchovich P.J., Stein K., Woods S.W. (2002). Prospective diagnosis of the initial prodrome for schizophrenia based on the Structured Interview for Prodromal Syndromes: preliminary evidence of interrater reliability and predictive validity. *Am. J. Psychiatry*, **159**, 863–865.
164. Hambrecht M., Häfner H. (1997). Sensitivity and specificity of relatives' reports on the early course of schizophrenia. *Psychopathology*, **30**, 12–19.

165. Cohen R.Z., Seeman M.V., Gotowiec A., Kopala L. (1999). Earlier puberty as a predictor of later onset of schizophrenia in women. *Am. J. Psychiatry*, **156**, 1059–1064.
166. Remschmidt H. (2002). Early-onset schizophrenia as a progressive-deteriorating developmental disorder: evidence from child psychiatry. *J. Neural Transm.*, **109**, 101–117.
167. Keith S.J., Matthews S.M. (1991). The diagnosis of schizophrenia: a review of onset and duration issues. *Schizophr. Bull.*, **17**, 51–67.
168. Jackson H.J., McGorry P.D., Dudgeon P. (1995). Prodromal symptoms of schizophrenia in first-episode psychosis: prevalence and specificity. *Compr. Psychiatry*, **36**, 241–250.
169. McGorry P.D., McFarlane C., Patton G.C., Bell R., Hibbert M.E., Jackson H.J., Bowes G. (1995). The prevalence of prodromal features of schizophrenia in adolescence: a preliminary survey. *Acta Psychiatr. Scand.*, **92**, 241–249.
170. McGorry P.D., McKenzie D., Jackson J.H., Waddell F., Curry C. (2000). Can we improve the diagnostic efficiency and predictive power of prodromal symptoms for schizophrenia? *Schizophr. Res.*, **42**, 91–100.
171. Eaton W., Harrison G. (2001). Life chances, life planning and schizophrenia. A review and interpretation of research on social deprivation. *Int. J. Ment. Health*, **30**, 58–81.
172 Häfner H., Maurer K., Ruhrmann S., Bechdolf A., Klosterkötter J., Wagner M., Maier W., Bottlender R., Möller H.-J., Gaebel W., *et al.* (2004) Early detection and secondary prevention of psychosis: facts and visions. *Eur. Arch. Psychiatry Clin. Neurosci.*, **254**, 117–128.

CHAPTER

2

The Management of Early Psychosis

Patrick McGorry, Jane Edwards and Alison Yung

University of Melbourne, Parkville, Australia

INTRODUCTION

The onset of psychotic illnesses occurs most commonly in late adolescence or early adulthood. The emergence of the illness via a prodrome with the later advent of acute psychotic symptoms is typically an extremely disturbing experience for a young person, their family and friends, leading to a highly emotional and volatile environment. The way that a psychotic illness is first managed provides an opportunity to reduce the immediate and future harm associated with it, and to establish a positive basis for future care. This simple principle has been embraced in an increasing number of centres around the world and underpins the widespread reform process now under way [1].

High quality care has the potential to provide special benefits in young people with early psychosis. Late adolescence and early adulthood is a critical stage of psychological, social, educational and vocational development. Serious mental illness can cause very substantial disruption to these processes, leading to long-term functional disability and poor outcomes. Effective intervention in the initial phases of psychosis can help prevent the biological, psychological and social deterioration that can occur in the early years [2]. This chapter focuses particularly on the optimal care of the prepsychotic phase and the first episode of psychosis.

Challenges

Challenges for clinicians include the need to reduce the trauma associated with early psychosis and its treatment, while ensuring the safety of the patient and others. Management strategies should be broad in their

Early Detection and Management of Mental Disorders.
Edited by Mario Maj, Juan José López-Ibor, Norman Sartorius, Mitsumoto Sato and Ahmed Okasha.
 ISBN 0-470-01083-5.

approach, addressing not just the biological aspects of the illness but also the psychological and social components. Approaches to treatment should be flexible, so they can adapt to the diagnostic uncertainty that often characterizes early psychosis and recognize that the challenging behaviours of normal adolescence can accompany the abnormal behaviours resulting from the illness. Clinicians and the mental health system should be able to quickly address the specific needs of the patient and family, rather than applying a standard and inflexible model of care [3].

Failures in the care of young people with early psychosis have included:

- prolonged delays in accessing effective treatment, which all too often begins at a time of a severe crisis [4,5];
- provision of initial treatment which is traumatic and alienating [6];
- poor continuity of care;
- poor engagement of the patient in treatment [1].

Special Features of Early Psychosis

Some differences between individuals with early psychosis and those with chronic psychotic illness are summarized in Table 2.1.

Table 2.1 Special features of early psychosis

Compared to people with a chronic psychotic illness, those with early psychosis tend to be:

- much younger
- less informed about mental illness
- agitated or distressed by unfamiliar symptoms which can be frightening or bewildering
- unaware of mental health services that are available, and how they operate
- more likely to deny the existence of an illness and to have a sense of invulnerability
- exhibiting normal adolescent behaviours which can mask symptoms
- experiencing an illness which is still "evolving", making diagnosis more difficult
- uncertain about, or afraid of, treatment including medication and hospital admission
- not previously exposed to psychotropic medication and more susceptible to side effects.

WHY EARLY PSYCHOSIS?

The umbrella term "early psychosis" has been preferred to a narrower focus such as "first episode schizophrenia", both for clinical and research purposes, for several reasons [7]. First, it enables the prodromal period, the first episode of psychosis and the so-called "critical period" [8] of the early years post-diagnosis to be included in the management focus. Second, it allows for diagnostic flux and evolution to be handled [9]. Third, the clinical needs of patients with early psychosis, and their families, are very similar irrespective of diagnostic subtype. Finally, the negative prognostic expectations associated with a diagnosis of schizophrenia can be minimized by using a more prognostically neutral umbrella term for the clinical programme. The term schizophrenia still is used as a second-line statement, but is explained as no more than a descriptive syndrome, and as a diagnosis rather than a prognosis. This approach works well clinically and for a variety of research purposes.

PHASES OF ILLNESS

The course of psychotic illnesses can be divided into phases which reflect the evolution of signs and symptoms over time and the changing needs of patients and their families. The concept also highlights the prospects for recovery, establishes a sense of realistic optimism, and indicates to patients that the distress of the acute phase will have a limited duration. The notion that the content and intensity of treatment differs according to the phase or stage of illness, such that early psychosis requires different interventions from those used in late or established schizophrenia, is related to the concept of "staging" employed in the treatment of serious medical disorders, e.g. cancer and arthritis.

- Obvious symptoms of psychotic illness are often preceded by a lengthy *prodrome*, often lasting for years. The prodromal focus is the frontier for clinical research in early intervention and is becoming a possible therapeutic focus for the first time.
- Psychotic symptoms become apparent in the *acute phase*, which may include a brief initial crisis lasting days or weeks, or a late behavioural crisis may trigger entry to care following a prolonged period of untreated psychosis.
- *Recovery* should be expected following an acute episode of psychosis. The recovery process may take some time – usually months. Symptomatic recovery is more easily achieved than social or functional recovery in the short term.

- Once recovery has occurred, the individual often enters a phase of relative stability. Depending on the underlying cause of the initial episode, there may be a risk of acute psychosis recurring, especially during the critical period of the first 2–5 years post-onset.

The prodrome often involves subtle behavioural changes such as social withdrawal, loss of interest in school or work, deterioration of personal care, unusual behaviour or outbursts of anger. A similar prodrome can occur before subsequent relapses [10]. The recognition and management of this phase is discussed below.

During the acute phase, patients exhibit severe psychotic symptoms such as delusions, hallucinations, severely disorganized thinking and odd behaviour. They are often unable to care for themselves appropriately, and negative symptoms often become more severe as well. The person's behaviour is likely to be at its most disruptive or disturbing, prompting family, friends or others to seek assistance. Some people with a first episode of psychosis voluntarily seek help, but others do not see the need for intervention and choose not to accept assistance [11,12]. Delays are common around the world, often with serious consequences [4,13].

MODERN APPROACHES TO TREATMENT

The central message of the early intervention paradigm is clearly reflected in the very first guideline statement in the National Institute for Clinical Excellence (NICE) document: "Health professionals should work in partnership with service users and carers offering help, treatment and care in an atmosphere of hope and optimism" [14]. Realistic hope and optimism are key ingredients in the management of all potentially serious conditions and should be valued therapeutically. This represents a significant shift in the care of psychoses in general and schizophrenia in particular and should be extended to all phases of illness [15].

Modern approaches to the treatment of early psychosis also reflect the following issues:

- It is often difficult to make a precise diagnosis in patients with a first episode of psychosis. When an initial diagnosis is made, it will often be modified as time passes and more information becomes available [9].
- The early course of illness is a dynamic process, reflecting interactions between the vulnerability of individuals and the stressors that are present in their environments.
- The long-term outcome after a first episode of psychosis is variable, but recovery from acute symptoms should be expected.

- There is scope to apply a preventive model, to reduce the recurrence and/or severity of future psychotic illness.
- Optimal treatment for young people with early psychosis may differ markedly from that for older people with chronic psychotic illnesses, as discussed above.

THE PREPSYCHOTIC PHASE OF ILLNESS

Conceptual Issues

The rise of the early psychosis paradigm has enabled the prepsychotic phase of schizophrenia and related psychoses to come strongly into focus for the first time. Reacting to the pessimism intrinsic to the concept of schizophrenia and also to the damage wrought by a disorder for which effective treatments were lacking, an earlier generation of psychiatrists were attracted to the notion of prepsychotic intervention [16,17]. What remained a dream for decades is now starting to become a reality. This section describes principles and progress in the prospective detection, engagement and treatment of young people with incipient psychosis.

With the advent of widespread first-episode programmes, it has become possible to detect and engage a subset of young people who are subthreshold for fully fledged psychotic disorder, yet who have demonstrable clinical needs and other syndromal diagnoses, and who appear to be at incipient risk of frank psychosis [18,19].

The prepsychotic or prodromal phase needs to be clearly distinguished from the premorbid phase on the one hand and the first episode of psychosis on the other. To understand the potential advantages of prepsychotic intervention, it is important to explicate the concept of prodrome, a term which has only recently been widely used in schizophrenia. The period prior to clear-cut diagnosis has traditionally been referred to as the premorbid phase. However, this term has led to some confusion, because it actually covers two phases, not one, and has not been useful from a preventive perspective. Studies of the childhood antecedents of schizophrenia, while demonstrating significant but minor differences between controls and those who later developed schizophrenia, paradoxically highlighted the quiescence of the illness during this phase of life [20]. However, these studies and the findings of Häfner and colleagues [21] revealed that psychotic illnesses really begin to have clinical and social consequences after puberty, typically during adolescence and early adult life. The period of emergence of nonspecific symptoms and growing functional impairment prior to the full emergence of the more diagnostically specific positive psychotic symptoms constitutes the prodromal phase.

Table 2.2 Potential advantages of prepsychotic intervention

- An avenue for help is provided, irrespective of whether transition ultimately occurs, to tackle the serious problems of social withdrawal, impaired functioning and subjective distress that otherwise become entrenched and steadily worsen prior to the onset of frank psychotic symptoms.
- Engagement and trust are easier to develop and lay a foundation for later therapeutic interventions, especially drug therapy if and when required. The family can be similarly engaged and provided with emotional support and information outside of a highly charged crisis situation.
- If psychosis develops, it can be detected rapidly and duration of untreated psychosis minimized, and hospitalization and other lifestyle disruption rarely occur. A crisis with behavioural disturbance or self-harm is not required to gain access to treatment.
- Comorbidity, such as depression and substance abuse, can be effectively treated and the patient therefore gets immediate benefits. If psychosis worsens to the point of transition, the patient enters first episode in better shape with less distress and fewer additional problems.
- The prospective study of the transition process is enabled, including neurobiological, psychopathological and environmental aspects. Patients are less impaired cognitively and emotionally, and are more likely to be fully competent to give informed consent for such research endeavours.

The fact that a very substantial amount of the disability that develops in schizophrenia accumulates prior to the appearance of the full positive psychotic syndrome and may create a ceiling for eventual recovery in young people is a key reason for attempting some form of prepsychotic intervention (Table 2.2). Other benefits include the capacity to research the onset phase of illness and examine the psychobiology of progression from the subthreshold state to fully fledged disorder. More proximal risk factors such as substance use, stress, and the underlying neurobiology can also be uniquely studied. The delineation of this discrete phase, the boundaries of which are often difficult to map precisely, is of great heuristic and practical value. Whether prodrome is the best term for it is, however, a matter for debate [10,18,22]. A number of obstacles to intervention during this phase should also be noted (Table 2.3).

The "Close-in" Strategy

The development of an alternative high-risk strategy with a higher rate of transition to psychosis, a lower false positive rate and shorter follow-up period than the traditional genetic studies has been central to progress in very early preventive interventions for psychosis. Bell proposed that

TABLE 2.3 Obstacles to prepsychotic intervention

- False positive rate for early psychosis remains substantial. Are falsely identified individuals helped or harmed by involvement in clinical strategies? Receiving treatment at this time may heighten stigma or personal anxiety about developing psychosis or schizophrenia. If exposed to drug therapies, especially antipsychotic medications, adverse reactions may occur without benefit in false positive cases.
- If the false positive rate is improved, then the accurate detection rate may conversely decrease. This is a mathematical feature of the screening process, even when this is based on encouraging help-seeking for this group. Even with enrichment or successful screening, most of the "cases" will still emerge from the low-risk group. The solution may be two- or three-step sequential screens with a continuous entry mechanism. Even if there is a ceiling for the proportion of cases that can be detected and engaged at this phase, there will still be some advantages.
- We are unable to distinguish between false positives and false false positives (in the latter case a true vulnerability exists though it has not yet been fully expressed) [10].
- Lessons from early intervention in cancer, coronary heart disease and stroke have not yet been translated to psychosis and schizophrenia.

"multiple-gate screening" and "close-in" follow-up of cohorts selected as being at risk of developing a psychosis would minimize false positive rates [23]. Multiple-gate screening is a form of sequential screening that involves putting in place a number of different screening measures to concentrate the level of risk in the selected sample. In other words, an individual must meet a number of conditions to be included in the high-risk sample, rather than just one, as in the traditional studies. Close-in follow-up involves shortening the period of follow-up necessary to observe the transition to psychosis by commencing the follow-up period close to the age of maximum incidence of psychotic disorders. In order to improve the accuracy of identifying the high-risk cohort further, Bell also recommended using signs of behavioural difficulties in adolescence as selection criteria. This also allows the approach to become more clinical, to move away from traditional screening paradigms and to focus on help-seeking troubled young people, who are therefore highly "incipient" and frankly symptomatic. To maximize the predictive power as well as enabling the engagement of the patient to be well justified on immediate clinical grounds, the timing is critical. Patients should really be as "incipient" as possible, yet this is difficult to measure and consistently sustain. Transition rates in samples may therefore vary on this basis and also because of variation in the underlying proportions of true and false positives who enter the sample. It should be emphasized that young people involved in this strategy have clinical problems and help is being sought either directly by them or on their behalf by concerned relatives.

Developing Criteria for At-risk Mental States and Ultra-high Risk

The ideas expressed by Bell [23] were first translated into practice in Melbourne, Australia in 1994 at the Personal Assessment and Clinical Evaluation (PACE) Clinic [24]. This approach has now been adopted in a number of other clinical research programmes across the world (e.g. 25–27). These studies have been referred to as "ultra-high-risk" (UHR) studies to differentiate them from the traditional high-risk studies that rely on family history as the primary inclusion criteria. Intake criteria for such studies were initially developed from information gleaned from literature reviews and clinical experience with first-episode psychosis patients and have been evaluated and refined in the PACE Clinic over the past eight years. Although the UHR studies ostensibly seek to identify individuals experiencing an initial psychotic prodrome, infallible criteria have not yet been developed towards this end. In addition, "prodrome" is a retrospective concept that can only be applied once the full illness develops. Therefore, criteria used in these studies are collectively referred to as at-risk mental state (ARMS) criteria [28,29] or "precursor" signs and symptoms [30], while the UHR criteria are the operationally defined subset which accurately predicts transition. This terminology does not imply that a full threshold psychotic illness such as schizophrenia is inevitable, but suggests that an individual is at risk of developing a psychotic disorder by virtue of his/her current mental state. This terminology is more conservative than the use of the term prodrome which, as mentioned, can only be accurately applied in retrospect if and when the disorder in question fully emerges. Additionally, the ARMS concept acknowledges current limitations in our knowledge and understanding about psychosis. This frankness is arguably superior in an ethical sense, and it should be noted that participants in this approach are voluntary and help-seeking, i.e. they are concerned about changes in their mental state and functioning and are requesting some assistance to address these changes. Indeed, in many cases, the young people are concerned about the possibility that they may be developing a psychotic disorder.

UHR criteria currently in operation at the PACE Clinic require that the person falls into one or more of the following groups: (a) attenuated psychotic symptoms group (they have experienced subthreshold, attenuated positive psychotic symptoms during the past year); (b) brief limited or intermittent psychotic symptoms (BLIPS) group (they have experienced episodes of frank psychotic symptoms that have not lasted longer than a week and have spontaneously abated); or (c) trait and state risk factor group (they have a first-degree relative with a psychotic disorder or the identified client has a schizotypal personality disorder and they have experienced a significant decrease in functioning during the previous year). Operationalized criteria are shown in Table 2.4. As well as meeting the criteria for at least one of these groups, subjects are aged between 14 and 30 years, have not experienced a previous psychotic episode and live in the Melbourne metropolitan area. Thus, the UHR criteria identify young people in the age range with peak incidence of onset of a psychotic disorder (late adolescence/early adulthood) who additionally describe mental state and functional changes that are suggestive of an emerging psychotic process and/or may have a strong family history of psychosis. Thus, the multiple-gate screening and close-in strategies recommended by Bell [23] have been translated into practice. Despite the paucity of knowledge about causal risk factors, clinical and functional changes have been utilized to fill this gap and connote increased levels of risk. Exclusion criteria are intellectual disability, lack of fluency in English, presence of a known organic brain disorder, and a history of a prior psychotic episode, either treated or untreated. It is recognized that some subthreshold cases, in particular those meeting BLIPS criteria, might meet criteria for DSM-IV brief psychotic disorder. However, such a diagnosis does not necessarily require the prescription of antipsychotic medication.

Criteria have also been developed to define the onset of psychosis in the UHR group (Table 2.4). These are not identical to DSM-IV criteria, but are designed to define the minimal point at which antipsychotic treatment is indicated. This definition of onset of psychosis might be viewed as somewhat arbitrary, but does at least have clear treatment implications and applies equally well to substance-related symptoms, symptoms that have a mood component – either depression or mania – and schizophrenia spectrum disorders. The predictive target is first-episode psychosis which is judged to require antipsychotic medication, arbitrarily defined by the persistence of frank/severe psychotic symptoms for over 1 week. Schizophrenia is a subset or subsidiary target, since although the majority of progressions from the ARMS ultimately fall within the schizophrenia spectrum (schizophreniform disorder or schizophrenia), a significant minority do not. In fact, the broader first-episode psychosis target is a more proximal and therapeutically salient one than schizophrenia, which can be considered a subtype to which additional patients can graduate distal to first-episode psychosis (as well as being one of the proximal categories). This logic applies to the early intervention field generally, where first-episode psychosis is a more practical, flexible and safer concept than first-episode schizophrenia (again best considered as a subtype).

The criteria described in Table 2.4 have been evaluated in a series of studies at the PACE Clinic between 1994 and 1996. Young people meeting the UHR criteria were recruited and their mental state was monitored over a 12-month period. At the end of the follow-up, 41% of the cohort had developed an acute

Table 2.4 Ultra-high-risk criteria according to Comprehensive Assessment of At-Risk Mental States (CAARMS) scores

Group 1: Attenuated psychotic symptoms

- Subthreshold psychotic symptoms: severity scale score of 3–5 on Disorders of Thought Content subscale, 3–4 on Perceptual Abnormalities subscale and/or 4–5 on Disorganized Speech subscales of the CAARMS; plus
- Frequency scale score of 3–6 on Disorders of Thought Content, Perceptual Abnormalities and/or Disorganized Speech subscales of the CAARMS for at least a week; or
- Frequency scale score of 2 on Disorders of Thought Content, Perceptual Abnormalities and Disorganized Speech subscales of the CAARMS on more than two occasions; plus
- Symptoms present in the past year and for not longer than five years.

Group 2: Brief limited or intermittent psychotic symptoms (BLIPS)

- Transient psychotic symptoms: severity scale score of 6 on Disorders of Thought Content Subscale, 5 or 6 on Perceptual Abnormalities subscale and/or 6 on Disorganized Speech subscales of the CAARMS; plus
- Frequency scale score of 1–3 on Disorders of Thought Content, Perceptual Abnormalities and/or Disorganized Speech subscales; plus
- Each episode of symptoms is present for less than one week and symptoms spontaneously remit on every occasion; plus
- Symptoms occurred during last year and for not longer than five years.

Group 3: Trait and state risk factors

- First-degree relative with a psychotic disorder or schizotypal personality disorder in the identified patient (as defined by DSM-IV); plus
- Significant decrease in mental state or functioning, maintained for at least a month and not longer than 5 years (reduction in Global Assessment of Functioning (GAF) scale of 30% from premorbid level); plus
- The decrease in functioning occurred within the past year and has been maintained for at least a month.

Transition to first-episode psychosis or acute psychosis criteria

- Severity scale score of 6 on Disorders of Thought Content subscale, 5 or 6 on Perceptual Abnormalities subscale and/or 6 on Disorganized Speech subscales of the CAARMS; plus
- Frequency scale score greater than or equal to 4 on Disorders of Thought Content, Perceptual Abnormalities and/or Disorganized Speech subscales; plus
- Symptoms present for longer than one week.

psychosis and had been started on appropriate antipsychotic treatment [18,19]. This occurred despite the provision of minimal supportive counselling, case management and selective serotonin reuptake inhibitor (SSRI) medication, if required. The primary diagnostic outcome of the group who developed an acute psychosis was schizophrenia (65%) [19].

The high transition rate to psychosis indicates that these criteria accurately identify young people with an extremely high risk of developing a psychotic disorder within a short follow-up period. These results cannot be easily generalized to the wider population as a whole or even to individuals with a family history of psychosis who are asymptomatic. Participants at the PACE Clinic are a selected sample, characterized perhaps by high help-seeking characteristics or other nonspecific factors. The sample undoubtedly includes only a minority of those who proceed to a first episode of psychosis, and a possibly unstable proportion of false positives, depending on sampling and detection factors, which in turn are difficult to define and measure, but which can affect the base rate of true positives in the sample. Hence the transition rate may vary and needs to be validated and monitored, because the UHR criteria are not the only variable involved. However, these criteria are now being utilized in a number of other settings around the world, with preliminary results indicating that they predict equally well in the USA, the UK and Norway as in Melbourne, Australia [26,27,31].

Intervention Research

The first randomized controlled trial (RCT) specifically developed around the needs of the UHR population, with the aim of preventing or delaying the onset of psychosis, or at the very least ameliorating presenting symptoms, was conducted in Melbourne between 1996 and 1999. This was felt to be required because of the high transition rate in an earlier study, which occurred despite comprehensive supportive care and active treatment of presenting syndromes (such as depression) and problems. In the RCT, the impact of a combined intensive psychological (cognitive) treatment plus very low dose atypical antipsychotic (risperidone) medication (specific preventive intervention, SPI; $n = 31$) was compared with the effect of supportive therapy (needs-based intervention, NBI; $n = 28$) on the development of acute illness in the high-risk group. At the end of the 6-month treatment phase, significantly more subjects in the NBI group had developed an acute psychosis than in the SPI group ($p = 0.026$). This difference was no longer significant at the end of a post-treatment 6-month follow-up period ($p = 0.16$), though it did remain significant for the risperidone-adherent subgroup of cases. This result suggests that it is possible to delay the onset of acute psychosis in the SPI group compared to the NBI group. Both groups experienced a reduction in global psychopathology and improved functioning over the treatment and follow-up phases compared with entry levels [32]. Longer-term follow-up of the participants in this study is now taking place and a replication is under way. Other centres [27,33] have also carried out randomized trials in this phase with similar encouraging findings.

Current Clinical Guidelines

While this phase of illness remains a research focus and further evidence on appropriate and safe interventions must be developed, patients with this pattern of symptoms and functional impairment may still seek help, especially where proactive first-episode psychosis programmes are available. How should they be treated?

The global aim of treatment in this phase is to reduce the symptoms with which the young person presents when first referred, and, if possible, to prevent these symptoms from worsening and developing into acute psychosis. A stress-vulnerability model of the development of psychosis usefully underpins the treatment approach, incorporating medical and psychological strategies. Treatment options should be discussed with patients and their families and reviewed regularly as mental state changes unfold over the course of treatment, and as new evidence becomes available. The following points are based on a draft set of international clinical practice guidelines for early psychosis [1]:

- While the onset of psychiatric disorders of all types peaks in adolescence and early adult life, the possibility of psychotic disorder should be carefully considered in any young person who is becoming more socially withdrawn, performing more poorly for a sustained period of time at school or at work, or who is becoming more distressed or agitated yet unable to explain why. Assessment and regular monitoring of mental state and safety in a context of ongoing support represent the minimal standard here. This should be carried out in a home, primary care or office-based setting in order to reduce stigma. Current syndromes such as depression, substance abuse and problem areas such as interpersonal, vocational and family stress should be appropriately managed where these are present. This level of care essentially represents good general mental health care for young people.
- Young people meeting specific criteria (ARMS) for UHR have a substantially (up to 30–40%) higher risk of transition to psychosis within 12 months *even with* good quality psychosocial intervention. They invariably have significant levels of symptoms, moderate levels of disability and distress, and often a significant risk of suicidal behaviour.
- If these young people are actively seeking help for the distress and disability associated with their symptoms, they need to be engaged, and offered regular assessment and support, specific treatment for manifest syndromes such as depression, anxiety or substance abuse, and family education and support. If they are not seeking help, regular contact with family members is an appropriate strategy. Information should be provided in a flexible, careful but clear way about risks for psychosis and other mental disorders as well as about existing syndromes and

problems. Nearly always, as help-seekers, usually with subthreshold positive symptoms, they are aware of the risk of worsening of the problem, which is a good way of explaining the psychosis risk. Many will have family members with psychosis. Education must be individually tailored. Once again, such intervention should ideally be carried out in a home, primary care or low-stigma office-based setting. At present there is no general indication for the use of treatments aimed specifically at the reduction of risk of psychosis, such as cognitive therapy for psychosis, atypical antipsychotics or experimental neuroprotective drug strategies. The evidence that such treatments are effective remains preliminary. More data are required on the replicability of initial studies, and the risk/benefit ratio of various interventions.

- More specifically, *no antipsychotic medications* should be used *unless* the person meets criteria for a DSM-IV psychotic disorder with a duration of over one week, unless rapid deterioration is occurring, severe suicidal risk is present and antidepressants have proven ineffective (assuming depression is present), or aggression or hostility are increasing and pose a risk to others. In the latter two situations, it is likely that inpatient care and observation will be required. If antipsychotics are considered, atypical medications should be used in low doses and considered as a "therapeutic trial" for a time-limited period. If there is benefit and resolution of symptoms on 6-week review, the medication should be continued for a further 6–12 months, after all risks have been explained and understood, and the patient is willing. After this, an effort should be made to withdraw the medication, provided the patient agrees and there has been a complete symptomatic and social recovery. If symptoms return when the medications are withdrawn, the patient may, if he/she elects to do so, recommence the medications, provided the longer-term risks have been clearly explained and understood. If the patient has not responded to one atypical antipsychotic, another may be tried, as long as the above indications still pertain.

Research Guidelines

- Further research is undeniably required to determine which treatment strategies may be effective in reducing the current burden of symptoms and disability in "at-risk mental states" and further in reducing risk for progression to frank psychosis and a diagnosis of a persistent psychotic disorder, most commonly schizophreniform disorder or schizophrenia.
- Such research must meet the highest ethical standards for medical research; no more and no less than is required for early intervention research in other medical fields. Patients must be fully competent, give

true informed consent, and be free to withdraw from such research at any time. Non-participation in research should in no way affect access to clinical care if this is desired and judged to be appropriate. Any potential sources of harm to the patient in such research must be minimized such as reducing stigma. In fact minimizing stigma is a key consideration to providing clinical care to such patients, irrespective of whether they participate in research. For example, if a specialized clinical service is established for "at-risk" patients, it should be a primary care setting and/or possess a generic title if possible. Ultimately, engaging patients during this phase of illness has the potential to reduce stigma even if psychosis does supervene, since duration of untreated psychosis (DUP) can be reduced to minimal levels, and hospitalization and disruption to lifestyle are usually markedly less. This reduces the extent of labelling and consequent stigma.

- If research in this phase is carried out in non-Western cultures, it should be led or heavily informed by local clinicians and researchers, so that culturally normal experiences and behaviours are not mislabelled as pathological psychosis. In fact, this is the key task in Western cultures too. However, it is presumed that the risks may be higher when cross-cultural factors come into play. In multicultural developed societies this problem must also be carefully addressed.

CONTEXT FOR MANAGEMENT OF FIRST-EPISODE PSYCHOSIS

Aims of Treatment

Intervention in the acute phase of first-episode psychosis has a number of aims, including those listed in Table 2.5. Although some strategies have immediate or short-term aims, all interventions should help build a foundation for sustained recovery. The fundamental aim of treatment in early psychosis is to assist patients to return to their normal lives as early as possible.

Prevention of future harm is an important aim. Long-term outcomes will be compromised if the young person experiences persistent negative symptoms, persistent positive symptoms, suicidal impulses or substance abuse. It has been suggested that the experience of psychosis is itself "toxic" to the brain [34], although this hypothesis has been challenged [35]. Psychological consequences of psychosis include a loss of self-esteem and confidence, developmental stagnation, and secondary disorders such as depression and post-traumatic stress disorder. Social costs of psychosis include disruption of family networks, peer networks, sexual relationships,

TABLE 2.5 Aims of intervention in first-episode psychosis

Overall aims
- Ensure the safety of the individual and others.
- Reduce symptoms of psychosis and disturbed behaviour.
- Build a sustainable therapeutic relationship with the individual and carers.
- Develop a management plan to aid recovery from the acute episode.

Specific aims
- Monitor the patient's status.
- Prevent harm.
- Minimize trauma.
- Reduce delay in treatment.
- Provide optimal medication to target positive symptoms and disturbed behaviour.
- Prevent or treat negative symptoms and coexisting problems such as depression, mania, anxiety or panic attacks and substance abuse.
- Instil realistic hope.
- Provide an acceptable explanatory model, with education about psychosis and its treatment, including time to recovery.
- Support the family to relieve their distress and improve family functioning.
- Promote adjustment and psychosocial recovery.
- Promote functional recovery.
- Promote continuity of care and adherence to treatment.
- Promote early recognition of further episodes, and identify factors that precipitate or perpetuate episodes.
- Facilitate access to other services in the mental health, general medical and social service systems.

education and vocation, as well as the risks of institutionalization and homelessness [36].

Engagement and collaboration with the patient, family members and other caregivers should begin in the acute phase, as they are often highly motivated to participate in treatment during this time of crisis.

Models of Care

Our experience is based on work carried out in the Early Psychosis Prevention and Intervention Centre (EPPIC) [37] in Melbourne, Victoria, as well as the work of many people around the world. The EPPIC catchment area has a total population of about 850,000, of whom 200,000 are aged 15 to 29 years, the period of peak onset of psychotic disorders. Development of a specialized service for a large catchment area is one approach to the provision of early psychosis services. An increasing number of such centres now exist around the world [1], and provide local examples of evidence-based care of early psychosis. Some other Australian mental health services have established specialized sub-units to provide a focus on early psychosis, but in many services there is still no administrative or clinical structure specifically for this crucial group of patients [38].

Nevertheless, many of the principles of managing people with early psychosis may be applied regardless of the service structure that has been adopted, though a special focus and structure does make this more achievable and sustainable. They are based on recognizing the special characteristics of such patients and applying current standards of optimal care.

CRISIS MANAGEMENT, ENTRY TO CARE AND ENGAGEMENT

First "Episode" Psychosis: An "Avoidable Crisis"?

The onset of a first episode of psychosis often represents a crisis, with the patient and family experiencing considerable trauma and multiple losses. In a small number of cases the onset is very acute and a hitherto completely well person descends into a florid phase of illness which can truly be called an "episode". Much more commonly, the so-called "episode" is largely an artefact of late presentation. The episode or crisis could have been prevented, since the patient presents after a considerable period of significant symptoms and impaired function, plus several attempts by himself or his family to seek help [39,40]. However, as any clinician knows, there are a number of obstacles to the early detection and treatment of first episode cases (Table 2.6). Typically, an additional critical event such as an overdose or aggressive incident will have been necessary for a new patient to gain access to specialist assessment and care. This means that intervention usually needs to occur within a broad framework of crisis intervention.

What is the optimal standard of care following detection and diagnosis? Clinical practice guidelines on the treatment of schizophrenia from the Royal Australian and New Zealand College of Psychiatrists [41] state that comprehensive and sustained intervention should be assured during the early years following diagnosis. The long-term course of illness is strongly influenced by what occurs in this "critical period" [8], and patients should not have to prove they are chronically ill before they gain consistent or "tenured"access to specialist care.

A flexible diagnostic approach by mental health services can assist in optimizing care. It is possible to recognize the syndrome of psychosis and

TABLE 2.6 Obstacles to the early detection and treatment of early psychosis [42]

- The incidence of a first episode of psychosis is relatively low, making it difficult for primary care clinicians to maintain a high level of vigilance and clinical expertise.
- Patients are often concerned about the consequences of referring themselves to mental health services, and might be unwilling to participate when they are referred by concerned families or carers.
- Clinicians are often faced with a dilemma of when, and how assertively, to intervene. This is a particular problem when young people with prodromal features are suffering considerable distress and disability but do not yet fulfil the criteria for a psychotic illness.
- Even when psychosis is apparent and intervention is clearly warranted, there are often delays. First, there may be reluctance to act on the part of some doctors, due to misplaced therapeutic nihilism, especially if the clinical picture resembles schizophrenia. Second, the health system is usually reactive rather than proactive, and often uses a narrow definition of "serious mental illness" based on patients having established disability or immediate risk. In such a system, emerging first-episode psychosis might not be regarded as "serious" enough, or patients might be considered too difficult to engage or not in need of assertive follow-up, despite the serious risks inherent in such an approach.

provide full assessment, appropriate treatment and systematic follow-up for young people, despite inevitable initial uncertainty about the underlying causes (e.g. the role of drugs), the precise diagnostic subtype and the longer-term prognosis. The descriptive diagnosis of schizophrenia in particular was poorly designed for early intervention and should not be the sole focus for service provision around onset and the critical period. Derived within tertiary settings, it is still most useful in those environments, though it clearly can be recognized elsewhere.

Help-seeking, Recognition and Referral

While many patients with an emerging psychotic illness present to a primary care professional (for example, a general practitioner, GP) before their eventual entry to treatment [43], help-seeking can be delayed for a number of reasons:

- Specific features of psychosis can include suspiciousness, persecutory ideas, social withdrawal and lack of insight.
- Young people may have difficulty understanding and interpreting psychotic experiences and mental health problems, and their adolescent cognitive bias of "invulnerability" can delay help-seeking.

- Lack of knowledge in the general community about psychosis, combined with the continuing stigma associated with seeking care for mental health problems, adds to the barriers. Shame is a key barrier to seeking help.
- Comorbid problems, such as substance use, depression and social anxiety, may interfere with a person's ability to recognize the need for assistance and to access mental health services.
- It is a fundamentally difficult step to trust a stranger to share and help with intensely personal problems. If this can be gradually overcome, management usually proceeds well.

Recognition of a problem by GPs, other primary health workers or care providers is a key step in the path to psychiatric care, but it depends partly on the skill, experience, knowledge and interest of the practitioner. The subtlety of symptoms in the early stages of psychosis, and distinguishing the symptoms from "normal" adolescent behaviour, can make recognition difficult even for skilled mental health professionals. A high index of suspicion assists recognition.

Even after a psychiatric disorder has been recognized, some patients are still not referred to an appropriate mental health service. Psychotic patients are more likely to be referred, usually because of the extent of behavioural changes and disability associated with psychosis, but this is not inevitable.

Once referred to a mental health service provider, young people with early psychosis can still be rejected, particularly if the service system is under-resourced. In such a situation, services are effectively rationed, with resources typically restricted to the existing case load of "old friends", those patients with chronic, established and clearly diagnosed illness, rather than focusing on the challenging and time-consuming referrals of obviously ill young people who nevertheless lack a clear diagnosis. This system behaviour is anti-preventive and demands chronicity and severity as criteria for initial and sustained access. Although a consequence of under-resourcing and rationing, it stands in stark contrast to service responses to cancer, diabetes and heart disease, where early intervention is held at a premium.

Mobile Detection and Engagement: One Solution to Delay and Poor Access

The barriers to early detection described above can be overcome. The Youth Access Team (YAT) at EPPIC provides one example of how entry to care, initial assessment and engagement of patients, as well as home-based care and assertive outreach, can be provided. Although YAT is part of a comprehensive early psychosis programme, this model can be successfully introduced within more generic service systems. For example, a similar model operating in Stavanger, Norway, the early detection (ED) team, has helped to reduce the duration of untreated psychosis dramatically [31].

YAT is a multidisciplinary mobile assessment, crisis intervention and community treatment team [1,43]. It operates 24 hours a day, 7 days a week to provide assessment for young people aged 15–29 years who present with a suspected first episode of psychosis. Whenever required, it also provides intensive home-based treatment for patients and families with early psychosis.

YAT is the first point of contact for all young people and referrers seeking help, providing a triage service. Referrals are accepted from any source, with the majority received by telephone. Possible outcomes from the telephone triage system include provision of information, referring to more appropriate agencies, allocation to the YAT team for non-urgent further assessment, or organization of an urgent assessment.

After receiving basic details, if there is a reasonable suspicion that the individual is experiencing emerging psychosis, then the person is accepted for further assessment. The philosophy is inclusive, rather than exclusive. It is considered preferable to assess all young people who may have a psychosis, in order to identify as many true cases as possible, even if this involves seeing many with other psychiatric disorders. This roughly translates into a ratio of 2:1, i.e. total cases seen: cases with "true positive" first-episode psychosis.

The flexibility of the YAT service allows for monitoring of young people who are not yet in acute crisis. Engagement can occur over several weeks, assisting the young person to recognize the need for treatment and to become motivated to attend regular outpatient appointments. YAT also facilitates alternatives to inpatient admission, for example through assistance with transport to a low-stigma outpatient centre or the provision of home-based treatment in appropriate cases. Young people who may be in the prodromal phase of psychosis are referred to EPPIC's PACE Clinic, a specific programme which provides structured, longer-term follow-up of individuals considered at high risk of progressing to psychotic illness. Several clinics of this type have developed around the world in recent years [44].

Psychoeducation and support for families at such a time of crisis is an essential component during the engagement phase. Information from families can be invaluable in initial assessment and triage. Engagement of families as early as possible will assist in monitoring the patient and providing continuing care, and also facilitate direct support to the family at a time of considerable distress.

Engagement

Engagement of patients is a critical step in the process of triage and assessment, but barriers often exist, including denial of illness or symptoms such as suspiciousness and social withdrawal. The first contact of patients and families with a mental health service is highly influential, as it lays the foundation for future interactions.

Engagement in first-episode psychosis usually occurs in parallel with assessment and initial treatment, and may require contact with a number of clinicians. Careful planning and organization can assist in reducing the fragmentation of care. Repeated assessment by a range of people from different components of a service – such as the 24-hour community assessment team, an inpatient unit and then a case manager – not only hampers engagement but is also unwieldy and inefficient.

Some patients with first-episode psychosis will have resisted attempts to seek treatment on their behalf by the time they come into contact with a mental health service. They might have increased risk of violence or self-harm, and have been exposed to adverse experiences during their pathway to care. The traumatizing effects of such experiences can interfere with trust and engagement, and the development of a therapeutic alliance, and can also further undermine the patient's fragile social structures.

Engagement is usually more successful if the initial contact occurs prior to a major crisis, while the person retains some awareness that "something is not quite right".

TABLE 2.7 Engagement techniques – a summary [1]

- Recognize that the patient may be nervous, wary or not want to see health professionals.
- Be aware that psychosis might distort patients' interactions and their ability to process information.
- Listen carefully to patients and take their views seriously.
- Acknowledge and respect patients' viewpoints.
- Identify common ground.
- Consider appropriate body language when interviewing patients who may be paranoid, aroused or manic (sit side-by-side, avoid too much eye contact, allow personal space).
- Be helpful, active and flexible.
- Carefully explain the procedures involved in physical or other assessments.
- Gather information gradually, at the same time as fostering a close relationship.
- Introduce key players who will take part in the patient's management.
- Provide good continuity of care and good communication between professionals.

General principles of engagement and developing a therapeutic alliance should be applied, such as warmth, empathy and respect. Dispelling fears and establishing trust are particularly important in first-episode psychosis. Clinicians need to balance a respect for patients' interpretations of their psychotic experiences with the need to communicate their clinical judgment and advice about treatment. Initial contacts can be emotionally charged. Severely disturbed or agitated patients can provoke reactions in clinicians that undermine engagement, as they attempt to control the situation – for example, the use of criticism, implied threats, or alliance with other carers for whom the patient has little respect.

Engagement requires a calm, reassuring, professional and friendly manner, with a commitment to flexibly negotiating the best initial outcome. Time invested at this early stage can help develop rapport and encourage the patient to help develop options for dealing with his/her concerns. Simple techniques may be very effective in gaining trust and cooperation (Table 2.7).

ASSESSMENT, INVESTIGATIONS AND DIAGNOSIS

Aims of Assessment

Comprehensive assessment of biological, psychological and social factors in a patient with a first episode of psychosis should:

- define the influences which predisposed to, precipitated and may perpetuate the episode;
- allow a proper formulation of the patient's condition, treatment options, likely responses, risks, available supports, likelihood of treatment compliance and prognosis [42].

An incomplete or inadequate assessment is likely to result in incorrect decisions. Other consequences can include a failure to engage the individual, to understand the patient, the family and their needs, and to provide continuity of care.

Diagnosis

Initial assessment will not necessarily lead to a firm diagnosis. However, a delay in determining the precise diagnosis does not mean that symptomatic treatment also has to be delayed.

The onset of psychosis is often characterized by slowly evolving and fluctuating symptoms which are closely related to psychosocial stressors or developmental issues [42]. Symptoms of early psychosis can mimic nonpsychotic disorders commonly seen in adolescence, such as adjustment disorders or emergent personality or mood disorders. Confirmation of psychosis may be difficult, particularly if delusions are not particularly bizarre or if patients deliberately conceal the changes they are experiencing.

Timing and Location of Assessment

Preliminary assessment will be required when a young person first presents with a suspected psychosis. The extent of the initial assessment will be influenced by factors such as the urgency of intervention (based on the severity of symptoms and safety issues) and the extent to which the person and family can be engaged. It might be impossible to safely and effectively assess people in an acute psychotic state until they have been adequately contained, perhaps in an emergency department or inpatient setting. In other less acute situations, thorough assessment is more appropriately conducted in the person's home, in a community-based clinic or in some other community location that is acceptable to them. In less urgent situations, this can be carried out over a series of meetings spread over several days or even weeks. Home-based assessments are particularly valuable in early psychosis for a variety of reasons.

Antipsychotic-free Period

Ideally, assessment of a first episode of psychosis should be completed before any antipsychotic medications are administered. Whether managed at home or in hospital, an antipsychotic-free period of at least 24 hours allows clinicians to make repeated assessment of the evolving mental state, gather further clinical information and conduct some routine biological investigations. It also reduces the potential for premature and inappropriate diagnostic interventions or treatment. An antipsychotic-free period allows time for psychoeducation on the nature of the problem and the need for treatment, emphasizing that decisions about treatment are thoughtful and considered.

An antipsychotic-free period is particularly valuable when:

- time is needed for symptoms of a drug intoxication or withdrawal to lessen;
- symptoms of psychosis are vague or transient;
- symptoms are subtle or denied by the patient.

In these circumstances, premature prescription of antipsychotics may mask the correct diagnosis.

An "antipsychotic-free" period does not mean that all other medications or interventions should be withheld. For example, benzodiazepines can be used to restore normal sleep and to reduce anxiety or agitation. Psychological and social treatments can be implemented, and the patient and family should receive intensive support and education.

Interviewing Young People with Early Psychosis

Power [42] described the approach to interviewing young people suspected of having an early psychotic disorder. Establishing rapport should begin with putting the patient at ease by spending time with introductions and explanations of one's role, acknowledging, listening carefully, respecting the patient's viewpoint, and trying to identify common ground. At the same time, the patient's appearance, responsiveness, attention span, affect, level of anxiety, agitation, hostility and unpredictability can be observed, as well as movements, communication, responses and willingness to engage.

Attention should be given to the setting of the interview (for example, seating arrangements) and use of body language to minimize confrontation, particularly with paranoid, anxious or manic patients. The interviewer should be positioned side-by-side with the patient, avoiding direct face-to-face contact, and yet allowing adequate "personal space" for an agitated person to move around. With patients who are highly aroused or hostile, more than one clinician should be present. The clinician should be able to reach the door, and retreat from a situation should it escalate. One should avoid stating a position if there are not the resources to support it.

Once the interview is established, the patient's view of recent experiences may be explored with open-ended questions, which allow patients to provide their own account. At the same time, thought form, stream and content, evidence of perceptual disturbances and level of insight can be assessed. Empathic language should be simple and attuned to the focus of distress or suffering ("that must be awful/very distressing", *not* "I know how you feel/I understand what it's like"), and any immediate fears about treatment should be identified and dealt with.

Specific interview techniques include the "Colombo technique" of adopting an excessively naïve stance and asking a series of very basic questions to evoke greater disclosures from a cautious or guarded patient.

At the end of the interview, provide initial feedback to the patient together with options for the next step, and link these ideas with the problem areas that have been identified by the patient, e.g. "I can't get to sleep... I don't feel comfortable with my friends... I can't concentrate at work".

The Mental State Examination in Early Psychosis

- The mental state can vary considerably in response to different settings and to different staff members.
- Some patients retain a considerable ability to control their symptoms.
- Patients can learn quickly to conceal some psychotic phenomena – for example, to avoid treatment or a prolonged stay in hospital.
- Patients with paranoid psychosis may be more willing to reveal information to visiting clinicians or research staff than their treating clinicians.
- Clinical signs can vary significantly depending on the time of day, with signs of depression being more common in the morning and mania escalating in the late evening.

For these reasons, it is useful to conduct a series of assessments by different clinicians, each contributing to a comprehensive assessment summary. This should be arranged in a way that maintains the patient's sense of continuity of care and preserves one or two clinicians as primarily responsible for care.

Regular formal reviews of mental state should be undertaken during an episode of acute psychosis. Most of the mental state examination can be conducted in a routine manner, except that patients with a first episode of psychosis may describe phenomena that are less well formed than in patients with chronic disorders, especially if they are of recent onset, and may be less well "schooled" in providing descriptions.

Phase of Psychosis

It is useful to determine the rate of emergence of the psychosis and where in the cycle the patient is being assessed. In the early phase of a rapidly developing florid psychosis, patients are often perplexed and frightened and have fleeting and poorly formed delusions. Patients presenting for the first time after a prolonged episode of untreated psychosis often have clearly formed delusions or interpretations of psychotic phenomena.

Insight

The level and quality of insight should be explored [45]. Insight is a complex and somewhat controversial feature which involves several elements, including:

- awareness of changes in mental functioning;
- awareness that the changes are the symptoms of a mental illness;
- awareness that the illness requires treatment.

Insight varies markedly between patients and seems to have only a partial association with the severity or phase of psychosis. Insight can vary in a patient within a single interview, depending on the level of arousal and mood state. A suspicious guarded presentation may imply reduced insight, while a frank denial of symptoms may reflect a complete lack of awareness of any change, or merely concealment in the context of fear of the consequences of disclosure.

Negative Symptoms

Negative symptoms in first-episode psychosis appear to be more responsive to treatment than in subsequent episodes. Many are secondary (a response to symptoms) rather than primary (an inherent part of the illness). Assessment of negative symptoms is important in determining the treatment and the prognosis.

Cognitive Function

Careful serial assessment of cognitive function should be performed both in the acute phase and later recovery, because it is closely correlated with level of psychosocial function.

Comorbidity

Coexisting or comorbid features are common in patients with first-episode psychosis and are associated with worse outcomes. Alcohol and drug abuse are common, occurring in up to 70% of cases [46,47].

Substance use should be assessed, including a description of the type, amount, frequency and method of use, the reasons for use and the effects of use, particularly during the time that psychotic symptoms started to develop. Patients' attitudes towards substance use and their motivation to cease should be explored. Patients tend to deny substance use initially, but then give more accurate accounts as they start to recover. Urine drug screens can provide a more objective assessment. Patients and families may focus on substance use as a less stigmatizing explanation for the psychotic episode.

Disorders that are less commonly associated with early psychosis, but need to be identified, include obsessive–compulsive disorder, affective disorders such as depression and anxiety disorders (including panic disorder and social phobia), eating disorders and medical conditions. The onset and course of these disorders and their relationship to the emergence of psychosis should be assessed.

Secondary Morbidity

Additional problems, such as depression and post-traumatic syndromes, can arise as a direct result of experiencing a psychotic episode [1]. Factors contributing to such secondary morbidity include:

- terrifying delusions or hallucinations that lead to post-traumatic stress disorder;
- fear and demoralization;
- disruption to personal development;
- loss of self-esteem and confidence;
- the development of an unwanted and feared "possible self";
- disruption of relationships with family and friends.

Social and Educational Assessment

Assessing the level of psychosocial function prior to the onset of illness is essential in order to determine the duration of the prodrome, the presence of any premorbid limitations in functioning, the degree of current impairment, and the level of functional recovery that should be expected. The assessment should be based on sources such as educational reports, work references and collateral information from relatives.

Assessing the home environment, the family dynamics and the adaptive response of the family to the illness can help define the stressors faced by the patient and family. This is best done through home visits "*in vivo*". It can also identify any cultural factors which should be considered when developing psychosocial interventions for the patient.

Risk Assessment

Risk assessment tends to focus on the risk of physical harm to the patient or to others, but other aspects of risk should also be considered, including neglect of any dependents, victimization by others, nonadherence to treatment and absconding. Prompt and regular formal risk assessments are required, and the results should be communicated to other staff and carers involved in treatment and supervision. New patients are "unknown quantities'' for clinicians, and the first priority is to ensure that the patient and his or her environment are safe [42].

Suicide

The importance of assessing suicide risk in the first interview cannot be overstated [42]. Up to 23% of patients with first-episode psychosis experience suicidal thoughts and about 15% have attempted suicide in the past. The risk persists in patients with chronic psychotic illness. Suicide is the leading cause of premature death in patients with schizophrenia, and the incidence of completed suicide among patients with schizophrenia is 10–13% [11].

The early stages of a psychotic disorder are a time of high risk. During the assessment process, suicidal thoughts and intent can often be explored near the end of the interview once some rapport has been established. For example:

- Explore how distressing the patient's experiences have been.
- How does the person usually cope with emotional distress?
- Ask whether the patient has ever considered life unbearable.
- Discuss the factors that can motivate suicide in psychosis, and how they can be reduced by effective treatment.
- Negotiate ways for patients to seek help should they become suicidal.

Suicidal thoughts are often transient and therefore need constant monitoring. Thoughts of suicide are the best predictor of a subsequent suicide attempt. It is vital to note that:

- There is a greater risk of suicide following, rather than preceding, the active phase of the illness, perhaps associated with greater awareness of the illness that has been experienced and its potential consequences. This is why a positive and optimistic attitude to prognosis is crucial at this stage.
- Hopelessness can still occur when the rest of the mental state is restored to a relatively normal state.

Suicide is influenced by a broad range of social, biological and psychological factors. Table 2.8 outlines some specific general risks and protective factors to consider during the assessment process.

Patients considered at high risk for suicide should be hospitalized, with precautions such as close, 24-hour one-to-one observation, and removal of any means of self-harm. It is important to optimize the treatment of psychotic and depressive symptoms, and to address suicidal thoughts directly with an empathic and supportive approach. Among outpatients, the frequency of visits may need to be increased (even to daily home visits)

TABLE 2.8 Factors to consider in assessing suicide risk in early psychosis

Recent experience of suicide
- Recent death of a relative or close friend by suicide.
- Recent history of suicidal behaviour (particularly in the last 6 months).

Suicide-related cognitions
- Detail and lethality of plans to self-harm.
- Preparations and access to lethal means.
- Impulsivity.
- Regards suicide as the only "logical" solution.

Mental status factors
- Self-destructive command hallucinations.
- Nihilistic delusions.
- Delusions and hallucinations which result in dangerous behaviours or a desire to escape, such as a belief in an ability to fly or that one is indestructible, delusions of guilt, delusions of persecution.
- Recent deterioration in mental state.
- Degree of subjective distress and level of hopelessness.
- Severity of depression or anxiety, including symptoms such as self-criticism.
- Alcohol and drug abuse.
- Increasing insight into the nature of the illness.

Withdrawal and isolation
- May be influenced by severity of illness.

Recent significant stressors
- Multiple stressors or ongoing exposure to stressors.
- Recent discharge from an inpatient unit.

Supports and help-seeking capacity
- Availability of supervision and support.
- Potential for compliance with medications or with protective management plans.
- Degree of openness with carers and the clinician about current mental state.
- Capacity to self-manage impulses.

Reasons for living and barriers to self-harm
- Potential of future goals and success.
- Ongoing responsibilities to others, e.g. children.
- Cultural and religious factors.
- Fear of death and physical suffering/pain.

Protective mental state features
- Apathy – "deficit" features.
- Disorganized thinking which limits the ability to implement actions for suicide.
- Lack of insight which can reduce the distress associated with symptoms.

---

during higher-risk periods, including the time shortly after discharge from hospital. Other useful strategies may include:

- providing frequent reassurance and encouragement;
- providing clear explanations and feedback about the temporary nature of the distressing experiences;

- ensuring consistency of messages from staff;
- ensuring continuity of care.

Aggression and Violence

The risks of aggression and violence associated with psychosis are probably overestimated by the community. However, such risks do exist and cannot be ignored [48]. Aggressive or highly agitated behaviour is sometimes the key factor which finally motivates families and others to seek help, and an appropriate response by mental health services is vital.

The clinical features of the episode of acute psychosis, including the degree of agitation and the nature of hallucinations and delusions, should be considered in assessing the risk of violence. General risk factors for violence in psychotic disorders include a history of violence in the past, substance abuse and the presence of neurological impairment [12]. However, clinical features of the illness are a better short-term predictor of violence in the acute episode.

The use of safety precautions, such as the availability of extra staff, is essential in dealing with potentially violent people. Outlined below are some issues in managing crisis situations before a full assessment is possible, and in community settings, which are less secure than a hospital environment.

A history of prior violence is one of the best predictors of future violence. Gaining as much history as possible from other sources before approaching the patient, for example family, friends and police, is an important step [49]. Check for specific current threats or evidence of impulsivity, whether there is an obvious precipitant to this episode, the individual's main concerns or needs, and whether he or she has access to a weapon or other means of causing harm.

A number of behaviours can suggest actual or impending aggression, including:

- loud, clipped or angry speech;
- pacing;
- angry facial expression;
- refusal to communicate;
- threats or gestures;
- physical or mental agitation;
- restlessness;
- persecutory ideation;
- delusions or hallucinations with violent content;
- people themselves reporting violent feelings.

Some useful techniques in first dealing with an agitated young person who may be experiencing an episode of acute psychosis or other disturbed behaviour are outlined in Table 2.9.

Once the situation has eased and some rapport has been established, it may be possible to start assessing the immediate risks that the individual will attempt to harm himself or herself, or harm others.

Knowledge of local mental health legislation will be required in these circumstances, particularly if a judgement is made that the individual requires involuntary hospital admission.

At this time of crisis it is important to consider establishing a productive relationship with the family, if present, and use them constructively in resolving the situation. If their presence exacerbates the situation, then they should be asked tactfully to withdraw.

TABLE 2.9 Approaching an acutely agitated young person with early psychosis [49]

- Ensure that adequate back-up is available in case the situation escalates. Alert police or other security personnel if appropriate and, if possible, have them located unobtrusively close by.
- If your safety or that of others is directly threatened, then withdraw rather than persist.
- Maintain as much privacy as is possible while ensuring a safe environment.
- If in a room, ensure you can reach the door but do not block the exit from the young person (angry people may rather leave than resort to violence).
- Consider removing clothing (such as ties or necklaces) which could be used to grasp you, or items such as pens or other objects which could be used as weapons.
- Approach in a calm, confident manner.
- Avoid sudden or violent gestures and adopt a relaxed, non-threatening posture.
- Avoid prolonged eye contact (staring).
- Do not confront the person physically or "tower over them" (for example, if they are seated).
- Do not humiliate or ignore the person.
- Allow the individual ample "personal space".
- Use an empathic, non-confronting manner, emphasizing your desire to help.
- Do not turn your back.
- Focus on the immediate situation – the "here and now" – and the immediate needs of the individual, rather than dwelling on the past.
- Try not to give ultimatums.

Unintentional Harm to Others

People experiencing an acute psychotic illness might cause unintentional harm to others, particularly by neglecting the physical or emotional needs of children or others under their care. Assistance may be needed from child protection or family welfare services.

Neglect and Death

Other causes of illness and death in young people with psychosis include [42]:

- exposure to high-risk lifestyles such as homelessness, with a greater risk of accidental death, assault or murder;
- exposure to human immunodeficiency virus (HIV) infection;
- excess cigarette smoking;
- substance abuse.

Death from physical complications of early psychosis is rare, but it is necessary to monitor physical status, including nutritional status and hydration.

Victimization by Others

There is a need to protect inpatients (and outpatients if possible) against violence, intimidation, harassment or exploitation by others. Younger people are more vulnerable, and harassment and intimidation may be subtle and unreported. Highly vulnerable patients should be identified from the outset and protected, for example by one-to-one care.

Biomedical Investigations

It is necessary to conduct a careful physical and mental state examination in a young person with a first episode of psychosis as a first step in excluding other medical conditions that could contribute to the symptoms [42]. Such conditions include head injury, temporal lobe epilepsy, infection or malignancy of the central nervous system, and some endocrine and metabolic disorders.

Only a small percentage of young patients with a first episode of psychosis are found to have an organic cause for their illness. Often this can be detected from clinical examination, so routine laboratory or radiological investigations in otherwise healthy young people rarely detect significant abnormalities – i.e. the yield is low. However, if systematic investigations

TABLE 2.10 Recommended and optional investigations in first-episode psychosis [42]

Recommended before commencing antipsychotic medication
- Urine tests: drug screen, urine microscopy
- Full blood examination, erythrocyte sedimentation rate
- Renal function tests (electrolytes, urea, creatinine)
- Serum calcium and phosphate
- Liver function tests
- Thyroid function tests
- Fasting glucose
- Serum lipids
- Electrocardiogram

As early as possible
- Computed tomography brain scan or, ideally, magnetic resonance imaging
- Neurocognitive assessment

Optional, depending on clinical indications
- Electroencephalogram
- Urine tests: pregnancy test, urinary porphyrins
- Blood tests: pregnancy test, nutritional indices (e.g. vitamin B12, folate, iron); autoantibody screens, hepatitis screens, HIV and syphilis screens, copper studies
- Chest X-ray
- Echocardiogram

are not carried out at this stage, it is unlikely they will be conducted in the future. A physical examination and laboratory investigations can also assess the effect of the psychosis and its treatment on general health.

In the early phase of psychosis, young people with little or no experience of medical procedures can be anxious and suspicious of physical examinations and investigations. Reassurance and careful explanations of the procedures and the results are essential.

Measuring vital signs and a brief neurological examination are useful as part of the first community-based assessment, followed by a more complete physical examination in a clinic or hospital, if appropriate, when laboratory investigations are being carried out.

Recommended and optional investigations are listed in Table 2.10. By far the most useful investigation is a urine drug screen. Substance use is common in this group of patients, and regular screening will establish the role of drug abuse in the presentation or perpetuation of psychosis. Tests to assess other general medical needs of patients should be considered, depending on factors such as their age, exposure to physical risks and findings on physical examination.

A computed tomography (CT) brain scan is recommended, but it is usually preferable to wait until the psychosis has settled, so patients can tolerate and cooperate with the procedure. Urgent CT and magnetic resonance imaging

(MRI) scans are recommended only when there is a strong indication of an organic cause for the psychosis. The clinical significance of abnormalities found on CT and MRI scans in first-episode patients is often unclear [50].

The value of a routine electroencephalogram (EEG) is questionable. However, EEGs should be used if there is a history of epilepsy, birth trauma, head injury, mental handicap or significant findings on CT or MRI.

Psychosis is typically associated with a range of neuropsychological deficits, particularly in attention, information processing, verbal memory and learning. These deficits are apparent even during the first episode. Neuropsychological testing may be useful in determining the prognosis and in guiding approaches to psychological and social interventions. However, accurate neuropsychological testing is usually difficult while a patient is experiencing acute psychotic symptoms and it is unlikely to assist in making a diagnosis.

Review of cardiac function, including an electrocardiogram, is now indicated in patients who are being considered for antipsychotic medications, particularly clozapine, which are known to have adverse cardiovascular side effects. The findings may influence the choice of medication. Other examinations may be necessary depending on the particular medication that is being considered [11].

PRINCIPLES OF MEDICATION IN THE ACUTE PHASE

Antipsychotics

The efficacy of antipsychotics as a first-line treatment for psychosis has been well established, and earlier treatment is associated with an improved prognosis [34,51]. In young people with early psychosis, relatively low doses of antipsychotics are usually effective in controlling hallucinations, delusions, thought disorder and bizarre behaviour. Low doses minimize the risk of distressing side effects, particularly extrapyramidal symptoms [3].

However, it takes at least 10–14 days for antipsychotic medication to have a significant effect on symptoms, and 6 weeks or longer for a maximum response to be obtained. "Impatient" prescribing, with rapid increases in dosage or changes of medication, will not shorten the treatment course or the length of the acute phase, but will increase the risk of poor compliance in the future and of relapse. McEvoy *et al.* [52] demonstrated that there is a threshold effect for antipsychotic action. In their study, the mean threshold dose was 2 mg/day of haloperidol for first-episode cases and 4 mg/day for multi-episode cases. Once this dose, located just on the brink of precipitation of extrapyramidal side effects, or an equivalent dose of other antipsychotics, is achieved, there is probably no additional benefit from further increases. This strategy is quite feasible in routine clinical practice, as shown by Power *et al.* [46]. These doses have been confirmed by more recent studies with atypical and typical antipsychotic medications [53,54] and landmark positron emission tomography (PET) studies, which have clarified the biological basis for appropriate dosing strategies [55]. There is a general consensus, though challenged still by some, that atypical antipsychotics should be used as first-line therapy, largely on the basis of better safety and tolerability [1,14,41,56].

As discussed above, it is ideal to avoid prescribing antipsychotics for the first 24–48 hours in a young person with a first episode of psychosis, in order to allow a more accurate assessment of the symptoms.

Benzodiazepines

Benzodiazepines relieve agitation, anxiety and sleep disturbance and are well tolerated. They act rapidly, in contrast to antipsychotics. Benzodiazepines can be used to relieve a young person's distress during any planned antipsychotic-free period. Benzodiazepines should be regarded as a short-term measure to be used only during the first few weeks of an acute episode, then sporadically as needed, rather than as long-term therapy.

Other Drugs

When syndromes of mania and major depression are prominent or persistent, then antidepressants and antimanic agents will be required.

Treatment of Side Effects

Medications might be required to treat the extrapyramidal and cholinergic side effects which occur more commonly with the older "typical" antipsychotics [11]. Decisions about medications for side effects depend on the severity and degree of distress associated with the side effect and on the availability of other potential strategies, including lowering the dose of the antipsychotic or switching to an alternative.

Some principles in the use of antipsychotic medication are summarized in Table 2.11.

TABLE 2.11 Principles in the use of antipsychotic medication in early psychosis [3]

- If possible, let the patient (and family) participate in the decision to choose an antipsychotic, however...
- Use novel or "atypical", second-generation antipsychotics as first-line treatment [14,41,57].
- Inform the patient (and family) about the goals of the antipsychotic treatment.
- Inform about the acute and long-term side effects and possible impairment of subjective well-being.
- Monitor side effects closely, especially extrapyramidal symptoms, subjective dysphoria, weight gain and cognitive dysfunction.
- Give repeated psychoeducation about efficacy, tolerability and safety of the antipsychotic.
- Avoid polypharmacy with antipsychotics. Use of more than one antipsychotic should generally be avoided, but concurrent use of a benzodiazepine in the short term, and antidepressant or mood stabilizer in the long term, is commonly necessary and beneficial.
- Avoid multiple or indeterminate prescriptions.
- Use the minimal effective dose to minimize side effects.
- Do not change dose or type of medication impulsively. Wait for at least 3 weeks to assess the response to a given dose or medication change.
- Use for appropriate duration (for example, 1–2 years for antipsychotics).
- Discontinue gradually (4–6 months).
- Follow up after discontinuation (especially in first 3–6 months).

Medication Adherence and Route of Administration

A patient's initial experience of medication can have a powerful influence on short-term and long-term adherence to treatment [3]. Nonadherence can be considered the norm, rather than the exception [58]. Adherence is influenced by several factors, including:

- attitudes towards illness;
- insight;
- concerns about the effects of medication.

An investment in addressing these issues in the early stages of treatment can have a worthwhile long-term impact.

Administering medication can be considered as a process of negotiation between clinicians, the patient and the family. Identifying and dealing with anxieties and specific fears about medication empowers patients, which in turn encourages greater adherence [3].

Premature use of depot medications can be interpreted as a "soft option" which blames the patient for noncompliance. Depot medications are justified as second-line therapy in a small minority of cases, for specific reasons such as extreme denial, demonstrated inability to adhere despite good educational and psychosocial support, or severe risks associated with relapse. Long-acting depot medications are not usually prescribed for acute psychotic episodes, because they take months to reach a stable therapeutic level and are eliminated very slowly [11]. As a result, there is relatively little control over the amount of medication the patient is receiving, and it is difficult to titrate the dose to strike a balance between side effects and therapeutic effects. Long-acting injectable forms of novel antipsychotic medications are now becoming available and may change the current pattern of use somewhat.

Choice of Antipsychotic

Many clinical practice guidelines (e.g. 14,41) state that the treatment of choice for most patients is now the novel ("atypical") antipsychotics, such as olanzapine, risperidone, quetiapine, ziprasidone, aripiprazole and amisulpride. This is supported by a recent meta-analysis by Davis *et al.* [57], challenging earlier views which questioned these guidelines [59]. The benefits of atypical antipsychotics are particularly marked in first-episode patients. Although there is little evidence that novel antipsychotics are more efficacious than the conventional antipsychotics in the treatment of positive symptoms, they may have greater efficacy for negative and neurocognitive symptoms. It is now clear that novel antipsychotics are much better tolerated and produce fewer motor side effects, including, and crucially, tardive dyskinesia. However, the atypicals do have some disturbing side effects of their own, notably weight gain and metabolic/endocrine complications, and hence need to be carefully monitored, particularly in the medium to long term. Nevertheless, because patients are generally more likely to feel better and therefore to take these medications than the older drugs, their real-world effectiveness may prove to be much greater than suggested by efficacy studies. The Clinical Antipsychotic Trials of Intervention Effectiveness (CATIE) study in the USA [60] is expected to throw light on this issue. Conventional antipsychotics in low doses may still have a role to play in a small proportion of patients; however, the indications are shrinking progressively.

Dosage

Current clinical practice strongly favours the initial use of low doses of antipsychotics in patients with a first episode of psychosis [14,41,56], with slow titration to higher doses if required. Guidelines from the American Psychiatric Association [11] also emphasize the importance of selecting a dose that is effective but not likely to cause serious side effects. Patients should be monitored during low-dose therapy for several weeks, requiring clinicians to be patient and avoid the temptation to prematurely escalate the dose for patients who are responding slowly.

Titration of the dose is based on symptom response. Information on symptoms should be gathered from the patient, other members of the treatment team, and the family to provide a longitudinal perspective, as well as through formal assessments of mental state. The use of rating scales can help quantify changes in the severity of symptoms over time.

"Treatment Resistance"

Failure to respond to medication, sometimes termed "treatment resistance", is not always due to a failure of the medication itself or an inadequate dose. The lack of response might be explained by factors such as nonadherence, unusual metabolism of the medication or poor absorption [11]. If nonadherence is a problem, then more intensive and sophisticated psychoeducation treatment can be helpful, as can administering the medication in liquid oral form or parenterally if ultimately essential (and if appropriate formulations are available).

If the patient has complied with treatment for an adequate time but psychotic symptoms have failed to improve, then alternative treatment approaches should be considered. If the patient can tolerate a higher dose without significant side effects, then raising the dose for a limited period, such as 4–6 weeks, can be tried, although it is rarely beneficial [11]. If this does not result in an adequate response, a second atypical antipsychotic medication should be considered.

A trial of clozapine should be considered for patients who have positive (and perhaps negative and cognitive) symptoms that do not fully respond to an adequate trial of at least one and probably two other antipsychotic medications within the first few months of treatment. Clozapine treatment requires patients to be free of special risk factors such as cardiac arrhythmia, and to be willing and able to cooperate with regular monitoring, including blood tests for haematological side effects and glucose intolerance, and cardiac monitoring. Cognitive–behaviour therapy may also be a useful adjunctive strategy, when positive symptoms are persistent [61].

Continuation of Antipsychotic Therapy

There may be pressure from patients and their families to discontinue antipsychotic medication once acute psychotic symptoms start to improve.

However, the rate of relapse after a first episode is relatively high in the absence of continued medication [11,41,62]. Between 40% and 60% of untreated patients relapse within a year after recovery from the initial acute psychotic episode [62]. Microrelapses may be even more common [63], yet most authorities stop short of advocating long-term medication for all patients who have had a single episode of psychosis [64].

At least one year of maintenance treatment with antipsychotic medication is recommended once symptoms remit after a first episode. This may be longer than current practice in some services, but is recommended because the deterioration and losses following a relapse may be severe. Careful monitoring for an extended period (months) after medication withdrawal is highly recommended in such cases.

PSYCHOSOCIAL ASPECTS OF CARE IN FIRST-EPISODE PSYCHOSIS

Clinical practice guidelines [1,14,41] stress that psychosocial interventions should be routinely available for all patients with early psychosis and provided by appropriately trained mental health professionals who have enough time to devote to the task. Elements can include family interventions, psychological therapies such as cognitive-behavioural therapy, and vocational rehabilitation.

Family Support and Intervention

It is essential to attend to the immediate needs of family and friends of young people with a first episode of psychosis. Many young people with early psychosis still live with their parents, and families are the main source of their care during the prodromal and early acute phases. Families require an accessible and flexible service, which acknowledges their role and contribution to care. A crisis intervention model can be used, based on education, to reduce carers' stress and confusion while maximizing their support for the patient [65].

Education

Education about psychosis is essential from the earliest stages of a psychotic disorder. Strategies to deliver effective education should be integrated within the culture of the mental health service, and targeted to families and other carers as well as the patient.

The type and intensity of education must be adapted to the phase of the illness and the capacity of the family and the patient to interpret it. In the earliest stages of a psychotic disorder, at a time of uncertainty, distress and sometimes fear, patients and their carers can be particularly receptive to information about what is occurring, why it is happening and what can be done. "Normalizing" the experience – stressing that it is not unique and that it is familiar to health care professionals – is reassuring. Reassurance can also be provided through clear messages that they are in no way to blame for the illness, the health system is ready to assist, that the current distress will be rapidly relieved and that eventual recovery is to be expected. Repeated delivery of educational messages may be needed, particularly in the acute stage. Even when they are acutely psychotic, patients usually understand pragmatic information about their care, and may find it less threatening to be given information than to feel excluded from the information flow [66]. As the patient's acute disturbance starts to settle, then more comprehensive educational strategies can be implemented.

Challenges to education in the first episode of psychosis include the following:

- an uncertain diagnosis and prognosis;
- the normal defensive processes of patients and families in a time of crisis;
- the impact of psychotic symptoms;
- secondary morbidity such as depression;
- cognitive impairment associated with some psychotic illnesses;
- the stigma of mental illness and self-trauma;
- other life stresses and lack of social supports.

Mental health professionals can become desensitized to the impact of an episode of acute psychosis. They need to remain focused on the needs of families, as they face a daunting illness with unfamiliar treatments and systems of care, perhaps after many months or even years of coping alone through a traumatic prodromal period. There is a need to be sensitive to transcultural and language issues.

Families often experience considerable blame and guilt as they search for a reason for the illness. Explaining psychosis using traditional illness models can ease the burden, by describing the roles of neurotransmitter changes and other biological features of psychosis. It is sometimes best to defer any detailed examination of precipitating and perpetuating factors until the acute episode has settled, to avoid perceptions that the family may be to blame.

Table 2.12 Possible fears of families about treatment

- Clinicians will overtly or covertly blame the family for the illness.
- Clinicians will automatically admit the person to hospital without consultation.
- Clinicians will fail to provide adequate follow-up after the assessment process.
- The young person will be turned into a "zombie" by medication.
- The young person will never forgive the family for contacting the service.

Emotional Aspects

Families often move through phases similar to those of the psychotic episode:

- During the prodrome and early stages of a psychotic episode, families might experience some denial and attempt to minimize the problem, until they acknowledge that "something is not quite right" and seek help.
- After psychosis has been identified, they can experience a period of grief and distress. A crisis often precipitates first contact with mental health services and the provision of a diagnosis, although the contact with services might initially be ambivalent. Once the patient is in "the system", families can be faced with an avalanche of bureaucratic procedures and jargon.
- As the patient moves towards recovery, families develop some sense of coping, confidence and adaptive functioning, while recognizing that professional help will not always be unlimited. There is a realignment of roles and expectations within the family, accompanied by concerns about the possibility of relapse.

Some fears of families about treatment are listed in Table 2.12. Such fears can remain unstated. It is vital to allay them with emotional support and strategic information, which may need to be repeated by different people at different contacts.

Psychological Interventions in First-Episode Psychosis

Psychological interventions can help to reduce the severity of acute psychotic symptoms [12]. Patients generally require an environment which provides low stimulation and high levels of support. Empathy and concern for the distress of the patient and family is essential, even though interaction with a floridly psychotic person might be difficult.

TABLE 2.13 Reasons for psychological interventions in early psychosis

- To develop a therapeutic alliance
- To promote adherence to medication
- To provide emotional support in the face of disturbing subjective experiences and stigma
- To specifically target individual symptom complexes, comorbidities and maladaptive schemas
- To reduce treatment resistance
- To enhance coping and adaptation
- To improve cognitive functioning
- To improve interpersonal relationships, which may be independently problematic or have been disrupted by illness
- To promote vocational recovery
- To provide support and care to family members including siblings
- To reduce risks of suicide and aggression
- To prevent relapse

Psychological interventions are essential for many reasons in early psychosis [67] (Table 2.13).

In the acute phase, cognitive strategies can be brought into play quite rapidly to:

- facilitate discussion about distressing symptoms;
- obliquely challenge patients' thoughts and assumptions about themselves and the future;
- enhance self-esteem;
- facilitate discussion about stigma.

Individual interventions based on cognitive–behavioural approaches can hasten and consolidate the resolution of psychotic symptoms [68]. They assist patients to recognize their symptoms, label them appropriately, deal with secondary affective features, and use various distraction or desensitization techniques. More specific targeting of delusional beliefs and hallucinations may also help attenuate these features before they become too deeply entrenched. The second to fourth week of medication is probably a crucial time for introducing cognitive–behavioural techniques which "challenge" the patient's delusions and hallucinations, as it is at this stage that most patients start to develop some insight into their psychotic experiences. Cognitively oriented therapies can also help to facilitate recovery over the subsequent 6–12 months of care [69] as well as focusing on specific clinical foci such as suicide risk and persistent positive symptoms [70,71].

HOME-BASED TREATMENT IN EARLY PSYCHOSIS

Choice of Treatment Setting

Patients should be cared for in the least restrictive setting that is likely to be safe and to allow for effective treatment [11]. It should not be assumed that every patient with a first episode of psychosis will require admission to hospital.

Hospital admission is indicated for patients who are thought to pose a serious threat of harm to themselves or others, who are unable to care for themselves, or who have general medical or psychiatric problems that are not safely or effectively treated in a less intensive setting [11]. Even when psychotic patients are not at risk, the hospital may sometimes be the preferred setting, because patients can be carefully observed during a period of assessment, and then medication can be introduced while they are closely monitored for the development of any adverse side effects. This is much less likely and available than in previous eras.

The three most common reasons for admission to hospital in a first episode of psychosis [3] are:

- concerns about safety;
- sustained refusal to accept community assessment or treatment;
- lack of appropriate family and social support.

Alternative treatment settings such as partial hospitalization, home care, family crisis therapy, crisis residential care and assertive community treatment can be considered for patients who do not need formal hospitalization but require more intensive services than can be expected in a typical outpatient setting. If resources are available and the person's family or carers are coping, then treatment can be initiated safely in the community. This avoids the anxiety, loss of control, increased stigma and trauma which can all too frequently accompany hospitalization.

The first experience of treatment for early psychosis can strongly influence future attitudes to all types of therapy and the mental health system in general. Effective home-based care is likely to be regarded favourably by patients, enhance the therapeutic alliance, improve adherence with medication and other interventions, and facilitate follow-up care.

General Principles

Kulkarni [72] has outlined the following features of home-based care required in early psychosis.

The Individual and the Illness

Severe psychotic illness in itself is not a barrier to successful home-based treatment. Clinical experience suggests it is the dangerousness of the symptoms, rather than their intensity, that determines whether patients will require hospitalization. Suicidal and homicidal thoughts, as well as hostility directed towards family members that is driven by delusions, will encourage hospital admission rather than home-based care. Access to firearms and other weapons needs to be assessed.

Illicit substance abuse, particularly of cannabis and amphetamines, can precipitate and perpetuate psychosis. The family needs to be able to prevent access to illicit drugs during the acute phase of the illness.

The role of the patient in the family and compliance with treatment need to be evaluated. A shared illness model involving patients, their families and clinicians can be useful but is not always necessary for success. It is more useful to reach agreement on management strategies and their implementation rather than the possible reasons for the onset of psychosis.

The Family

The needs and capabilities of the family must be carefully assessed, as they will be the primary caregivers. Families of hospitalized patients are usually of secondary importance in mental health care systems, but in home-based care their welfare and health are more important. Work schedules, the availability of family members and their resources in terms of extended family or friends are important issues.

Poor family interactions and pre-existing family problems may be exacerbated during this time of disruption and stress. However, high expressed emotion can be of value – provided the hostility and critical components are not pronounced – as people with families that might otherwise be considered "over-involved" tend to remain engaged in treatment and recover more quickly than people with distant, disengaged families.

Containment is an important ingredient of treatment in acute psychosis. The family must be empowered to enforce containment, for example by confiscating car keys. There is a need to avoid "splitting" the family on the best course of action for containment.

Implementation and explanation of clear management plans to the family is very important, particularly as early family reactions to a psychotic illness can involve confusion, guilt, denial and emotional numbing. They must receive an unambiguous message about the likelihood of a favourable outcome and recovery from the acute phase.

Table 2.14 is a checklist for the initiation of home-based treatment, from the family perspective.

TABLE 2.14 Checklist for the initiation of home-based treatment.

- Family member requires treatment.
- Family member is not able to attend appointments at community-based services.
- Clinician's and family's risk assessment indicates that home-based treatment is a safe option.
- The collective resources of the treating team and the family enables provision of the required treatment.
- Family understands the tasks involved in home-based treatment.
- Family is willing to take on home-based treatment.
- Good communication can be facilitated through qualified interpreters when needed.

Treating Team

A team treating a patient at home is working in a very different environment from that in a hospital or clinic. They are "guests" in the patient's home, and need to respect power relationships within the family. Challenges they must face include:

- a loss of control over the working environment;
- a lack of access to medical equipment;
- diminished access to colleagues;
- safety issues.

The work requires great flexibility, and staff treating acutely ill patients at home need to be experienced and confident as they make decisions about the safety of the patient and family, and monitor diverse aspects of treatment.

Staffing numbers in a home-based treatment service need to be high enough to allow up to three visits each day. There is a risk of staff "burn-out" from the high demands, so integrating home care into larger systems may help to spread the load and provide greater flexibility. A larger team which provides both home-based intervention and continuing care can ensure continuity of care, with follow-up from the same clinicians. The risk of this approach is that the focus and priority for home-based care can get lost.

Confidentiality issues may arise when the family are functioning as primary carers, and it may be difficult to provide sufficient privacy for therapeutic interventions. Families will have little interaction with others in the same situation, and will depend on the treating team for information and education. The treating team must ensure that all aspects of management are covered. There are usually well-established protocols for assessment and treatment in hospital and clinic settings, but they may be undermined by the flexibility essential in providing home-based care.

Specific Strategies

Treatment Package

All participants in home-based treatment need a structured management plan. A "treatment package" can be used to provide a written timetable which outlines step-by-step treatment plans. In addition, it will reinforce expectations about the course of the acute episode of psychosis and the likelihood of recovery. Treatment packages should be formulated individually with the patient and carers, avoid jargon, and be based on pragmatism and optimism. The plan also provides a reminder of standard protocols to the treating team. An example is shown in Table 2.15.

Plans for the recovery phase and further follow-up can be developed at the same time, reinforcing signals to patients and their families about the expected progress.

Medication Management

Sedation of the patient is usually needed in the hyperacute phase of psychosis to quickly reduce anxiety. This is especially important to allow an

Table 2.15 Home based care: crisis and acute phase (adapted from 72)

Initial phase – commonly 2–7 days

- Formulation and delivery of the individual "package" of care.
- Provision of a clear visiting schedule by the treatment team.
- Medication (usually sedative, e.g. temazepam), then choice of an appropriate atypical antipsychotic.
- Organize blood tests, X-rays etc., to check physical health.
- Assessment of troubling symptoms.
- Discussion with family on helping them to cope and gathering information about the patient prior to the illness.
- Get to know the patient and family, and allow them to get to know the treating team.
- Liaison with patient's general practitioner.

Acute phase – commonly 7–10 days

- Monitor type and dose of antipsychotic medication.
- Treating team to initially administer medication, then hand over to family with clear verbal and written instructions.
- Team to monitor pulse, blood pressure and response to medication.
- Discuss with patient and family the nature of psychosis and how medications work.
- Deal with issues of leave from work and organize certificates.

anxious and vigilant family to rest and "re-group". Sedating benzodiazepines such as temazepam are useful in this phase and can be used during the day if necessary, as well as at night.

Decisions about the choice of antipsychotic medication in these circumstances are very important. It is essential to prevent any dangerous side effects as constant clinical monitoring is not available. The treating team should carry emergency kits of anticholinergic medication with intravenous and intramuscular injection equipment, as well as other emergency medications and resuscitation equipment. Antipsychotics which possess a "gentle" onset of action and yield fewer side effects are preferable to drugs which carry a high risk of extrapyramidal side effects. This essentially means atypical antipsychotics. As with all first-episode patients, the initial doses of antipsychotics should be low and increased slowly, relying on benzodiazepines in the short term to assist with rapid symptomatic relief.

Physical Investigations

Physical investigations which are part of the routine assessment of patients with first-episode psychosis may be more difficult to organize in home-based treatment, but should not be overlooked. Some pathology services collect samples at home, and specialized tests such as CT and MRI can usually be organized on an outpatient basis.

Psychosocial Issues

Stressors and the patient's method of coping with them need to be addressed early in a first episode of psychosis. These can include psychosocial stressors, abuse of substances in response to stress, and sleep deprivation, which worsens emerging psychotic symptoms.

Ideally, home-based treatment will lead to more rapid reintegration into the community, with much less of the secondary morbidity often associated with hospitalization. However, patients who have been treated mainly at home may be unwilling to participate in formal recovery programmes and are more likely to use denial as a recovery style. General community-based programmes for specific skills training or other socialization needs may be more appropriate than "psychiatric" day programmes.

Need for Hospitalization

If hospitalization becomes necessary during a period of home treatment, it should not be viewed as a "failure". The treatment team has the opportunity to facilitate a non-traumatic hospital admission, and then provide follow-up after discharge.

Outcomes of Home-based Therapy

Fitzgerald and Kulkarni [73] reviewed 18 patients who received home-based treatment for a first episode of psychosis. Thirteen were managed exclusively at home, without the need for hospital admission. The level of social support, not the severity of psychopathology, was the main factor determining whether home care was possible. In serious mental disorders generally, where indicated, home-based care is at least as effective as inpatient care, reduces family burden, and improves consumer satisfaction and retention in services [74].

INPATIENT TREATMENT IN EARLY PSYCHOSIS

Criteria for Hospital Admission

Despite the best efforts of a treating team, many patients with a first episode of psychosis will:

- be unwilling or unable to engage in a comprehensive assessment process;
- need urgent intensive care in hospital to minimize serious risks of self-harm or violence.

Criteria for admission will depend on the structure of the mental health service, including factors such as the availability of intensive outreach teams. If good outreach teams exist, then admission can be reserved primarily for risk management. At EPPIC, about one half of patients avoid hospitalization during the first three months of treatment and, when hospitalization does occur, it is usually for relatively short periods (typically 7–14 days). If involuntary admission is required, then it should not be viewed as a failure but as an aid to ensuring appropriate levels of care and treatment [46].

Goals of Inpatient Care in Early Psychosis

Treatment in hospital aims to reduce the severity of psychotic symptoms, and promote the remission of psychosis through the use of thorough

Table 2.16 Some goals of inpatient care in first-episode psychosis

- Ensure safety.
- Provide comprehensive assessment.
- Provide effective treatment with the lowest possible doses of medication to minimize the side effects.
- Minimize the trauma of admission to a psychiatric unit.
- Instil hope and an expectation of recovery.
- Provide counselling and support to assist the patient come to terms with the illness and hospitalization.
- Involve the family in assessment, treatment and discharge planning.
- Provide information about psychosis and treatment for the patient and family.
- Involve a case manager as soon as possible, to facilitate engagement with the community team and continuity of care.
- Involve a general practitioner in care as soon as possible.
- Provide activities and group programmes which are appropriate for young people and promote supportive social interactions.

assessment, careful and selective use of medication, supportive nursing and a broad range of biological, psychological and social interventions. Ideally, inpatient staff and the patient's outpatient doctor and case manager should begin planning for discharge very early in the admission, actively involving the young person and family in the process. Some goals of inpatient care are listed in Table 2.16.

Addressing Concerns about Hospitalization

When patients with a first episode of psychosis are admitted to an inpatient unit, they may be concerned that they:

- will forfeit basic rights;
- will be incarcerated indefinitely;
- will be injected with chemically-restraining medications;
- will be assaulted;
- are not unwell like other patients in the unit [42].

It is possible to address most of these concerns by providing patients with clear choices about their options, ensuring they have access to second opinions and legal assistance, and explaining their rights of appeal if they are subject to involuntary treatment. Most patients subsequently regard their period of hospitalization as a positive event which assisted them to recover.

It is particularly useful for the clinician who first had contact with the patient to accompany the patient and family to hospital, provide a sympathetic description of the hospital process, introduce them to hospital staff, and ensure a full orientation to the inpatient unit and its policies. If possible, avoid transport to hospital by ambulance or the police. Although police admissions are often uneventful and well managed, they have the potential to be traumatizing for the patient. Continued feedback and debriefing to the family is essential before, during and after admission.

Families also have concerns about hospitalization, particularly if it occurs involuntarily. If this is the case, it is important to ensure the family understands that:

- the final decision to admit as an involuntary patient is taken by the treating team, not the family, and this will be explained to the patient;
- if the situation continued, the family would have become increasingly exhausted, which would have hampered their capacity to provide care;
- without short-term intensive care, the patient would have become more unwell, resulting in an even longer period of time before recovery;
- staff are aware of many other cases where inpatient care enabled treatment to be initiated very effectively;
- inpatient care is only for the short term, and the treating team will be involved once the patient comes home again.

Models of Inpatient Care

EPPIC has a 16-bed inpatient unit devoted to the treatment of young people with early psychosis. Such a unit is unusual, being one of a handful of such specialized facilities around the world. As with other components of the EPPIC model, the principles adopted within the unit are not unique and can be applied in other less specialized inpatient settings, including the treatment of patients with early psychosis as part of a general psychiatric service. This is generally facilitated by physically demarcating a section of the unit as the "early psychosis wing". This sends a potent message, which is otherwise lost, to patients and staff that their management and prognosis is substantially different from patients with more established illnesses. Other models of care emphasize residential alternatives to inpatient care [75], but these models still require back-up from traditional inpatient services where the special needs of early psychosis patients are not responded to.

Inpatient care in early psychosis focuses on symptom reduction and containment [1]. It emphasizes brief admissions in order to prepare patients for community treatment in the home or through an outpatient case management service. There needs to be close integration between different elements of the service, with staff members working across the different components of the programme and a case manager being assigned immediately on entry to the early psychosis service. The median length of stay in the EPPIC inpatient unit is 9 days (mean 13 days), and 6 days for subsequent (re)admissions.

Low doses of antipsychotics are standard practice during the acute phase. Disturbed behaviour is managed by targeted nursing interventions, liberal use of benzodiazepines as "antipsychotic-sparing" agents, and minimizing the use of potentially traumatic interventions such as seclusion and restraint.

Favourable Hospital Environment

Attention to the hospital environment can make the period of hospitalization a more positive experience for patients. For example, flexible visiting times will encourage continued contact between the patient, family and friends. Personal comfort and respect for individual privacy should be encouraged, with an emphasis on small but important details such as diet, access to and safety of personal possessions, access to phones, and provision of accurate information about the expected length of stay. Staff can help to demystify and humanize the experience of hospitalization, rather than the opposite.

A specific unit for young patients with psychosis is ideal, but not always achievable. Exposure to older patients with chronic mental illness can be a distressing and demoralizing experience. Staff can become desensitized to the typical environment of an acute psychiatric unit, but should not underestimate how frightening and distressing it can be for young people and their families.

Calm but sociable wards facilitate recovery, and distraught but disorganized patients benefit from a ward environment that reduces environmental chaos [66]. In the absence of a specialized early psychosis unit, in addition to the demarcation of specific early psychosis beds, it may be possible to provide a meaningful activity programme in as relaxed an atmosphere as possible for inpatients away from the ward, aimed at reducing negative symptoms, encouraging the development of social skills and improving self-esteem. This can begin the process of patients gradually developing more insight, acquiring coping strategies and resuming responsibility before being discharged.

Staff in an early psychosis inpatient unit must strive to allow flexibility in their management of patients, with considerable tolerance of "normal" adolescent behaviour and an effort to accept frustration, anger and other emotions as normal reactions to illness. Such flexibility must be balanced by the need to maintain safety. It often necessitates a compromise in the desire of staff to "control" all aspects of patients' behaviour and to "win" each potential confrontation. This approach is more dependent on the culture of the unit than on a high level of resources.

The ward, which should be of modest size (12–16 beds maximum), should not be locked, but a small lockable intensive care area should be available for aggressive patients and for those who are at high risk of absconding when safety is an issue. At least one nurse should be on duty for each four patients. With patients at high risk of self-harm, one-to-one nursing is preferable to placing the patient in a locked area with agitated or aggressive patients. A policy of low-dose antipsychotic therapy and avoidance of excessive sedation is adopted in order to enhance the outcomes for patients, but it adds to the demands on nursing staff. However, night-time sedation with benzodiazepines should be freely available.

Ward routines should be less rigid than in other units. For example, there should be flexibility as to when patients get out of bed each day, when they eat, and when they have visitors. Family members or friends should be able to stay overnight on the ward if this assists in reducing anxiety and distress. This is the mirror-image of the home-based care model.

Whenever possible, treatment, including medication, should be negotiated with patients rather than imposed without discussion. For example, patients are allowed some time and actively assisted to gain control over their behaviour wherever possible, before involuntary use of medication. Openness to negotiation increases the prospects for engagement with staff and for long-term compliance.

On their first admission, patients should be given a tour of the unit with a clear statement about the rules of the ward, including respect for others. Specific fears can be addressed with information, explanation and reassurance. Staff can clarify the reason for admission, the likely course and duration of treatment, and the plans for discharge.

Managing Risks of Harm to Self and Others in Hospital

Aggression and Violence

Minimizing the risks and impact of violence is an increasing challenge for staff in acute inpatient wards [3]. Because of a trend to admit only the most acutely disturbed patients and for short periods, some wards are becoming "anti-therapeutic" environments where both staff and patients feel unsafe.

Limited staffing and poor building design can increase the risks to staff in inpatient units [42]. A volatile mix can develop in busy, noisy units with groups of young and unfamiliar patients confined by involuntary hospitalization and agitated by their psychotic experiences or mood disturbances.

TABLE 2.17 Response to aggression in an inpatient unit

- Distinguish between normal "adolescent" behaviour and symptoms of psychosis.
- Redirect energy through sport activities, walks with staff or other physical activity.
- Exert a high degree of self-control despite anxiety in the face of aggressive behaviour.
- Check what the patient wants: the issue might have arisen from difficulty with a simple request such as access to a phone.
- Avoid looking or becoming nervous: stay calm and self-confident.
- Recognize real threats and withdraw when appropriate: don't be a hero, and have the confidence to exit safely.
- Use a calm voice at low volume to convey simple messages.
- Adopt a non-threatening posture with some eye contact but avoid staring.

New arrivals can find their worst fears about hospital confirmed and become insecure and threatened. A vicious cycle develops as the therapeutic alliance breaks down, escalating confrontation and further increasing the risk of violence. Careful attention to staff morale, improving the quality of the inpatient milieu, and specific staff training in aggression management (especially preventive strategies) can help improve the situation.

Some aspects of dealing with aggressive patients were addressed above. Some additional techniques are outlined in Table 2.17.

Self-harm and Suicide

Assessment of the risks of self-harm and suicide were addressed in detail above. High risk of suicide is often a factor in deciding to admit a patient to hospital. Accurate risk assessment, close monitoring, removal of means of self-harm and optimal treatment (including psychological therapies as well as medication) are key steps in maintaining safety while on the ward. Formal classification of patients to different levels of nursing observation and severity will assist in this process.

Observation, Seclusion and Restraint

Use of more intensive nursing categories on an open ward can greatly reduce the need for seclusion or restraint of patients, which should be undertaken only after less restrictive alternatives have failed or when they are considered to have a low probability of success [11]. This is particularly important in first admission patients for obvious reasons. Clinicians must review secluded or restrained patients as often as needed to monitor any changes in physical or mental status and to comply with mental health legislation. Release from seclusion or restraint can be graded, as the risk of harm to self or others diminishes.

If seclusion is to be therapeutic, it should include prior orientation to the reality of being secluded, then reduction of sensory input, then reintegration back into the general ward environment [76]. Like other interventions, it should be patient-centred, with patients encouraged to exercise choice and enhance necessary coping skills.

In the early psychosis inpatient unit, an intensive care area should be used flexibly, and primarily to provide brief periods of "time-out" for patients. The period in the intensive care area may be as little as an hour. It provides a low-stimulation environment with limited contact with other patients, allowing irritability and aggression to abate in a safe environment.

Seclusion should be used rarely. It can be used if it is necessary to protect the person or others from an immediate or imminent risk to health or safety, or to prevent the person from absconding. The use of seclusion, and requirements for monitoring and reporting on seclusion, are governed by mental health legislation.

Transition to the Recovery Phase

An acute psychotic episode may be the event which precipitates entry to a mental health service, and inpatient services tend to focus exclusively on this phase. However, the service should ideally provide "seamless" integrated care, following patients through the early and late stages of recovery. Achieving such an integrated approach remains a challenge. If it results in more effective care, then it should be possible to extract greater value from existing resources: integrated care from acute illness to recovery does not necessarily require more resources.

A culture of realistic optimism will recognize that most young people with early psychosis will recover from the initial acute episode but remain at risk of relapse, particularly if they adhere poorly to long-term treatment or are re-exposed to stressors, including substance misuse. A positive transition from acute care to longer-term care will help improve the chance that such a relapse does not occur or that, if it does, the individual seeks help early.

CONCLUSIONS

Improved recognition and optimal treatment of early psychosis continue to develop rapidly. Current issues for research are likely to produce new information on issues including:

- more accurate identification of young people at risk of developing a psychotic illness;
- the neurobiological basis of early psychosis and the onset of acute episodes;
- the most effective way to use existing and new pharmacological interventions;
- the delivery of effective family-based intervention;
- treatment of comorbidity, particularly substance abuse;
- psychological interventions in the pre-psychotic, acute and recovery phase;
- the optimal response to a delayed recovery from the acute phase;
- interventions during the recovery phase to minimize the risk of relapse, substance abuse and suicide, and maximize social and vocational recovery.

This chapter has focused particularly on the prepsychotic period, the process of successfully initiating treatment and the management of the initial episode of illness. Expert management of the subsequent "critical period" of the first two to five years of illness is a third and crucial focus in early psychosis, and, while not covered here in detail, is receiving increasing attention [8]. Social and vocational recovery should constitute the primary goal, building on the symptomatic resolution usually achieved during the initial phase of treatment.

ACKNOWLEDGEMENT

This chapter has drawn upon an array of source documents, treatment manuals, oral input and feedback and an accumulation of clinical wisdom from a large number of people. Special appreciation goes to Tony James, Daryl Wade, Peter Burnett, Lisa Phillips, numerous international colleagues and particularly our young patients and their families.

REFERENCES

1. Edwards J., McGorry P.D. (2002). *Implementing Early Intervention in Psychosis: A Guide to Establishing Early Psychosis Services*. Dunitz, London.
2. Birchwood M., Macmillan J.F. (1993). Early intervention in schizophrenia. *Aust. N. Zeal. J. Psychiatry*, **27**, 374–378.
3. Kulkarni J., Power P. (1999). Initial treatment of first-episode psychosis. In: McGorry P.D., Jackson H.J. (eds) *The Recognition and Management of Early Psychosis. A Preventive Approach*. Cambridge University Press, Cambridge, pp. 184–205.

4. Bottlender R., Moller H.J. (2003). The impact of the duration of untreated psychosis on short- and long-term outcome in schizophrenia. *Curr. Opin. Psychiatry*, **16** (Suppl. 2), S39–S43.
5. Garety P., Jolley S. (2000). Early intervention in psychosis. *Psychiatr. Bull.*, **24**, 321–323.
6. McGorry P.D., Chanen A., McCarthy E., Van Riel R., McKenzie D., Singh B.S. (1991). Posttraumatic stress disorder following recent-onset psychosis. An unrecognised post-psychotic syndrome. *J. Nerv. Ment. Dis.*, **179**, 253–258.
7. McGorry P.D. (1995). A treatment-relevant classification of psychotic disorders. *Aust. N. Zeal. J. Psychiatry*, **29**, 555–558.
8. Birchwood M., Fowler D., Jackson C. (eds) (2000). *Early Intervention in Psychosis: A Guide to Concepts, Evidence and Intervention*. John Wiley & Sons Ltd, Chichester.
9. McGorry P.D. (1994). The influence of illness duration on syndrome clarity and stability in functional psychosis: does the diagnosis emerge and stabilise with time? *Aust. N. Zeal. J. Psychiatry*, **28**, 607–619.
10. Yung A.R., McGorry P.D. (1996). The initial prodrome in psychosis: descriptive and qualitative aspects. *Aust. N. Zeal. J. Psychiatry*, **30**, 587–599.
11. American Psychiatric Association (1997). *Practice Guidelines for the Treatment of Patients with Schizophrenia*. American Psychiatric Association, Washington, DC.
12. Jarry M., Andrews G., Hunt C. (1997). *Management of Mental Disorders, World Health Organization Treatment Protocol Project*, 2nd edn. World Health Organization Collaborating Centre for Mental Health and Substance Abuse, Darlinghurst, NSW.
13. Norman R.M.G., Malla A.K. (2001). Duration of untreated psychosis: a critical examination of the concept and its importance. *Psychol. Med.*, **31**, 381–400.
14. National Institute for Clinical Excellence (NICE) (2002). *Schizophrenia: Core Interventions in the Treatment and Management of Schizophrenia in Primary and Secondary Care. Clinical Guideline 1.* NICE, National Collaborating Centre for Mental Health, London.
15. Harrison G., Hopper K., Craig T., Laska E., Siegel C., Wanderling J., Dube K.C., Ganev K., Giel R., van der Heiden W., *et al.* (2001). Recovery from psychotic illness: a 15- and 25-year international follow-up study. *Br. J. Psychiatry*, **178**, 506–517.
16. Meares A. (1959). The diagnosis of prepsychotic schizophrenia. *Lancet*, **i**, 55–59.
17. Sullivan H.S. (1927). The onset of schizophrenia. *Am. J. Psychiatry*, **6**, 105–134.
18. Yung A.R., Phillips L.J., McGorry P.D., Hallgren M.A., McFarlane C.A., Jackson H.J., Francey S., Patton G.C. (1998). Can we predict onset of first episode psychosis in a high-risk group? *Int. Clin. Psychopharmacol.*, **13** (Suppl. 1), S23–30.
19. Yung A.R., Phillips L.J., Yuen H.P., Francey S.M., McFarlane C.A., Hallgren M., McGorry P.D. (2003). Psychosis prediction: 12 month follow up of a high risk ("prodromal") group. *Schizophr. Res.*, **60**, 21–32.
20. Jones P., Rodgers B., Murray R., Marmot M. (1994). Child development risk factors for adult schizophrenia in the British 1946 birth cohort. *Lancet*, **344**, 1398–1402.
21. Häfner H., Nowotny B., Löffler W., an der Heiden W., Maurer K. (1995). When and how does schizophrenia produce social deficits? *Eur. Arch. Psychiatry Clin. Neurosci.*, **246**, 17–28.
22. Phillips L.J., Yung A.R., Yuen H.P., Pantelis C., McGorry P.D. (2002). Prediction and prevention of transition to psychosis in young people at incipient risk for schizophrenia. *Am. J. Med. Genet.*, **114**, 929–937.

23. Bell R.Q. (1992). Multiple-risk cohorts and segmenting risk as solutions to the problem of false positives in risk for the major psychoses. *Psychiatry*, **55**, 370–381.
24. Yung A.R., McGorry P.D., McFarlane C.A., Patton G.C. (1995). The PACE clinic: development of a clinical service for young people at high risk of psychosis. *Australas. Psychiatry*, **3**, 345–349.
25. Cornblatt B., Lencz T., Correll C., Authour A., Smith C. (2002). Treating the prodrome: naturalistic findings from the RAP Program. *Acta Psychiatr. Scand.*, **106** (Suppl. 413), 44.
26. Miller T.J., McGlashan T.H., Rosen J.L., Somjee L., Markovich P.J., Stein K., Woods S.W. (2002). Prospective diagnosis of the initial prodrome for schizophrenia based on the Structured Interview for Prodromal Symptoms: preliminary evidence of interrater and predictive validity. *Am. J. Psychiatry*, **159**, 863–865.
27. Morrison A.P., Bentall R.P., French P., Walford L., Kilcommons A., Knight A., Kreutz M., Lewis S.W. (2002). Randomised controlled trial of early detection and cognitive therapy for preventing transition to psychosis in high-risk individuals. Study design and interim analysis of transition rate and psychological risk factors. *Br. J. Psychiatry*, **181** (Suppl. 43), s78–s84.
28. McGorry P.D., Singh B.S. (1995). Schizophrenia: risk and possibility. In: Raphael B., Burrows G.D. (eds) *Handbook of Studies on Preventive Psychiatry*. Elsevier, Amsterdam, pp. 491–514.
29. Yung A.R., McGorry P.D. (1997). Is pre-psychotic intervention realistic in schizophrenia and related disorders? *Aust. N. Zeal. J. Psychiatry*, **31**, 799–805.
30. Eaton W.W., Badawi M., Melton B. (1995). Prodromes and precursors: epidemiological data for primary prevention of disorders with slow onset. *Am. J. Psychiatry*, **152**, 967–972.
31. Larsen T.K., Friis S., Haahr U., Joa I., Johannessen J.O., Melle I., Opjordsmoen S., Simonsen E., Vaglum P. (2001). Early detection and intervention in first-episode schizophrenia: a critical review. *Acta Psychiatr. Scand.*, **103**, 323–334.
32. McGorry P.D., Yung A.R., Phillips L.J., Yuen H.P., Francey S., Cosgrave E.M., Germano D., Bravin J., Adlard S., McDonald T., *et al.* (2002). Randomized controlled trial of interventions designed to reduce the risk of progression to first episode psychosis in a clinical sample with subthreshold symptoms. *Arch. Gen. Psychiatry*, **59**, 921–928.
33. Miller T.J., Zipursky R.B., Perkins D., Addington J., Woods S.W., Hawkins K.A., Hoffman R., Preda A., Epstein I., Addington D., *et al.* (2003). The PRIME North America randomized double-blind clinical trial of olanzapine versus placebo in patients at risk of being prodromally symptomatic for psychosis. II. Baseline characteristics of the "prodromal" sample. *Schizophr. Res.*, **61**, 19–30.
34. Wyatt R.J. (1991). Neuroleptics and the natural course of schizophrenia. *Schizophr. Bull.*, **17**, 325–351.
35. Ho B.-C., Alicate D., Ward J., Moser D.J., O'Leary D.S., Arndt S., Andreasen N.C. (2003). Untreated initial psychosis: relation to cognitive deficits and brain morphology in first-episode schizophrenia. *Am. J. Psychiatry*, **160**, 142–148.
36. McGorry P.D. (1992). The concept of recovery and secondary prevention in psychotic disorders. *Aust. N. Zeal. J. Psychiatry*, **26**, 3–17.
37. McGorry P.D., Edwards J., Mihalopoulos C., Harrigan S., Jackson H.J. (1996). The Early Psychosis Prevention and Intervention Centre (EPPIC): an evolving system of early detection and optimal management. *Schizophr. Bull.*, **22**, 305–326.

38. McGorry P.D., Yung A.R. (2003). Early intervention in psychosis: an overdue reform: An introduction to the Early Psychosis Symposium. *Aust. N. Zeal. J. Psychiatry*, **37**, 393–398.
39. Lincoln C., McGorry P.D. (1999). Pathways to care in early psychosis: delay and decline? In: McGorry P.D., Jackson J.J. (eds) *The Recognition and Management of Early Psychosis: A Preventive Approach*. Cambridge University Press, New York, pp. 51–80.
40. Skeate A., Jackson C., Birchwood M., Jones C. (2002). Duration of untreated psychosis and pathways to care in first-episode psychosis. *Br. J. Psychiatry*, **181**, s73–s77.
41. McGorry P.D., Killackey E., Elkins K., Lambert M., Lamter T. (2003). Summary Australian and New Zealand clinical practice guideline for the treatment of schizophrenia (2003). *Australas. Psychiatry*, **11**, 136–147.
42. Power P., McGorry P.D. (1999). Initial assessment of first-episode psychosis. In: McGorry P.D., Jackson H.J. (eds) *The Recognition and Management of Early Psychosis. A Preventive Approach*. Cambridge University Press, Cambridge, pp. 155–183.
43. Yung A.R., Phillips L.J., Drew L.T. (1999). Promoting access to care in early psychosis. In: McGorry P.D., Jackson H.J. (eds) *The Recognition and Management of Early Psychosis. A Preventive Approach*. Cambridge University Press, Cambridge, pp. 81–114.
44. McGorry P.D., Yung A.R., Phillips L.J., Cadenhead K., Sharma T. (in press). Clinical service models for intervention in the prepsychotic phase: towards effective and safe strategies for earliest intervention in psychotic disorders. *Schizophr. Bull.*
45. McGorry P.D., McConville S.B. (1999). Insight in psychosis: an elusive target. *Compr. Psychiatry*, **40**, 131–142.
46. Power P., Elkins K., Adlard S., Curry C., McGorry P., Harrigan S. (1998). An analysis of initial treatment of first episode psychosis. *Br. J. Psychiatry*, **172** (Suppl. 33), 71–76.
47. Strakowski S.M., Tohen M., Stoll A., Faedda G.L., Mayer P.V., Kolbrener M.L., Goodwin D.C. (1993). Comorbidity in psychosis at first hospitalisation. *Am. J. Psychiatry*, **150**, 752–757.
48. Humphries M.S., Johnstone E.C., Macmillan J.F., Taylor P.J. (1992). Dangerous behaviour preceding first admissions for schizophrenia. *Br. J. Psychiatry*, **161**, 501–505.
49. NSW Health, Centre for Mental Health (2002). *Mental Health for Emergency Departments – A Reference Guide Pocket Version*. NSW Health, Sydney.
50. Lubman D.I., Velakoulis D., McGorry P.D., Smith D.J., Brewer W., Stuart G., Desmond P., Tress B., Pantelis C. (2002). Incidental radiological findings on brain magnetic resonance imaging in first-episode psychosis and chronic schizophrenia. *Acta Psychiatr. Scand.*, **106**, 331–336.
51. Loebel A.D., Leiberman J.A., Alvir J.M.J., Mayerhoff D.I., Geisler S.H., Szymansky S.R. (1992). Duration of psychosis outcome in first episode schizophrenia. *Am. J. Psychiatry*, **149**, 1183–1188.
52. McEvoy J.P., Hogarty G.E., Steingard S. (1991). Optimal dose of neuroleptic in acute schizophrenia. A controlled study of the neuroleptic threshold and higher haloperidol dose. *Arch. Gen. Psychiatry*, **48**, 739–745.
53. Merlo M.C.G., Hofer H., Gekle W., Berger G., Ventura J., Panhuber I., Latour G., Marder S.R. (2002). Risperidone, 2 mg/day vs. 4 mg/day, in first-episode,

acutely psychotic patients: treatment efficacy and effects on fine motor functioning. *J. Clin. Psychiatry*, **63**, 885–891.

54. Lieberman J.A., Tollefson G., Tohen M., Green A.I., Gur R.E., Kahn R., McEvoy J., Perkins D., Sharma T., Zipursky R., *et al.* (2003). Comparative efficacy and safety of atypical and conventional antipsychotic drugs in first-episode psychosis: a randomized, double-blind trial of olanzapine versus haloperidol. *Am. J. Psychiatry*, **160**, 1396–1404.
55. Kapur S., Zipursky R., Jones C., Remington G., Houle S. (2000). Relationship between dopamine D_2 occupancy, clinical response, and side effects: a double-blind PET study of first-episode schizophrenia. *Am. J. Psychiatry*, **157**, 514–520.
56. National Early Psychosis Project Clinical Guidelines Working Party (1998). *Australian Clinical Guidelines for Early Psychosis.* National Early Psychosis Project, University of Melbourne, Melbourne.
57. Davis J.M., Chen N., Glick I.D. (2003). A meta-analysis of the efficacy of second-generation antipsychotics. *Arch. Gen. Psychiatry*, **60**, 553–564.
58. Nosé M., Barbui C., Tansella M. (2003). How often do patients with psychosis fail to adhere to treatment programmes? A systematic review. *Psychol. Med.*, **33**, 1149–1160.
59. Geddes J., Freemantle N., Harrison P., Bebbington P. (2000). Atypical antipsychotics in the treatment of schizophrenia: systematic overview and meta-regression analysis. *Br. Med. J.*, **321**, 1371–1376.
60. Stroup T.S., McEvoy J.P., Swartz M.S., Byerly M.J., Glick I.D., Canive J.M., McGee M.F., Simpson G.M., Stevens M.C., Lieberman J.A. (2003). The National Institute of Mental Health Clinical Antipsychotic Trials of Intervention Effectiveness (CATIE) project: schizophrenia trial design and protocol development. *Schizophr. Bull*, **29**, 15–31.
61. Garety P.A., Fowler D., Kuipers E. (2000). Cognitive-behavioral therapy for medication-resistant symptoms. *Schizophr. Bull.*, **26**, 73–86.
62. Robinson D.G., Woerner M.G., Alvir J.M.A., Geisler S., Koreen A., Sheitman B., Chakos M., Mayerhoff D., Bilder R., Goldman R. *et al.* (1999). Predictors of relapse following response from a first episode of schizophrenia or schizoaffective disorder. *Arch. Gen. Psychiatry*, **56**, 241–247.
63. Gitlin M., Nuechterlein K., Subotnik K.L., Ventura J., Mintz J., Fogelson D.L., Bartzokis G., Aravagiri M. (2001). Clinical outcome following neuroleptic discontinuation in patients with remitted recent-onset schizophrenia. *Am. J. Psychiatry*, **158**, 1835–1842.
64. Carpenter W.T. (2001). Evidence-based treatment for first-episode schizophrenia? *Am. J. Psychiatry*, **158**, 1771–1773.
65. Gleeson J., Jackson H.J., Stavely H., Burnett P. (1999). Family intervention in early psychosis. In: McGorry P.D., Jackson H.J. (eds) *The Recognition and Management of Early Psychosis*. Cambridge University Press, New York, pp. 376–406.
66. Aitchison K.J., Meehan K., Murray R.M. (1999). *First Episode Psychosis*. Dunitz, London.
67. Gleeson J.F.M., McGorry P.D. (2004). *Psychological Interventions in Early Psychosis: A Treatment Handbook*. John Wiley & Sons Ltd, Chichester.
68. Lewis S., Tarrier N., Haddock G., Bentall R., Kinderman P., Kingdon D., Siddle R., Drake R., Everitt J., Leadley K., *et al.* (2002). Randomised controlled trial of cognitive–behaviour therapy in early schizophrenia: acute-phase outcomes. *Br. J. Psychiatry*, **181** (Suppl. 43), s91–s97.

69. Jackson H.J., McGorry P.D., Edwards J., Hulbert C., Henry L., Francey S., Cocks J., Power P., Harrigan S., Dudgeon P. (1998). Cognitively oriented psychotherapy for early psychosis (COPE): preliminary results. *Br. J. Psychiatry*, **172** (Suppl. 33), 93–100.
70. Power P.J.R., Bell R.J., Mills R., Herrman-Doig T., Davern M., Henry L., Yuen H.P., Khademy-Deljo A., McGorry P.D. (2003). Suicide prevention in first episode psychosis: the development of a randomised controlled trial of cognitive therapy for acutely suicidal patients with early psychosis. *Aust. N. Zeal. J. Psychiatry*, **37**, 414–420.
71. Edwards J., Maude D., Herrman-Doig T., Wong L., Cocks J., Burnett P., Bennett C., Wade D., McGorry P. (2002). A service response to prolonged recovery in early psychosis. *Psychiatr. Serv.*, **53**, 1067–1069.
72. Kulkarni J. (1999). Home-based treatment of first-episode psychosis. In: McGorry P.D., Jackson H.J. (eds) *The Recognition and Management of Early Psychosis. A Preventive Approach*. Cambridge University Press, Cambridge, pp. 206–225.
73. Fitzgerald P., Kulkarni J. (1998). Home-oriented management program for people with early psychosis. *Br. J. Psychiatry*, **172** (Suppl. 33), 39–44.
74. Joy C.B., Adams C.E., Rice K. (2000). Crisis intervention for people with severe mental illness. *Cochrane Database Systematic Reviews*, **2**, CS001087.
75. Bola J.R., Mosher L.R. (2002). At issue: predicting drug-free treatment response in acute psychosis from the Soteria project. *Schizophr. Bull.*, **28**, 559–575.
76. Farrell G.A., Dares G. (1996). Seclusion or solitary confinement: therapeutic or punitive treatment? *Aust. N. Zeal. J. Ment. Health Nursing*, **5**, 171–179.

CHAPTER

3

Children of Persons with Schizophrenia: An Overview of Empirical Research

Allan F. Mirsky and Adrienne K. Elliott

National Institute of Mental Health, Bethesda, MD, USA

INTRODUCTION

Schizophrenia is the most serious of mental disorders, leading to significant, although not always persistent, impairments in functioning in approximately 1% of the population [1]. From an evolutionary perspective, schizophrenia has been conceptualized as either a disadvantageous by-product of human brain evolution or an evolutionarily advantageous outcome [2]. In terms of day-to-day living, untreated schizophrenia has a clear deleterious effect on functioning, with seemingly minimal social or occupational advantage. Despite significant impairment, particularly in moderate to severe cases, some people with schizophrenia find partners and have children, most likely prior to their first psychotic episode. The offspring of these individuals are at increased risk for developing psychiatric disorders, including schizophrenia, because of both genetic and environmental factors. These risks may be exacerbated by the greater likelihood that schizophrenic women will have children with men who are also suffering from a psychiatric disorder [3].

The diathesis–stress model proposed by Meehl in 1962 [4] has been widely accepted as the most comprehensive explanation for the development of psychosis. Data gathered over the past 100 plus years provide strong support for the notion that both genetic vulnerability and environmental stressors play a role in the development of schizophrenia spectrum disorders. These factors either enhance or compromise the development of personality in a complex, multi-directional fashion. The latter point is illustrated in the case of the Genain sisters, a group of

Early Detection and Management of Mental Disorders.
Edited by Mario Maj, Juan José López-Ibor, Norman Sartorius, Mitsumoto Sato and Ahmed Okasha.
 ISBN 0-470-01083-5.

monozygotic quadruplets concordant for schizophrenia but discordant for the severity and onset of their illness [5]. Despite identical genetic load, a combination of environmental idiosyncrasies and differential treatment by their parents has apparently either enhanced or diminished the expression of their genetic vulnerability [6,7]. Similarly, their genetic endowment appears to have interacted with the environment to affect outcome. For example, two of the girls were considered more attractive and less frail than the others, and consequently were treated as healthier and more likely to succeed. The less attractive girls were seen as more inept, even "retarded", and were treated by their parents accordingly [8]. In reality, this pairing of the twins was probably unfounded, as one of the "less attractive" girls was actually more functional than her parents' treatment would suggest [8]. More in-depth data gathered from the Genain quadruplets will be discussed in a later part of this chapter, with the main point here being that genetic and environmental factors seem to have additive and reciprocal effects. This reality complicates efforts to identify and separate the effects of genetic and neurobehavioural disease markers.

Another challenge to researchers looking for disease predictors involves disentangling prodromal signs from premorbid indicators [9]. For example, social isolation in adolescence may be a prodromal sign of schizophrenia whereas this same variable may be viewed as a premorbid indicator if present in early childhood. Longitudinal studies have been particularly helpful in identifying predictors of illness, although categorizing these predictors as prodromes versus premorbid indicators is difficult. The strength of longitudinal studies is that they allow for a comprehensive assessment of high-risk children over the life course, prior to the emergence of full-blown psychosis. Converging evidence from these studies strongly suggests that neurodevelopmental processes are involved in the aetiology of schizophrenia; that is, antecedents of schizophrenia spectrum disorders are evident as early as infancy and continue to evolve over the course of childhood.

Although investigations indicate a link between genetic factors and subsequent development of psychosis, not all vulnerable persons go on to develop schizophrenia or spectrum disorders. Correctly predicting which high-risk individuals will actually go on to develop schizophrenia always involves a degree of error. Specificity is the probability of concluding that someone is affected by a disorder when he or she is truly not (false positive rate), while sensitivity refers to the probability of concluding that someone is affected with a disorder when he or she actually is (true positive rate). The sensitivity and specificity of particular indicators is an important aspect of discerning whether or not an indicator will be useful. Classifying someone as likely to develop schizophrenia when this is not the case could result in costly and perhaps damaging intervention efforts, because of labelling, stigmatizing, etc. Conversely, underestimating who is likely to develop the disorder would lead to a higher preponderance of individuals being deprived of needed early intervention. This chapter provides an overview of empirical research related to children who are at high risk for developing schizophrenia, those children who are the offspring of a schizophrenic parent (or parents). Consideration will be given to genetic factors thought to be important in the development of schizophrenia, identification of possible predictors and their relative usefulness, and intervention strategies that may be suitable for high-risk children.

GENETIC DIATHESIS

Understanding the genetic underpinnings of schizophrenia has been an important area of research for decades and has been studied using a wide variety of methods, including linkage and association studies, longitudinal assessments of high-risk children, and twin studies. The possible importance of genetic factors was noted as early as 1895 by Koller, who reported an aggregation of psychiatric disorders in families, with psychoses showing the strongest genetic link (as cited in 10). In his 1907 psychiatry text, Kraepelin noted, referring to dementia praecox: "defective heredity is a very prominent factor..." (as cited in 11). Adoption studies in the 1960s and 1970s offered further clarification of genetic factors by quantifying the significant incidence of schizophrenia spectrum disorders in high-risk children who were not being raised by their biological parents [12,13]. More recent investigations suggest that the risk of developing schizophrenia in the offspring of affected mothers is approximately 10%, while the chances of becoming schizophrenic are roughly 50% if one's identical twin has the disorder [14]. For children with two schizophrenic parents, the risk of developing the disorder is 40% [15].

Linkage and Association Studies

In terms of the genetics of schizophrenia, additive and interactive genes are thought to increase the possibility of developing the disorder, although this outcome is not inevitable even with the requisite genetic combination. Linkage studies, which assess genetic factors within families, have suggested that mutations on chromosomes 6p, 8p and 11q are possible contributors to the development of the disorder [16–18]. Association studies offer another method for uncovering the genetic underpinnings of schizophrenia by looking at disease markers in unrelated persons or animals [19]. One example of an association study using an animal model comes from Joober *et al.* [20]. Using mouse genetics and quantitative trait locus (QTL) analysis, they explored mouse prepulse inhibition, which refers to "an inhibition of the startle response when a low-intensity stimulus, the prepulse, preceded the startling stimulus (by 30–500 ms)" [20]. Deficits in prepulse inhibition are associated with attentional problems and other cognitive deficits, both of which are observed in persons with schizophrenia [21]. Based on this work, Joober and colleagues have uncovered two candidate genes in mice, which may be related to sensorimotor gating deficits in humans [20]. With the mapping of the human genome, future breakthroughs in understanding the aetiology of schizophrenia are surely on the horizon. Deciding how to apply this information in a useful and ethical manner remains a continuing area of debate, one that will be addressed briefly later in this chapter.

High-risk Studies

Longitudinal investigations of children who are statistically more likely to develop schizophrenia became popular during the 1950s and continue to offer rich clinical data today. In 1952, Barbara Fish launched the New York Infant High-risk Study, the first formal investigation of children born to schizophrenic mothers [22]. Based on her work, Fish theorized that the vulnerability seen in children of schizophrenic mothers was related to defective neural integration, which could be detected in infancy [23]. Fish described pandysmaturation (PDM), which was thought to be a marker for this neurointegrative defect [24]. PDM is characterized by slowed skeletal growth, "transient lags" in development during the first two years of life, and an abnormal profile where more complex developmental tasks are achieved while relatively simple tasks are failed [23]. Since Fish launched her study, many other high-risk studies have been initiated, such as the Copenhagen High-risk Project [25], the National Institute of Mental Health (NIMH) Israeli High-risk Study [26], the New York High-risk Project [27] and the Jerusalem Infant Development Study [28], among others. A brief overview of these first-generation high-risk studies follows; other sources provide more exhaustive reviews [23–31].

Copenhagen High-risk Study

In 1962, Mednick and Schulsinger launched the Copenhagen High-risk Project [25]. They based their investigation on the hypothesis that preschizophrenic children inherit an overly sensitive autonomic nervous system, which leads to an avoidance of excessively stressful environments [32]. Participants in this study were between the ages of 9 and 20 at the start of the investigation and were identified through central social and medical registers as having severely schizophrenic mothers. A control group of low-risk children matched for age and socioeconomic status was also included. From their sample, Mednick *et al.* [32] found that children of schizophrenic mothers were predisposed to schizophrenia spectrum disorders, not just to schizophrenia. This predisposition was more likely to be transmitted by mothers whose schizophrenia began at an earlier age and by mothers who had multiple relatives with schizophrenia, making for a larger genetic load [32]. Follow-up investigations shed light on personality variables that appear to predict future schizophrenia in high-risk individuals [33]. Although prior research with the Copenhagen subjects did not identify any premorbid differences in personality variables, a 25-year follow-up suggested that personality variables could distinguish paranoid preschizophrenic subjects from high-risk individuals who did not become ill [33]. Specifically, on a modified version of the Minnesota Multiphasic Personality Inventory (MMPI), paranoid preschizophrenics had deviant scores on the psychoticism scale, the paranoid schizophrenia scale, and a scale measuring unusual thoughts and experiences [33]. They also endorsed items that were indicative of psychotic processes, withdrawal and social aversion [33]. Earlier results from the Copenhagen study suggest that 5% of children of paranoid schizophrenic mothers were schizophrenic at age 24, whereas 29% of the offspring of non-paranoid schizophrenics had the disorder [34].

NIMH Israeli High-risk Study

Another investigation, the NIMH Israeli High-risk Study, overseen by Rosenthal and colleagues, was initiated in 1965 [35]. This study provided a unique opportunity to evaluate the stress–diathesis model of schizophrenia. As mentioned previously, this model proposes that the development of schizophrenia includes genetic vulnerability (diathesis) and environmental contributors (stress). In the Israeli study, school-age children with a schizophrenic parent (high-risk children), who were being raised either by professional child-care workers on a kibbutz or in a traditional family setting, were included. Control groups included non-high-risk children being reared on a kibbutz or by their own parents in a nuclear family. One goal of this investigation was to assess whether reduced exposure to a schizophrenic parent would yield better outcome [35]. Results indicated that children with clear neurobehavioural deficits and poor social competence were at greatest risk for later development of schizophrenia spectrum illness [36], and that children reared on the kibbutz developed psychiatric disorders at more than double the rate of high-risk children raised in traditional families [37]. In a follow-up study at age 30, high-risk kibbutz cases were significantly more likely to have an Axis I diagnosis as compared to children reared by a schizophrenic parent [38]. Several possible environmental factors unique to the kibbutz environment were implicated in this finding, including the stressful and demanding nature of this setting [39].

New York High-risk Project

The New York High-risk Project, initiated by Erlenmeyer-Kimling and colleagues in 1971, included children between 7 and 12 years of age who were the offspring of at least one schizophrenic parent [40]. Comparison groups included offspring of parents with affective disorder and children of psychiatrically healthy parents. A follow-up conducted when the offspring were approximately age 27 showed that the best predictor of adult psychosis, hospitalization and dysfunction was having a schizophrenic parent [41].

Attentional difficulties have been of interest to high-risk researchers and consistently emerge as a possible neurobehavioural marker in such studies. In the New York High-risk Project, more than a quarter of high-risk children showed problems with attention by age 7 and these difficulties persisted into adolescence and adulthood [42]. Attention deficits measured at the onset of adolescence yielded approximately 78% correct classification of future schizophrenia spectrum disorders, with a sensitivity of 67% and a specificity of 79% [43]. This is considerably better than the prediction afforded by looking at genetic vulnerability alone. While attentional deficits appear to be a promising indicator, Cornblatt *et al.* [43] urge caution and note that the specificity of this predictor has not yet been demonstrated in studies comparing adolescents with attention deficit disorder versus those with a schizophrenic parent.

The sensitivity and specificity of other neurobehavioural markers has also been investigated in the New York High-risk Project. Sensitivity for predicting schizophrenia spectrum disorders was 83% for verbal memory deficits and 75% for gross motor skills [44]. According to the authors, attention deviance appears to be a less sensitive predictor than the aforementioned ones, although it is associated with fewer false positives. A combination approach using an assessment of verbal memory, gross motor skills, and attention deviance offered the best predictive possibility [44]. This combination yielded a 10% false positive rate, 46% positive predictive validity and 83% overall accuracy [44]. One specific type of attention, the ability to shift attention from one aspect of a stimulus to another, has also been assessed in high-risk individuals. The Wisconsin Card Sorting Test (WCST) [45], a measure of mental flexibility or shifting attention, did not distinguish young adult offspring of schizophrenic parents from controls in the Israeli High-risk study [38]. However, in the New York High-risk Project, young adults with a schizophrenic parent had a profile similar to that seen in schizophrenic patients, albeit in milder form [46]. Future investigations designed to assess performance on varied attentional tasks might allow for further refinement of this predictor and might also help to distinguish children and adolescents with attention deficit from those who are at high risk for developing schizophrenia.

Jerusalem Infant Development Study

In 1973 another longitudinal study was launched by Marcus and colleagues, the Jerusalem Infant Development Study [47]. This investigation offered further evidence in support of Barbara Fish's neurointegrative deficit theory [24]. Between 1973 and 1976, pregnant women in Jerusalem who either had schizophrenia or were married to a man with the disorder were recruited for the study [47]. Control subjects included pregnant women with a history of affective disorders, personality disorders, neuroses or no psychiatric history. The researchers found that a subgroup of high-risk children had poor motor and sensorimotor performance during their first year, and although prenatal, perinatal and postnatal complications could not fully account for these differences, such insults had a more significant effect on these children [47]. High-risk children also exhibited perceptual and attentional difficulties in childhood [48]. Although motoric signs were evident, perceptual–cognitive functioning was more closely associated with parental diagnosis of schizophrenia [48]. Follow-up in adolescence suggested that a significant number of these children continued to show poor neurobehavioural functioning and poor psychiatric adjustment [49]. As adolescents, they also showed evidence of poor peer relationships, immaturity and unpopularity [50]. Such difficulties were especially evident in opposite-sex interactions [50]. The findings from the Jerusalem High-risk Study provide support for a neurodevelopmental model of schizophrenia spectrum disorders and suggest that neurobehavioural signs are measurable across development.

Twin Studies

Twin studies offer further evidence that genes and environment are implicated in the development of schizophrenia. The chances of becoming schizophrenic are roughly 50% if one's identical twin has the disorder [14] and 12% if one's non-identical twin has it [51]. Lack of complete concordance is typically attributed to environmental factors such as obstetric complications, family factors and other psychosocial stressors. Guidry and Kent [52] define environment more broadly to include that of the developing nervous system. They suggest that lack of complete concordance may be related to the inheritance pattern: "Schizophrenia may be explained parsimoniously by a germline mutation in a gene related to neurodevelopment, followed by a somatic mutation during brain development" [52]. This theory is thought to account for the variability in symptom expression, from mild symptoms to spectrum disorders to full-blown schizophrenia, in the relatives of schizophrenic patients. Other data suggest that being in a family where there are dizygotic twins is associated with an increased rate of schizophrenia in their relatives [53]. Klaning *et al.* [53] suggest that the same genes involved in dizygotic twinning may be involved in the transmission of schizophrenia. In their investigation of Danish subjects, they found a 35% increase in the rate of schizophrenia in the siblings of dizygotic twins whereas rates in relatives of monozygotic schizophrenic persons were comparable to that seen in siblings of singletons with the disorder [53].

While twin studies have provided a unique opportunity to assess genetic diathesis in the development of schizophrenia, an extraordinary group of monozygotic female quadruplets, all concordant for schizophrenia, have been the subject of a 39-year investigation [7]. The likelihood of four monozygotic twins all developing schizophrenia has been estimated by Rosenthal to be about one in 1.5 billion [54]. Despite identical genetic endowment, the onset and severity of their symptoms was highly varied. The Genain quadruplets, Nora, Iris, Hester and Myra, grew up in a mid-Western town in the USA where they were local celebrities as children, singing and dancing under the watchful eye of their mother [6]. Their father, who exhibited odd behaviour, intrusiveness, illogical thinking and suspiciousness, is the suspected genetic contributor to the girls' schizophrenic illness [6]. In 1963, Rosenthal published an extensive review of the family's history and functioning [54]. Since then various follow-up studies have been published, most recently in 2000. This report included data gathered when the quadruplets were 66 years old [7]. Because of significant dementia, Iris could not be tested during the most recent follow-up, but Nora, Myra and Hester were able to participate. Using neuropsychological data gathered at age 27 and 51 for comparison, it appeared that cognitive performance was generally stable, and in some cases improved, at age 66. Of all the sisters, Myra's illness was perceived to be the least severe. She had the most education, was the only sister to marry, had two children, and showed signs of illness at a later age [7]. Mirsky *et al.* [7] reported that, at age 66, Myra showed the best performance on 6 of 13 neuropsychological measures, including the WCST. Hester, who was assumed to have the most severe form of schizophrenia and showed prodromal symptoms as early as age 11, had the lowest scores on 5 of the 13 measures, including the WCST [7]. Compared to their mean performance at age 27, the women all showed some improvement in their scores on the Continuous Performance Test (CPT), a measure of sustained attention, suggesting that the symptoms of schizophrenia are not necessarily chronic and unremitting [7]. As of this writing, Iris and Hester have died, both in their early 70s, and Nora and Myra continue to live in the community where they were born.

Summary

Data gathered from linkage and association studies, high-risk investigations and twin studies are consistent with Kraepelin (see 11) and Koller's (see 10) speculations nearly 100 years ago that schizophrenia is a heritable disorder. Linkage and association studies have been useful in suggesting possible genetic contributors. For example, linkage studies suggest that mutations on chromosomes 6p, 8p and 11q may be involved [16–18]. High-risk studies have contributed significantly to the notion that schizophrenia is a neurodevelopmental disorder, as evidenced by the presence of social and biobehavioural anomalies spanning from infancy through adulthood [49]. Consistent with cross-sectional investigations, these studies also strongly suggest that attentional impairments are a potentially important predictor of later development of schizophrenia and spectrum disorders [42]. Based on data from the New York High-risk Project, verbal memory, gross motor skills and attention deviance predict schizophrenia with a sensitivity of 46%, specificity of 10% and 83% overall accuracy [44]. Finally, twin studies offer further evidence that genes and environment influence the disease process, although concordance is not found even in monozygotic twins [14]. Guidry and Kent [52] speculate that this lack of concordance may be related to variability in the environment of the developing neuronal system.

HIGH-RISK INDICATORS

In addition to aiding efforts to understand the genetic diathesis of schizophrenia, investigations of children with a schizophrenic parent have helped to elucidate other potential predictors, some of which were mentioned previously. While useful, such efforts have been challenging primarily because so much about schizophrenia is still unknown. Early theories proposed between 1940 and 1970 emphasized family patterns in the aetiology of schizophrenia. The so-called "schizophrenogenic life experience" and the "schizophrenogenic mother," initially proposed by Fromm-Reichmann [55], later evolved into the "schizophrenogenic family" [56,57]. These theories primarily focused on poor, inadequate and harsh parenting and confusing communication patterns as precursors. Although the concept of the schizophrenogenic parent is now largely rejected, stressful rearing environments do appear to influence aetiology. The latter may be particularly relevant to children being raised by a schizophrenic parent.

While several possible predictors have been proposed to identify individuals at risk, none of these variables seems specific enough to be highly accurate. Despite this, identifying potential indicators, even if their predictive accuracy is modest, has provided further evidence for the neurodevelopmental hypothesis and has shed light on several environmental and biobehavioural markers that, in conjunction with certain anomalous genes, may be involved in the aetiology of schizophrenia. Proposed predictors include children's social skills, personality variables, family variables, and obstetric complications. Biobehavioural markers, such as motor dysfunction, brain imaging anomalies and attention deviance have also been studied. Each of these variables will be briefly reviewed in the context of high-risk children. More extensive reviews have been published elsewhere [58–63].

Social Skills

Adult schizophrenics show evidence of social withdrawal, emotional detachment and impaired social cognition [64]. These behaviours have also been observed in preschizophrenic children. Litter and Walker [65] examined home videos of children who were later diagnosed with schizophrenia and their nonschizophrenic siblings. Between ages 5 to 7, preschizophrenic children showed more signs of negative affect, suggestive of poor emotional control [65]. Poor social skills have also been reported as a predictor of schizophrenia in studies of high-risk children [66]. In the New York High-Risk Project, social competence, affective flattening and smiling did not significantly differentiate high-risk subjects from controls in childhood but did so in adolescence [67]. In another high-risk investigation, adolescent offspring of schizophrenic parents could be distinguished from control subjects on the basis of poor peer relationships, especially with the opposite sex, immaturity and social rejection [50]. Teacher ratings of high-risk children have also been explored as predictors of later schizophrenia. In the Copenhagen High-Risk Project, preschizophrenic males were disruptive in class, inappropriate, anxious, lonely, rejected by peers, and more likely to have repeated a grade, while preschizophrenic females were nervous and withdrawn [68]. Social skills deficits, particularly in adolescence, appear to be a potentially useful predictor of later schizophrenia and can distinguish preschizophrenic individuals from healthy children. However, many other disorders are associated with poor social skills, making the specificity of this variable marginal.

Personality Variables

Personality traits have also been explored in high-risk samples. Given the odd, eccentric behaviour of persons with schizophrenia, Squires-Wheeler *et al.* [69] hypothesized that certain personality disorders, specifically schizoid, schizotypal and paranoid personality disorders, might be more prevalent in the adult offspring of schizophrenic parents. However, no such aggregation was found [69]. In a later follow-up with the same subjects, all from the New York High-risk Project, an experimental scale derived from the MMPI [70] was shown to be an effective predictor of schizophrenia-related psychoses [71]. This revised Schizophrenia Proneness scale predicted schizophrenia with over 95% accuracy. Positive predictive power was 40%, negative predictive power was over 97%, sensitivity was 37.5% and specificity was almost 98% [71]. Scores on this scale seem to offer significant promise as a relatively cost effective and efficient predictor, although the researchers caution that further refinement is needed [71].

Family Variables

Assuming other individuals or organizations are not raising them, high-risk children have the unique experience of being reared by a schizophrenic parent (or parents). As a result, family factors have been a source of interest, especially in high-risk studies. In a small retrospective study of adult children ($n = 9$) with a psychotic mother, themes of abuse and neglect, isolation, guilt and loyalty conflicts, dissatisfaction with mental health services, and efforts to seek social supports emerged [72]. Dunn also noted that many of these children were quite resilient: "As children, study participants described consciously overcoming feelings of shyness, feelings of being different from others, and fear of reprisal from their mother in order to put themselves in safe and affirming situations with peers or adults" [72]. In the New York High-risk Project, Erlenmeyer-Kimling and Cornblatt [40] noted several variables related to resilience, including a good parent–child relationship, good peer support in adolescence and physical attractiveness. In the Israeli High-risk Study, children reared by a schizophrenic parent had a better outcome than did children who were being raised by professional child-care workers on a kibbutz [35]. These findings offer some insight into factors that may protect high-risk children from developing schizophrenia and serve as a reminder that the majority of high-risk children do not have schizophrenia in adulthood.

Although the aforementioned findings offer some hope in terms of outcome, the family environment of high-risk children may be a useful predictor of later problems. In a British cohort study, schizophrenic mothers were three times more likely to identify their pregnancy as unwanted, a factor which is associated with later social and educational disadvantages [58]. In a longitudinal study, schizophrenic mothers seemed to provide less play stimulation, fewer learning experiences, and less emotional or verbal involvement as compared to depressed or healthy mothers [73]. In their review, Olin and Mednick concluded that poor family environment is a risk factor, especially for boys, and a good foster placement can serve as a protective factor for vulnerable children [62]. Other studies suggest that communication deviance (difficulty maintaining a shared focus) in the family and critical, intrusive parental attitudes are also risk factors for schizophrenia [74,75]. The latter findings are consistent with the work of Brown *et al.* [76] on expressed emotion in families with a schizophrenic member. The way family members relate to one another can either help or hinder children who are at risk for schizophrenia, depending on the quality and valence of the relationship.

Obstetric Complications

The significance of obstetric complications in the development of schizophrenia has led to some disagreement among researchers. In their 1978 review, McNeil and Kaij concluded that obstetric complications are not increased in the births of high-risk offspring [77]. A later meta-analysis arrived at a different conclusion: Sacker *et al.* found small but significant effect sizes indicating that "the risk of obstetric complications is increased in the births to parents with schizophrenia" [78]. Specifically, birth weights were lower, there were more birth complications and the baby's condition was poorer [78,79]. Schizophrenic women are thought to be at greater risk for complications because of the association between schizophrenia in young women and smoking, substance abuse and low socioeconomic status [78,79]. In addition to noting a higher incidence of obstetric complications in the births of schizophrenic mothers, complications have been explored as having a causal role in later development of schizophrenia in their offspring. Of all the obstetric variables studied, hypoxia shows the strongest association with later schizophrenia [80]. Compared to controls at low risk for schizophrenia, foetal hypoxia is associated with an increase in structural brain abnormalities in schizophrenic patients and their siblings [81]. Although hypoxia is associated with lower IQ, particularly in children with a schizophrenic parent, high-risk offspring and controls with suspected hypoxic insult did not significantly differ in overall IQ at the age of 7 [82].

Motor Dysfunctions

Neuromotor deficits have frequently been found in children who later develop schizophrenia, and are usually offered as further evidence of the neurodevelopmental theory [83,84]. Among high-risk children, neuromotor dysfunction was shown to be related to anxious/depressed behaviour and thought problems, although these dysfunctions did not distinguish high-risk children from children whose parents had another psychiatric illness or from children who were maltreated [85]. In the New York Infant Development Project, high-risk children who showed more delays in motor development during their first 2 years were more likely to be diagnosed with schizophrenia or spectrum disorders in adulthood [23]. Data from the NIMH Israeli High-risk Study [36] similarly offer evidence of poor motor coordination, hyperactivity, poor verbal abilities, and difficulties with perceptual tasks in adolescents who were later diagnosed with spectrum disorders. A follow-up study with the subjects from the Jerusalem Infant Development study found evidence of neuromotor deficits across development in preschizophrenic children [49]. Taken together, these results suggest that observable minor motor deficits are evident from as early as infancy and may be a useful biobehavioural marker for schizophrenia. As with other markers, the limitation is that motor abnormalities are not exclusive to schizophrenia spectrum disorders.

Brain Imaging Anomalies

Various methods have been used to assess the brain activity of schizophrenic patients, but the bulk of these studies have not included high-risk children. Nonetheless some relevant findings have emerged. Studies of the P300 event-related brain potential suggest that reduced P300 amplitude is correlated with disturbances in attention, effort, memory and information processing [63], although assessments of P300 amplitude in high-risk patients has yielded mixed results [86]. In a 1992 investigation, auditory event-related potentials (ERPs) distinguished high-risk children from controls and these differences were correlated with high-risk children's performance on a selective listening task [87]. In a review of neurobehavioural deficits in high-risk children, Erlenmeyer-Kimling [30] reported that children in the New York High-risk Project had no P300 or slow wave differentiation compared with control subjects.

Among discordant monozygotic twins, differences in corpus callosal anterior and middle segmental shape [88], differences in the size of the left anterior hippocampus and right hippocampus, and enlargement of the third and lateral ventricles have been observed [89]. High-risk children also have reduced left amygdala volume, smaller overall brain volume, and enlargement of the third ventricle [90]. Findings from high-risk studies are generally consistent with results seen in adult schizophrenics [30].

Attention Deviance and Other Cognitive Markers

Attention deficits have been shown to be highly characteristic of schizophrenic patients and their relatives. According to data gathered from the New York High-risk Project, attention deviance can be reliably detected in preschizophrenic children, and these deficits are stable and enduring over time [43]. In a 1992 review of attentional findings from the New York High-risk Project [42], the authors indicate that by at least the age of 7 more than a quarter of the high-risk sample had attention deficits. Similar attention deficits were also observed in low-risk children, but these problems persisted beyond childhood only in high-risk subjects [42]. Similar findings emerged from the NIMH Israeli High-risk Project, with adult schizophrenia spectrum cases showing greater attention difficulties at age 11 as compared to control groups [37]. Using samples of patients from Ireland, Israel and Washington, DC, Mirsky [91] found that schizophrenic patients performed most poorly on measures of attention, control subjects performed best, and relatives of ill patients, whether or not they had a psychiatric diagnosis, performed at an intermediate level. The ability to focus on environmental cues and respond appropriately, as well as the ability to sustain or maintain one's attention, were the most powerful discriminators of impaired attention in schizophrenic patients [91].

In addition to attention deficits, memory and neuromotor functioning seem to be particularly promising biobehavioural markers. Using a series of neuropsychological tests, Erlenmeyer-Kimling *et al.* [44] found that sensitivity for predicting schizophrenia spectrum disorders in high-risk children was 83% for verbal memory and 75% for gross motor skills. Attention deviance had a sensitivity of 58%, a specificity of 82% and an overall accuracy of 78%. Using all three variables (attention deviance, memory and gross motor skills) yielded a sensitivity of 50%, specificity of almost 90%, a 10% false positive rate, 46% positive predictive power, 90% negative predictive power, and an overall accuracy rate of 83% [44]. These findings offer particular promise with respect to developing useful screening batteries for high-risk children.

Summary

High-risk children show evidence of social skills deficits and poor peer relationships in childhood and in adolescence [50,65–68]. These deficits differentiate high-risk subjects from controls in adolescence but not in childhood [67]. With respect to personality variables, an experimental scale derived from the MMPI [70] predicted schizophrenia with over 95% accuracy and shows promise as a potentially useful screening measure [71]. Children raised by a psychotic parent report themes of abuse and neglect, isolation, guilt and loyalty conflicts, and dissatisfaction with mental health services [72]. Schizophrenic mothers provide less play stimulation, fewer learning experiences, and less emotional or verbal involvement as compared to depressed or healthy mothers [73]. These families are also characterized by a deviant communication style and critical, intrusive parental attitudes [74,75]. Hypoxia has also been implicated in the development of schizophrenia [80] and is associated with an increase in structural brain abnormalities in patients and their siblings [81].

High-risk children with delays in motor development during their first 2 years of life are more likely to be diagnosed with schizophrenia or spectrum disorders in adulthood [23] and they show evidence of poor motor co-ordination [36] across development [49]. Auditory ERPs have been shown to differentiate high-risk children from controls [87], although Erlenmeyer-Kimling reported that high-risk children in the New York High-risk Project did not differ from controls in measures of P300 or slow wave [30]. Finally, in terms of cognitive functioning, attention deviance has been consistently observed in preschizophrenic children and appears to be a stable and enduring phenomenon [43]. A battery of neuropsychological measures that assess attention deviance, memory and gross motor skills has been shown to predict schizophrenia with an overall accuracy rate of 83% [44] and seems to offer promise as a screening device.

INTERVENTIONS FOR HIGH-RISK CHILDREN

A major goal of studying children of persons with schizophrenia has been to develop screening and intervention tools. Such efforts are in their infancy, with the first early intervention study being initiated by Falloon [92] slightly over a decade ago. Genetic testing for children who may be at risk would be one means of early detection, although this information alone would not be sufficient and the specific genes involved have not yet been identified [93]. Furthermore, using genetic information for early detection is replete with ethical ramifications that are still being considered in the public arena. Another option would be to identify a set of prodromal symptoms and use those as a means of detecting at-risk individuals. Møller and Husby [94] identified two prodromal symptoms, "disturbance in self-perception", which is characterized by a sense of detachment or unreality, and "extreme preoccupation by and withdrawal to overvalued ideas". These symptoms may be useful in detecting at-risk persons. These experiential features were manifested in a number of behavioural dimensions, including quitting school or work, or major absenteeism; significant, observable shift in interests; social passivity and isolation; and marked and lasting changes in global appearance or behaviour [94]. Finally, identifying biobehavioural markers or indicators has yielded a rich body of literature but, with the exception of some neuropsychological findings, none of the identified markers offers the degree of sensitivity, specificity and predictive power needed for a useful screen.

A few intervention efforts have recently been launched, often based on the notion that shorter duration between first psychotic episode and subsequent treatment is associated with a better prognosis [95,96]. Improved access to care and increased education efforts have been shown to reduce treatment delay [95]. Other intervention options include pharmacological treatment with antipsychotics initiated during the prodromal phase or perhaps earlier. The risks of such intervention are significant: children may be more prone to side effects, including dyskinesias, and need careful monitoring [97]. The benefits of administering these medications, based on the possibility that they may develop schizophrenia, would need to be carefully weighed against the potential risks. Cornblatt's data from the Hillside Recognition and Prevention Project indicates that antidepressants in combination with a mood stabilizer and/or anxiolytic were as effective as antipsychotics in yielding clinical improvements among high-risk individuals [98]. One benefit of such an approach is that these medications have fewer negative side effects as compared to antipsychotics. Other intervention strategies include individual, group or family psychotherapy. For example, behavioural family therapy that includes education, communication skills training and problem solving has been shown to be helpful. Also effective is a group format that includes patients' relatives and addresses issues of problem solving, communication and expectations [99]. Finally, a controversial strategy proposes that family planning interventions be employed to prevent pregnancy in chronically ill female patients [100].

Although several early detection and intervention efforts have yielded promising results, as noted previously, they have also generated some controversy. Verdoux and Cougnard [101] note that there is no solid evidence that the duration of untreated psychosis is *causally* related to poor outcome. They also indicate that the threshold for *who* is actually in need of early intervention is unclear, as is the target population [101]. Data from high-risk studies might be useful in addressing some of these concerns. The Hillside Recognition and Prevention Program, which was launched in 1998, suggests that schizophrenia is preceded by a cluster of neurocognitive deficits, with actual psychosis emerging much later initially in the form of positive symptoms [98]. Based on findings from high-risk studies and the neurodevelopmental model, Cornblatt and the Hillside researchers [98] have identified a clinical entity that includes cognitive, academic and social impairments as well as disorganization and odd behaviour (CASID). If conclusions from genetic high-risk studies are correct – that early neurocognitive deficits play a causal role in schizophrenia – then Cornblatt [98] suggests that intervention efforts should be directed toward treating these deficits rather than waiting for prodromal symptoms to emerge. Mirsky and Duncan [102], Walker and Hochman [103] and others have made the same point in a recent volume on early intervention and prevention in schizophrenia [104].

CONCLUSIONS

We have reviewed the empirical literature on children of persons with schizophrenia, and have identified characteristics of such children that may qualify them as candidates for behavioural, environmental or pharmacological intervention. We have not yet found a biological marker that is unique to schizophrenia, and we must still begin our triage by asking whether there is a first-degree relative of the child with the disorder. From that point of view, we may not be much better off than Koller in 1895 or Kraepelin in 1907 [10,11]. Nevertheless, we now have well-controlled studies implicating genetic factors in the transmission of schizophrenia [14,15]; moreover, there are a number of candidate genes which we believe confer susceptibility to the disorder, including locations on chromosomes 6p, 8p and 11q [16–18]. A location in chromosome 6p (21.3) is of special interest to us, because a number of disorders in which impaired attention is a prominent symptom (schizophrenia, narcolepsy, attention-deficit/hyperactivity disorder, juvenile myoclonic epilepsy) have an abnormal gene in this HLA (human lymphocyte antigen) region of the chromosome [105].

Although most of us no longer believe in the concept of the schizophrenogenic mother or family, we can appreciate the impact of harsh treatment within the family [8] or from the community [39] on the severity of the disorder in a child at risk. So perhaps Fromm-Reichmann was not entirely wrong [55]. In addition, we now have superior behavioural methods (i.e. sophisticated assessments of attention, memory and motor skills) of identifying the one-in-ten at-risk child who is actually likely to develop a disorder. We know that we must proceed with some caution with respect to attention deficits, as there are other disorders in which compromised attention is seen [105].

Clearly, our progress in identifying a marker for schizophrenia is ultimately dependent upon our understanding the aetiology of the disorder, or disorders, that comprise the schizophrenia spectrum. As a potential contribution to the search for that holy grail (or grails) [104], we offer the modest suggestion that the final truth must implicate pathophysiological mechanisms in the brainstem, a main support of sustained attention [103].

REFERENCES

1. Sartorius N., Jablensky A., Korten A., Ernberg G., Anker M., Cooper J.E., Day R. (1986). Early manifestations and first-contact incidence of schizophrenia in different cultures: a preliminary report on the initial evaluation phase of the WHO Collaborative Study on determinants of outcome of severe mental disorders. *Psychol. Med.*, **13**, 59–76.
2. Polimeni J., Reiss J.P. (2003). Evolutionary perspectives on schizophrenia. *Can. J. Psychiatry*, **48**, 34–39.
3. Parnas J. (1988). Assortative mating in schizophrenia: results from the Copenhagen High-Risk Study. *Psychiatry*, **51**, 58–64.
4. Meehl P.E. (1962). Schizotaxia, schizotypy, schizophrenia. *Am. Psychol.*, **17**, 827–838.
5. DeLisi L.E., Mirsky A.F., Buchsbaum M.S., Van Kammen D.P., Berman K.F., Caton C., Kafka M.S., Ninan P.T., Phelps B.H., Karoum F., *et al.* (1984). The Genain quadruplets 25 years later – a diagnostic and biochemical follow-up. *Psychiatry Res.*, **13**, 59–76.
6. Mirsky A.F., Quinn O.W. (1988). The Genain quadruplets. *Schizophr. Bull.*, **14**, 595–612.
7. Mirsky A.F., Bieliauskas L.A., French L.M., Kammen D.P., Jonsson E., Sedvall G. (2000). A 39-year followup of the Genain quadruplets. *Schizophr. Bull.*, **26**, 699–708.
8. Mirsky A.F., Duncan-Johnson C.C. (1984). Nature versus nurture in schizophrenia – the struggle continues. *Integr. Psychiatry*, **2**, 137–141.
9. Parnas J. (1999). From predisposition to psychosis: progression of symptoms in schizophrenia. *Acta Psychiatr. Scand.*, **99** (Suppl. 395), 20–29.
10. Jablensky A. (1997). The 100-year epidemiology of schizophrenia. *Schizophr. Bull.*, **28**, 111–125.
11. DeLisi L.E. (1997). The genetics of schizophrenia: past, present, and future concepts. *Schizophr. Res.*, **28**, 163–175.
12. Heston L.L. (1966). Psychiatric disorders in foster home reared children of schizophrenic mothers. *Br. J. Psychiatry*, **112**, 819–825.
13. Rosenthal D. (1971). A program of research on heredity in schizophrenia. *Behav. Sci.*, **116**, 191–201.

14. Gottesman I.I., Shields J. (1982). *Schizophrenia: The Epigenetic Puzzle*. Cambridge University Press, Cambridge.
15. Gottesman I.I. (1991). *Schizophrenia Genesis*. Freeman, New York.
16. Pulver A.E., Lasseter V.K., Kasch L., Wolyniec P., Nestadt G., Blouin J.L., Kimberland M., Babb R., Vourlis S., Chen H., *et al.* (1995) Schizophrenia: a genome scan targets chromosomes 3p and 8p as potential sites of susceptibility genes. *Am. J. Med. Genet.*, **60**, 252–260.
17. Straub R.E., MacLean C.J., O'Neill F.A., Burke J., Murphy B., Duke F., Shinkwin R., Webb B.T., Zhang J., Walsh D., *et al.* (1995). A potential vulnerability locus for schizophrenia on chromosome 6p24-22: evidence for genetic heterogeneity. *Nature Genet.*, **11**, 287–293.
18. Wang S., Black D., Andreasen N., Crowe R.R. (1993). A linkage study of chromosome 11q in schizophrenia. *Arch. Gen. Psychiatry*, **50**, 212–216.
19. Sullivan P.F., Eaves L.J., Kendler K.S., Neale M.C. (2001). Genetic case–control association studies in neuropsychiatry. *Arch. Gen. Psychiatry*, **58**, 1015–1024.
20. Joober R., Boksa P., Benkelfat C., Rouleau G. (2002). Genetics of schizophrenia: from animal models to clinical studies. *Rev. Psychiatry Neurosci.*, **27**, 336–347.
21. Perry W., Geyer M.A., Braff D.L. (1999). Sensorimotor gating and thought disturbance measured in close temporal proximity in schizophrenic patients. *Arch. Gen. Psychiatry*, **56**, 277–281.
22. Fish B. (1957). The detection of schizophrenia in infancy. *J. Nerv. Ment. Dis.*, **125**, 1–24.
23. Fish B., Marcus, J., Hans S.L., Auerbach J.G., Perdue S. (1992). Infants at risk for schizophrenia: sequelae of a genetic neurointegrative defect. *Arch. Gen. Psychiatry*, **49**, 221–235.
24. Fish B. (1977). Neurobiologic antecedents of schizophrenia in children: evidence for an inherited, congenital neurointegrative defect. *Arch. Gen. Psychiatry*, **34**, 1297–1313.
25. Mednick S.A., Schulsinger F. (1965). Children of schizophrenic mothers. *Bulletin de L'Association Internationale de Psychologie Appliquée*, **14**, 11–27.
26. Mirsky A.F., Silberman E.K. (eds) (1985). The Israeli high-risk study. *Schizophr. Bull.*, **11**, 19–154.
27. Erlenmeyer-Kimling L., Cornblatt B. (1987). The New York high risk project – a follow-up report. *Schizophr. Bull.*, **13**, 451–461.
28. Marcus J., Hans S.L., Auerbach J.G., Auerbach A.G. (1993). Children at risk for schizophrenia – the Jerusalem infant development study, neurobehavioral deficits at school-age. *Arch. Gen. Psychiatry*, **50**, 797–809.
29. Cornblatt B., Obuchowski M. (1997). Update of high-risk research: 1987–1997. *Int. Rev. Psychiatry*, **9**, 437–447.
30. Erlenmeyer-Kimling L. (2000). The New York High-Risk Project: comorbidity for Axis I disorders is preceded by childhood behavioral disturbance. *J. Nerv. Ment. Dis.*, **188**, 751–756.
31. Cornblatt B., Erlenmeyer-Kimling L. (1984). Early attentional predictors of adolescent behavioral disturbances in children at risk for schizophrenia. In: Watt N.F., Anthony E.J., Wynne L.C., Rolf J.E. (eds) *Children at Risk for Schizophrenia: a Longitudinal Perspective*. Cambridge University Press, New York, pp. 198–211.
32. Mednick S.A., Parnas J., Schulsinger F. (1987). The Copenhagen High-Risk Project, 1962–86. *Schizophr. Bull.*, **13**, 485–495.

33. Carter J.W., Parnas J., Cannon T.D., Schulsinger F., Mednick S.A. (1999). MMPI variables predictive of schizophrenia in the Copenhagen High-Risk Project: a 25-year follow-up. *Acta Psychiatr. Scand.*, **99**, 432–440.
34. Jorgensen A., Teasdale T.W., Parnas J., Schulsinger F., Schulsinger H., Mednick S.A. (1987). The Copenhagen High-Risk Project: the diagnosis of maternal schizophrenia and its relation to offspring diagnosis. *Br. J. Psychiatry*, **151**, 753–757.
35. Nagler S., Mirsky A.F. (1985). Introduction: The Israeli High-Risk Study. *Schizophr. Bull.*, **11**, 19–29.
36. Marcus J., Hans S.L., Nagler S., Auerbach J.G., Mirsky A.F., Aubrey A. (1987). Review of the NIMH Israeli Kibbutz-City study and the Jerusalem Infant Development Study. *Schizophr. Bull.*, **13**, 425–438.
37. Mirsky A.F. (1988). Research on schizophrenia in the NIMH Laboratory of Psychology and Psychopathology, 1954–1987. *Schizophr. Bull.*, **14**, 151–156.
38. Mirsky A.F., Ingraham L.J., Kugelmass S. (1995). Neuropsychological assessment of attention and its pathology in the Israeli cohort. *Schizophr. Bull.*, **21**, 193–204.
39. Mirsky A.F., Duncan C.C. (1986). Etiology and expression of schizophrenia: neurobiological and psychosocial factors. *Annu. Rev. Psychol.*, **37**, 291–319.
40. Erlenmeyer-Kimling L., Cornblatt B. (1987). The New York High-Risk Project: a follow up report. *Schizophr. Bull.*, **13**, 451–461.
41. Erlenmeyer-Kimling L., Rock D., Squires-Wheeler E., Roberts S., Yang J. (1991). Early life precursors of psychiatric outcomes in adulthood in subjects at risk for schizophrenia or affective disorders. *Psychiatry Res.*, **39**, 239–256.
42. Erlenmeyer-Kimling L., Cornblatt B.A. (1992). A summary of attentional findings in the New York High-Risk Project. *J. Psychiatr. Res.*, **26**, 405–426.
43. Cornblatt B., Obuchowski M., Roberts S., Pollack S., Erlenmeyer-Kimling L. (1999). Cognitive and behavioral precursors of schizophrenia. *Develop. Psychopathol.*, **11**, 487–508.
44. Erlenmeyer-Kimling L., Rock D., Roberts S.A., Janal M., Kestenbaum C., Cornblatt B., Adamo U.H., Gottesman I.I. (2000). Attention, memory, and motor skills as childhood predictors of schizophrenia-related psychoses: the New York High-Risk Project. *Am. J. Psychiatry*, **157**, 1416–1422.
45. Grant D., Berg E. (1948). A behavioral analysis of degree of reinforcement and ease of shifting to new responses in a Weigl-type card sorting problem. *J. Exp. Psychol.*, **38**, 404–411.
46. Wolf L.E., Cornblatt B.A., Roberts S.A., Shapiro B.M., Erlenmeyer-Kimling L. (2002). Wisconsin Card Sorting deficits in the offspring of schizophrenics in the New York High-Risk Project. *Schizophr. Res.*, **57**, 173–182.
47. Marcus J., Auerbach J., Wilkinson L., Burack C.M. (1981). Infants at risk for schizophrenia. *Arch. Gen. Psychiatry*, **38**, 703–713.
48. Marcus J., Hans S.L., Auerbach J.G., Auerbach A.G. (1993). Children at risk for schizophrenia: the Jerusalem Infant Development Study. *Arch. Gen. Psychiatry*, **50**, 797–809.
49. Hans S.L., Marcus J., Nuechterlein K.H., Asarnow R.F., Styr B., Auerbach J.G. (1999). Neurobehavioral deficits at adolescence in children at risk for schizophrenia. *Arch. Gen. Psychiatry*, **56**, 741–748.
50. Hans S.L., Auerbach J.G., Asarnow J.R., Styr B., Marcus J. (2000). Social adjustment of adolescents at risk for schizophrenia: the Jerusalem Infant Development Study. *J. Am. Acad. Child Adolesc. Psychiatry*, **39**, 1406–1414.

51. Kaplan H.I., Saddock B.J. (1995). *Synopsis of Psychiatry*, 7th edn. Williams & Wilkins, Baltimore, MD.
52. Guidry J., Kent T.A. (1999). New genetic hypothesis of schizophrenia. *Med. Hypotheses*, **52**, 69–75.
53. Klaning U., Pedersen C.B., Mortensen P.B., Kyvik K.O., Skytthe A. (2002). A possible association between the genetic predisposition for dizygotic twinning and schizophrenia. *Schizophr. Res.*, **58**, 31–35.
54. Rosenthal D. (1963). *The Genain Quadruplets*. Basic Books, New York.
55. Fromm-Reichmann F. (1948). Notes on the development of treatment of schizophrenics by psychoanalytic psychotherapy. *Psychiatry*, **11**, 263–273.
56. Bateson G., Jackson D., Haley J., Weakland J. (1956). Toward a theory of schizophrenia. *Behav. Sci.*, **1**, 251–264.
57. Bateson G. (ed.) (1961). *Perceval's Narrative: A Patient's Account of his Psychosis, 1830–1832*. Stanford University Press, Stanford, CA.
58. Jones P. (1997). The early origins of schizophrenia. *Br. Med. Bull.*, **53**, 135–155.
59. Jones P., Cannon M. (1998). The new epidemiology of schizophrenia. *Psychiatr. Clin. North Am.*, **21**, 1–25.
60. Lewis D.A., Levitt P. (2002). Schizophrenia as a disorder of neurodevelopment. *Annu. Rev. Neurosci.*, **25**, 409–432.
61. Marenco S., Weinberger D.R. (2000). The neurodevelopmental hypothesis of schizophrenia: following a trail of evidence from cradle to grave. *Dev. Psychopathol.*, **12**, 501–527.
62. Olin S.S., Mednick S.A. (1996). Risk factors of psychosis: identifying vulnerable populations premorbidly. *Schizophr. Bull.*, **22**, 223–240.
63. Szymanski S., Kane J.M., Lieberman J.A. (1991). A selective review of biological markers in schizophrenia. *Schizophr. Bull.*, **17**, 99–111.
64. Platt J., Spivack G. (1972). Social competence and effective problem-solving thinking in psychiatric patients. *J. Clin. Psychol.*, **28**, 3–5.
65. Litter J., Walker E. (1993). Interpersonal behavior of preschizophrenic children: a study of home-movies. *Child Psychiatry Hum. Dev.*, **23**, 283–295.
66. John R.S., Mednick S.A., Schulsinger F. (1982). Teacher reports as a predictor of schizophrenia and borderline schizophrenia: a Bayesian decision analysis. *J. Abnorm. Psychol.*, **91**, 399–413.
67. Dworkin R.H., Cornblatt B., Friedmann R., Kaplansky L.M., Lewis J.A., Rinaldi A., Shilliday C., Erlenmeyer-Kimling L. (1993). Childhood precursors of affective vs. social deficits in adolescents at risk for schizophrenia. *Schizophr. Bull.*, **19**, 563–577.
68. Olin S.S., John R.S., Mednick S.A. (1995). Assessing the predictive value of teacher reports in a high risk sample for schizophrenia: an ROC analysis. *Schizophr. Res.*, **16**, 53–66.
69. Squires-Wheeler E., Skodol A., Adamo U.H., Bassett A.S., Cornblatt B.A., Roberts S.A., Erlenmeyer-Kimling L. (1993). Personality features and disorder in the subjects in the New York High-Risk Project. *J. Psychiatr. Res.*, **27**, 379–393.
70. Hathaway S.R., McKinley J.C. (1983). *Manual for Administration and Scoring of the MMPI*. National Computer Systems, Minnesota.
71. Bolinskey P.K., Gottesman I.I., Nichols D.S., Shapiro B.M., Roberts S.A., Adamo U.H., Erlenmeyer-Kimling L. (2001). A new MMPI-derived indicator of liability to develop schizophrenia: evidence from the New York High-Risk Project. *Assessment*, **8**, 127–143.
72. Dunn B. (1993). Growing up with a psychotic mother. *Am. J. Orthopsychiatry*, **63**, 177–189.

73. Goodman S.H. (1987). Emory University Project on Children of Disturbed Parents. *Schizophr. Bull.*, **13**, 411–423.
74. Goldstein M.J. (1987). The UCLA High-Risk Project. *Schizophr. Bull.*, **13**, 505–514.
75. Rund B.R. (1994). The relationship between psychosocial and cognitive functioning in schizophrenic patients and expressed emotion and communication deviance in their parents. *Acta Psychiatr. Scand.*, **90**, 133–140.
76. Brown G.W., Birley J.L.T., Wing J.K. (1972). Influence of family life on the course of schizophrenic disorders: a replication. *Br. J. Psychiatry*, **121**, 241–258.
77. McNeil T.F., Kaij L. (1978). Obstetric factors in the development of schizophrenia: complications in the births of preschizophrenics and in reproduction by schizophrenic parents. In: Wynne L.C., Cromwell R.L., Matthysse S. (eds) *The Nature of Schizophrenia*. John Wiley & Sons, New York, pp. 401–429.
78. Sacker A., Done D.J., Crow T.J. (1996). Obstetric complications in children born to parents with schizophrenia: a meta-analysis of case–control studies. *Psychol. Med.*, **26**, 279–287.
79. Bennedsen B.E. (1998). Adverse pregnancy outcome in schizophrenic women: occurrence and risk factors. *Schizophr. Res.*, **33**, 1–26.
80. Cannon T.D. (1997). On the nature and mechanisms of obstetric influences in schizophrenia: a review and synthesis of epidemiologic studies. *Int. Rev. Psychiatry*, **9**, 387–397.
81. Cannon T.D., van Erp T.G.M., Rosso I.M., Huttunen M., Lonnqvist J., Pirkola T., Salonen O., Valanne L., Poutanen V., Standertskjold-Nordenstam C. (2002). Fetal hypoxia and structural brain abnormalities in schizophrenic patients, their siblings, and controls. *Arch. Gen. Psychiatry*, **59**, 35–41.
82. Goldstein J.M., Seidman L.J., Buka S.L., Horton N.J., Donatelli J.L., Rieder R.O., Tsuang M.T. (2000). Impact of genetic vulnerability and hypoxia on overall intelligence by age 7 in offspring at high risk for schizophrenia compared with affective psychoses. *Schizophr. Bull.*, **26**, 323–334.
83. McNeil T.J., Harty B., Blennow G., Cantor-Graae F. (1993). Neuromotor deviation in offspring of psychotic mothers: a selective developmental deficiency in two groups of children at heightened risk? *J. Psychiatry Res.*, **27**, 39–54.
84. Neumann C.S., Walker E.F. (1996). Childhood neuromotor soft signs, behavior problems and adult psychopathology. *Adv. Clin. Child Psychol.*, **18**, 173–203.
85. Bergman A.J., Wolfson M.A., Walker E.F. (1997). Neuromotor functioning and behavior problems in children at risk for psychopathology. *J. Abnorm. Child Psychol.*, **25**, 229–237.
86. Pritchard W.S. (1986) Cognitive event-related potential correlates of schizophrenia. *Psychol. Bull.*, **100**, 43–66.
87. Schreiber H., Stolz-Born G., Heinrich H., Kornhaber H.H., Born J. (1992). Attention, cognition and motor preservation in adolescents at genetic risk for schizophrenia and control subjects. *Psychiatry Res.*, **44**, 125–140.
88. Casanova M.F., Sanders R.D., Goldberg T.E., Bigelow L.B., Christison G., Torrey E.F., Weinberger D.R. (1990). Morphometry of the corpus callosum in monozygotic twins discordant for schizophrenia: a magnetic resonance imaging study. *J. Neurol. Neurosurg. Psychiatry*, **53**, 416–421.
89. Suddath R.L., Christison G.W., Fuller Torrey E., Casanova M.F., Weinberger D.R. (1990). Anatomical abnormalities in the brain of twins discordant for schizophrenia. *N. Engl. J. Med.*, **322**, 789–794.
90. Keshavan M.S., Montrose D.M., Pierri J.N., Dick E.L., Rosenberg D., Talagala L., Sweeney J.A. (1997). Magnetic resonance imaging and spectroscopy in

offspring at risk for schizophrenia: preliminary studies. *Prog. Neuropsychopharmacol. Biol. Psychiatry*, **21**, 1285–1295.
91. Mirsky, A.F. (1996). Familial factors in the impairment of attention in schizophrenia: data from Ireland, Israel and the District of Columbia. In: Matthysse S., Benes D.F., Levy D., Kagan J. (eds) *Psychopathology – The Emerging Science of Mental Disorder*. Cambridge University Press, Cambridge, pp. 364–406.
92. Falloon I.R. (1992). Early interventions for first episodes of schizophrenia: a preliminary exploration. *Psychiatry*, **55**, 4–15.
93. Rutter M., Plomin R. (1997). Opportunities for psychiatry from genetic findings. *Br. J. Psychiatry*, **171**, 209–219.
94. Møller P., Husby R. (2002). The initial prodrome in schizophrenia: searching for naturalistic core dimensions of experience and behavior. *Schizophr. Bull.*, **26**, 217–232.
95. Johannessen J.O., McGlashan T.H., Larsen T.K., Horneland M., Joa I., Mardal S., Kvebaek R., Friis S., Melle I., Opjordsmoen S., *et al.* (2001). Early detection strategies for untreated first-episode psychosis. *Schizophr. Res.*, **51**, 39–46.
96. Christodoulou G.N. (1991). Prevention of psychopathology with early interventions. *Psychother. Psychosom.*, **55**, 201–207.
97. Remschmidt H., Schulz E., Herpertz-Dahlmann B. (1996). Schizophrenia psychoses in childhood and adolescence. *Dis. Manag.*, **6**, 100–112.
98. Cornblatt B. (2002). The New York High Risk Project to the Hillside Recognition and Prevention (RAP) program. *Am. J. Med. Genet. (Neuropsychiatr. Genet.)*, **114**, 956–966.
99. Montero I., Asencio A., Hernandez I., Masanet J., Lacruz M., Bellver F., Iborra M., Ruiz I. (2001). Two strategies for family intervention in schizophrenia: a randomized trial in a Mediterranean environment. *Schizophr. Bull.*, **27**, 661–670.
100. McCullough L.B., Coverdale J., Bayer T., Chervenak F.A. (1992). Ethically justified guidelines for family planning interventions to prevent pregnancy in female patients with chronic mental illness. *Am. J. Obstet. Gynecol.*, **167**, 19–25.
101. Verdoux H., Cougnard A. (2003). The early detection and treatment controversy in schizophrenia research. *Curr. Opin. Psychiatry*, **16**, 175–179.
102. Mirsky A.F., Duncan C.C. (2004). A neuropsychological perspective on vulnerability to schizophrenia, lessons from high-risk studies. In: Stone W.S., Faraone S.V., Tsuang M.T. (eds) *Early Clinical Intervention and Prevention in Schizophrenia*. Humana Press, Totowa, pp. 115–132.
103. Walker E., Hochman K.M., (2004). The nature and origin of socioemotional deficits in schizophrenia. In: Stone W.S., Faraone S.V., Tsuang M.T. (eds) *Early Clinical Intervention and Prevention in Schizophrenia*. Humana Press, Totowa, pp. 159–177.
104. Stone W.S., Faraone S.V., Tsuang M.T. (eds.) (2004). *Early Clinical Intervention and Prevention in Schizophrenia*. Humana Press, Totowa.
105. Mirsky A.F., Duncan C.C. (2001). A nosology of disorders of attention. In: Wasserstein J., Wolff L., LeFever F.F. (eds) Adult attention deficit disorder: brain mechanisms and life outcomes. *Ann. N. Y. Acad Sci.*, **931**, 17–32.

CHAPTER

4

Detection and Management of Bipolar Disorder in Children and Adolescents

Elizabeth Weller*, Roomana Sheikh‡, Joon Kang* and Ronald Weller§

**Children's Hospital of Philadelphia, PA, USA*
‡Drexel University College of Medicine, Philadelphia, PA, USA
§University of Pennsylvania, Philadelphia, PA, USA

INTRODUCTION

Bipolar disorder is a common and complex disorder that affects children and adolescents as well as adults. In the past, it was thought to be extremely rare in this age group [1]. Mood disturbance symptoms in adolescents were historically interpreted as normative and transient events of development. Recent epidemiological studies have provided significant evidence that both depression [2] and manic symptoms [3] are often observed in adolescents. Today, bipolar disorder is diagnosed even in preschool children. Diagnostic concepts are evolving and being refined for the younger population [4,5]. As a result, there have been an increasing number of federally funded projects on bipolar disorder in children and adolescents in North America. Also, recent epidemiological studies in Europe and Asia reflect the growing interest in paediatric bipolar disorder [6–9].

PREVALENCE OF BIPOLARITY IN CHILDREN: UNDERDIAGNOSIS, OVERDIAGNOSIS, MISDIAGNOSIS

Over the past two decades, the underdiagnosis and misdiagnosis of childhood bipolar disorder have been noted by several authors [10].

Early Detection and Management of Mental Disorders.
Edited by Mario Maj, Juan José López-Ibor, Norman Sartorius, Mitsumoto Sato and Ahmed Okasha.
 ISBN 0-470-01083-5.

Gammon *et al.* [11] interviewed 17 adolescent inpatients and their mothers using the Schedule for Affective Disorders and Schizophrenia for School-aged Children and Adolescents, Epidemiological Version (K-SADS-E), and found that 5 of the 17 adolescents (29%) satisfied DSM-III criteria for bipolar disorder or atypical bipolar disorder (bipolar II). These teenagers were not clinically diagnosed to have bipolar disorder.

Weller *et al.* [5] selected 157 case reports of children with severe psychiatric illnesses from English literature dating from 1809 to 1984. They then applied DSM-IIIR criteria to re-diagnose the selected 157 cases and found that mania had been underdiagnosed. In over 50% of the reviewed cases, the children could have easily fulfilled stringent criteria for mania. Instead, the children had been diagnosed to have other disorders such as schizophrenia or a behavioural disorder.

Data from adult studies support the idea of underdiagnosis and misdiagnosis during childhood. For example, 60% of bipolar adults report that their first symptoms occurred in childhood or adolescence, but there was a delay in diagnosis and treatment. In one report, the initial treatment for bipolar disorder was delayed an average of 10 years from the onset of symptoms [12].

It has been estimated that between one and two thirds of individuals with bipolar disorder do not receive appropriate treatment due to misdiagnosis [13]. Most adults see at least three physicians prior to being correctly diagnosed. Importantly, a misdiagnosis of unipolar depression (now referred to as major depressive disorder in DSM-IV-TR) may lead to induction of mania in depressed patients with bipolar disorder when they are treated with antidepressants [14–16].

Recently, a few investigators noted a tendency to overdiagnose paediatric bipolarity, possibly due to the lack of agreement on diagnostic criteria for bipolar disorder in children [17].

This change in diagnostic practice is reflected in practitioners' prescribing practices. A study conducted by Safer [18] examined the prescribing practices of child and adolescent psychiatrists in Baltimore, Maryland, in 1994. The author reviewed the active (1994) and closed (1988–1992) outpatient records of youths seen in four separate community mental health centres. Inpatient summaries of previously hospitalized youth were also reviewed. There was an increase in the use of medications typically used to treat mood disorders and in the use of multiple medications for both inpatients and outpatients in 1994. This change in practice mirrors that observed in adults.

Other researchers examined differences in the treatment practices for teenagers and prepubescent children in the inpatient setting. Patients under the age of 12 received more stimulants than teenagers, and lithium was prescribed to more patients over the age of 13 than to prepubescent children [19].

The changes in diagnostic trends and practices are reflected in epidemiological studies. Lifetime prevalence rates for bipolar disorder in children are dependent on the diagnostic concepts and the diagnostic instruments tailored to these concepts. For example, Carlson and Kashani [20] reported that 0.6% of 150 adolescents (14–16 years old) were diagnosed manic when severity and duration were both taken into account. However, 13.3% reported periods of at least two days in which they experienced four or more manic symptoms. While none of these adolescents exhibited sufficient impairment to meet criteria for a manic episode, three (1.5%) appeared to qualify for a diagnosis of bipolar II disorder or cyclothymia. These adolescents with manic symptoms exhibited high rates of comorbidity, and 70% were judged by the interviewers to need treatment [20]. In another study, Klein *et al.* [21] reported that 24% of patients with bipolar parents and 0% of the patients without bipolar parents had cyclothymia as assessed by the General Behavior Inventory, which had excellent correlation with interview-derived diagnosis, according to the authors.

Relatively recent prevalence rates, reported by Lewinsohn *et al.* [22], are rather similar to those reported in the Epidemiological Catchment Area study [23] and other recent epidemiological studies of adult samples [24]. These investigators studied a large, randomly selected community sample ($n = 1705$) that received diagnostic assessments during adolescence; a stratified subset was later assessed at the age of 24 ($n = 893$). In addition, direct interviews were conducted with all available first-degree relatives. Lifetime prevalence of bipolar disorder was 1%, the point prevalence of bipolar disorder was 0.64% and the 1-year incidence rate was 0.13%. Although most of these bipolar cases only met criteria for bipolar II disorder or cyclothymia, they exhibited considerable impairment, as well as high rates of attempted suicide, comorbidity and mental health care utilization, and a relatively chronic course. Less than 1% of adolescents with major depressive disorder "switched" to bipolar disorder by the age of 24. In addition, a subgroup was identified who reported distinct periods of elevated, expansive or irritable mood, but did not meet criteria for any form of bipolar disorder. These subjects also had considerable impairment. Lifetime prevalence for sub-syndromal bipolar disorder was approximately 5.7%. This was consistent with the findings of Carlson and Kashani [20], who also reported high rates of comorbidity and impairment (as indicated by the interviewers' judgement of need for treatment) in adolescents with manic symptoms, most of whom did not qualify for a bipolar disorder diagnosis.

These data highlight the clinical significance of even the milder and subthreshold forms of bipolar disorder in adolescence [22]. Adolescents with bipolar disorder had an elevated prevalence of bipolar disorder on follow-up at ages 19–23 years, while adolescents with sub-syndromal bipolar disorder groups had elevated rates of antisocial symptoms and borderline personality symptoms. Both groups showed significant impairments in psychosocial functioning and had higher mental health treatment utilization at the age of 24. The authors concluded that adolescent bipolar disorder showed significant continuity across developmental periods and was associated with adverse outcomes during young adulthood. Adolescent subsyndromal bipolar disorder was also associated with adverse outcomes in young adulthood, but was not associated with an increased prevalence of bipolar disorder. Due to high rates of comorbidity with other disorders, definitive conclusions regarding the specific clinical significance of subsyndromal bipolar disorder must await studies with larger numbers of "pure" cases.

In other recent surveys, the lifetime prevalence of bipolar I disorder among adolescents was estimated to be approximately 0.5% [2]. As of now, no national or international epidemiological study of bipolar disorder in children is available.

CLINICAL DESCRIPTIONS

This chapter will primarily focus on the manic/hypomanic phase of bipolar disorder. The clinical features of bipolar depression have yet to be addressed in the paediatric population. Despite the acceptance of a child and adolescent variant of bipolar disorder, the diagnosis continues to be controversial. Experts have not yet agreed on all diagnostic criteria and treatment methods. There are questions about the presence and duration of episodes and the hallmark symptoms of mania and hypomania.

The most common type of adult-onset bipolar disorder (classic presentation), with discrete episodes of depression and mania having a clear-cut onset and offset, appears to be less commonly seen in children. However, children and adolescents with full-blown bipolar illness have been described [11,25–30]. Children who exhibit discrete episodes of depression and mania respond well to lithium [31]. However, the natural course of paediatric bipolar disorder tends to be chronic and continuous rather than episodic and acute [32–35], and early onset bipolar disorder is associated with lithium resistance [36].

In a recent review of the past ten years of research on paediatric mania, Geller and Luby [37] concluded that childhood-onset mania is non-episodic, chronic, rapid-cycling and presents as mixed manic state. They emphasized, however, that the classic symptoms of mania remain the hallmark of the disorder and can be diagnosed even in children. Geller *et al.* [38] described developmental variants of five DSM-IV mania symptoms: euphoric mood, grandiosity, decreased need for sleep, racing thoughts and hypersexuality. They compared presentations of four of the five symptoms (manifestations of racing thoughts were similar in all age groups) in normal children, manic children and manic adults in an attempt to describe "paediatric age equivalents of adult symptoms of mania". At all ages, manic subjects appear to be the happiest of people, because of their infectious, amusing, elated affect. The authors recommend it is important to evaluate children's affect in relationship to historical features in exactly the way one evaluates the incongruity between the infectious elation of manic adult patients in the context of histories that include loss of family, unemployment and jail sentences. A common presentation for bipolar children is to harass teachers about how to teach the class; this harassment is often so intense that teachers telephone parents, begging them to ask their children to desist. These children may fail intentionally at school because they believe the courses are taught incorrectly. Another common grandiose manifestation in children as young as seven is to steal expensive items and be impervious to police officers who attempt to make them understand that what they have done is wrong and illegal. Similar to grandiose adults, grandiose children believe that stealing may be illegal for other people but not for them. Unlike patients with pure conduct disorder, manic children and adolescents, similar to bipolar adults, frequently know that stealing is a bad thing to do, but they believe that they are "above" the law. Common adolescent grandiose delusions are that they will achieve a prominent profession (e.g. lawyer) even though they are failing at school. Another example is that of a manic adolescent who, even in the absence of musical talent or ability to carry a tune, might practise all day with the belief that he or she can become a rock star. Unlike depressed patients, who have trouble falling asleep and lie in bed brooding, manic children have high activity levels in the bedroom prior to sleep, e.g. rearranging furniture for several hours. Manic adolescents will wait until parents are asleep and then go out "partying", whereas manic adults will party and work around the clock. Pressured speech is relatively similar at all ages in that the individual can be difficult or impossible to interrupt. Children and adolescents frequently describe racing thoughts in very concrete terms. For example, children state that they are not able to get anything done because their thoughts keep interrupting. Geller *et al.* [38] describe an adolescent who wished she had a button on her forehead to turn off her thoughts.

Also at all ages, minor perturbations in the environment can produce marked amounts of distractibility. Increased motor activity and goal-directed behaviours in children and adolescents frequently look like normal activities done in a profuse amount. The manic child may in a brief period of time make curtains, begin an illustrated book, rearrange furniture and make multiple phone calls. Involvement in pleasurable activities with a high level of danger is manifested in age-specific behaviours. Hypersexuality in children frequently begins when a child brought up in a conservative home without any history of sexual abuse or excessive exposure to sexual situations begins to use profanity and may tell a teacher to "f*** herself" and "give her the finger". Children may masturbate frequently, initially openly, and then, when told not to do it publicly, will simply make frequent trips to the bathroom to continue the stimulation. Children will begin to proposition teachers and make overt sexual comments to classmates. Adolescents develop romantic fantasies and delusions about teachers. Older children and adolescents will call the premium rate sex telephone lines, which the family discovers when the telephone bill arrives. Older adolescents will have multiple partners with unprotected sexual behaviours and frequently will feel an urgency to have sex. Geller *et al.* [38] give an example of an adolescent who wrote to her boyfriend, starting the letter with the sentence, "When are we going to f***?".

Interest in money appears in young children when they start their own businesses in school and when they begin to order multiple items, trips and plane tickets from advertised premium rate telephone numbers. Again, the family frequently does not discover this until items arrive at the house or telephone bills arrive. Across the age span, taking more dares is common. In older adolescents and adults, this frequently appears as wild driving, resulting in many speed and "driving under the influence" tickets. In children it manifests as grandiose delusions that they can fly out of the window.

Many investigators contend that irritability or prolonged aggressive temper outbursts rather than euphoria are the hallmarks of the disorder in children and adolescents [39]. However, episodic irritability can also be seen in depressed children and chronic irritability is common in attention-deficit/hyperactivity disorder (ADHD), oppositional defiant disorder and some variants of pervasive developmental disorder. Other investigators have suggested the episodic decreased need for sleep being a hallmark of bipolar disorder. Of all the symptoms of mania, decreased need for sleep is the one that has been shown to have pathophysiological significance [40,41]. Decreased need for sleep characteristic of mania should be distinguished from nonspecific insomnia (which is generally accompanied by feeling tired) or chronically decreased need for sleep that may be seen in ADHD. Also, stimulant-induced insomnia (generally early insomnia) needs to be ruled out.

Several investigators have implied that even relatively mild forms of bipolar disorder in adolescents are serious conditions that are associated with substantial impairment and comorbidity [42–45]. Although most of the bipolar cases only met criteria for bipolar II disorder or cyclothymia in Lewinsohn *et al.*'s study [22], they exhibited considerable impairment. During their most recent episode, a majority of these subjects reported impaired functioning in social situations, with family and at school, as well as a high degree of comorbidity. In particular, the bipolar subjects exhibited significantly elevated rates of comorbid anxiety disorders (especially separation anxiety and panic) and disruptive behaviour (especially ADHD). Moreover, the bipolar subjects were at least as impaired as the major depressive comparison group on every variable examined. Indeed, a greater proportion of bipolar subjects had attempted suicide compared to major depressive subjects. Also, bipolar subjects exhibited significantly greater impairment than the major depressive subjects on the Global Assessment of Functioning (GAF) at the second assessment and during the previous year. Finally, the bipolar subjects exhibited a relatively chronic course. The median duration of illness in this group was more than 4 years and these adolescents had already spent a median total of 28 months in an affective episode. Although more than half of these subjects had received some form of mental health treatment, only one had been treated with lithium. Many of these cases were not recognized as having a bipolar disorder by the mental health professionals with whom they had contact [22].

Akiskal [46] examined prodromal symptoms of childhood bipolar disorder and suggested that subtle presentations of mood regulation difficulties could be warning signs. He reported that many children diagnosed with bipolar disorder are described by their parents as having a difficult temperament since infancy. During childhood many of these behaviours may be ascribed to difficult temperaments, thus making it hard to conceptualize more severe difficulties as part of a potentially treatable disorder.

DIFFERENCES BETWEEN ADULT-, ADOLESCENT- AND CHILD-ONSET BIPOLAR DISORDER

The DSM-IV criteria for mania were developed from data on adults with bipolar disorder and do not consider the differences between bipolar adults and bipolar children and adolescents. Paediatric bipolar disorder has been described as atypical when compared to adult bipolar disorder. The similarities in the clinical presentation of adults with mixed states and preadolescents diagnosed with mania have been noticed. Several authors have drawn a comparison between the "virulent" form of the disorder in adults (with absence of discrete episodes) and the severe course observed in many pre-pubertal children [37,47,48].

Leibenluft *et al.* [40] suggested a phenotypic system of classifying juvenile mania consisting of a narrow phenotype, two intermediate phenotypes and a broad phenotype. Patients who meet the full DSM-IV diagnostic criteria for hypomania or mania (including the duration criterion and the presence of hallmark symptoms such as elevated mood or grandiosity) exhibit the narrow phenotype of juvenile mania. Patients with intermediate phenotype are those with clear episodes and hallmark symptoms, but a duration of episodes between 1 and 3 days, and those with demarcated episodes with irritable (but not elevated) mood. The broad phenotype is exhibited by patients who have a chronic, non-episodic illness that does not include the hallmark symptoms of mania but shares with the narrower phenotypes the symptoms of severe irritability and hyperarousal.

On 27 April, 2000, the National Institute of Mental Health (NIMH) Developmental Psychopathology and Prevention Research Branch, in collaboration with the Child and Adolescent Treatment and Prevention Intervention Research Branch, convened a small roundtable meeting to discuss research issues on the diagnosis of pre-pubertal bipolar disorder [49]. A proposal from this meeting was to categorize children with symptoms of bipolar disorder into two groups: (1) those who meet the DSM-IV criteria for bipolar I or II disorder and (2) those who do not meet the DSM-IV criteria but are severely impaired from mood and behavioural symptoms of bipolar disorder. Children who were in the latter group were categorized as suffering from bipolar disorder not otherwise specified (NOS) and further subdivided into four subcategories: (1) the signs and symptoms are present but do not last long enough to meet DSM-IV criteria; (2) the signs and symptoms are one short to fulfil the DSM-IV criteria; (3) signs and symptoms occur only in one setting, most typically at home; and (4) the symptoms are chronic, i.e. not episodic.

A few published studies have investigated the differences between child-onset and adolescent-onset bipolar disorder. Faraone *et al.* [50] recruited 68 children (12 years old or younger) and 42 adolescents (older than 13 years) who were hospitalized and met criteria for mania. Comparison groups were 527 non-manic referrals and 100 normal controls. With the exception of comorbidity with ADHD, there were more similarities than differences between the children and adolescents with mania. There was an inverse relationship between the rate of comorbidity with ADHD and age of onset of mania, i.e. higher in manic children, intermediate in adolescents with childhood-onset mania, and lower in adolescents with adolescent-onset mania. The authors concluded ADHD was more common in childhood-onset compared with adolescent-onset bipolar disorder and suggested ADHD may signal a very early onset of bipolar disorder in some cases.

In another study [51], adolescent-onset bipolar disorder was associated with a much higher risk for substance use disorder than childhood-onset bipolar disorder, which was not accounted for by conduct disorder or other comorbid psychopathology. In mid-adolescence, youth with adolescent-onset bipolar disorder were at significantly increased risk for substance use disorder relative to those with child-onset bipolar disorder (39% versus 8%, $p = 0.001$). Compared with those with child-onset bipolar disorder, those

TABLE 5.1 Differences in phenomenology related to age of onset in bipolar disorder (adapted from Carlson [52])

	Onset <10 years	Onset 10–25 years	Onset >30 years
Clear mood episodes	Absent	Present	Present
Comorbidity	>90%	50%	20%
Disruptive behaviour disorder	Very often	Sometimes	Never
Substance abuse	–	Often	Rare
Euphoric mania	Rare	Sometimes	Often
Psychomotor retarded depression	Rare	Yes	Yes
Confusion with schizophrenia	Rare	Often	Rare
Switch from major depressive disorder	Yes	Yes	Rare
Family history of mood disorder	Frequent	Frequent	Less frequent
Uncomplicated bipolar disorder	Rare	Common	Common
Rate of chronicity	High	5–10%	5%
Lithium response	Poor	Intermediate	Common

with adolescent-onset bipolar disorder had 8.8 times the risk for substance use disorder.

Table 5.1 summarizes the main differences among childhood-onset, adolescent-onset and adult-onset bipolar disorder.

DIFFERENTIAL DIAGNOSIS AND COMORBIDITY

The differential diagnosis of a manic episode may include a broad range of psychiatric conditions depending upon the age of the child. For example, sexual abuse is especially important in the differential diagnosis during the childhood years, because manic hypersexuality is often manifested in children by self-stimulatory behaviours including frequent masturbation. Thus, obtaining a careful history of whether the child could have been abused or exposed to adult sexual behaviours is important. Specific language disorders need to be differentiated from flight of ideas. Because of greater perceptual distortions in bipolar illness during adolescence, schizophrenia is a major differential diagnosis [53]. Differentiation is greatly aided by a family history of mania, which is more probable for bipolar disorder than schizophrenia [36].

Substance abuse begins to be an important comorbid condition during the teenage years and is to be considered in differential diagnosis [53,54]. For example, laughing fits may be due to smoking marijuana rather than being a manifestation of elation. Furthermore, very rapid cycling, which is according to some researchers a hallmark of child and adolescent bipolarity [38], can easily be mimicked by amphetamine highs followed by withdrawal "crashes". Hallucinogens can mimic the perceptual distortions of bipolar disorder [53,54].

Bipolar youths exhibit significantly higher rates of comorbid psychiatric conditions, including disruptive behaviour disorders (especially ADHD, conduct disorder and oppositional defiant disorder), anxiety disorders (especially separation anxiety and panic disorder) and eating disorders. The relationship between ADHD and mania is of interest. A very high comorbidity between paediatric bipolar disorder and ADHD has been reported. As many as 60–90% of the paediatric bipolar disorder cases have been diagnosed with concurrent ADHD [55,56,48]. Careful assessment is needed to clarify whether children have ADHD, bipolar disorder or both. There is an overlap of symptoms between mania and ADHD. These symptoms include increased motor activity, distractibility, rapid or pressured speech, impaired attention, racing thoughts and irritability.

Geller *et al.* [42] have suggested that ADHD is an age-dependent manifestation of bipolar disorder, as normal pre-pubertal children are more hyperactive than their post-pubertal counterparts. Thus, they assert that hyperactivity can be seen as the child analogue to the intense energy surges seen in the manic episodes of adults.

One prospective study [43] followed males who met, at the baseline assessment, criteria for mania+ADHD ($n = 15$), ADHD without mania ($n = 65$) or no psychiatric diagnosis ($n = 17$). These subjects were re-evaluated 6 years later. There were no group differences in the prevalence of Axis I or Axis II disorders, with the exception of alcohol abuse, which was higher in controls. Manic symptoms persisted in only one mania+ADHD subject, while three (5%) of the ADHD subjects had new onset of manic symptoms. There were no clear cases of bipolar disorder. Levels of service utilization or criminal behaviour did not differentiate the groups. However, global functioning was significantly lower at follow-up in the mania+ADHD group compared with controls. Although a pilot study in scope, the findings cast doubt on a link between manic symptoms associated with ADHD in childhood and follow-up bipolar disorder.

High levels of comorbidity with disruptive behaviour disorders have been observed in paediatric bipolar disorder. The overlap between paediatric bipolar disorder and conduct disorder is not surprising, considering that severe irritability with "affective storms" or aggressive temper outbursts is a common presentation [57]. This relationship was systematically examined by Biederman *et al.* [45] in 186 children and adolescents who met DSM-III-R diagnostic criteria for conduct disorder and mania on structured diagnostic interview. The investigators found that 116 subjects met criteria for conduct disorder, 110 for mania and 76 for both. The comorbid group represented 40% of subjects with an initial diagnosis of conduct disorder and 41% of subjects with an initial diagnosis of mania.

LONGITUDINAL COURSE OF THE DISORDER: OUTCOME STUDIES

The long-term outcome of children and adolescents with bipolar disorder has not been well studied. Results to date suggest that this is a recurrent illness with substantial morbidity. Adolescents with bipolar disorder are less responsive to treatment compared to bipolar adults [35,58,59].

Lewinsohn *et al.* [22] interviewed 893 adolescents and then reassessed them at the age of 24. At baseline, 18 had bipolar disorder, 14 had sub-syndromal bipolar disorder, and 275 had major depression. Out of the bipolar group, 27% had a recurrence by the age of 24. Only <1% of adolescents with major depression switched to bipolar disorder by the age of 24. Adolescents with bipolar disorder and sub-syndromal bipolar disorder had significant impairment in psychosocial functioning by the age of 24. However, none of the subjects with the sub-syndromal condition developed bipolar disorder during the 6-year follow-up period.

Strober *et al.* [60] investigated the course of bipolar disorder in a 5-year prospective study. Their sample consisted of 54 hospitalized bipolar adolescents. They reported a 96% recovery rate and a 46% relapse rate within 5 years. About 20% of the subjects attempted suicide. Carlson *et al.* [61] reported that pre-adolescent-onset manics were more likely to have fewer periods of remission compared to those with adolescent- or adult-onset mania in a 2-year period.

Geller *et al.* [62] followed the course of bipolar disorder in a prepubertal and early adolescent population and reported recovery and relapse rates at 6 months, 1 year and 2 years. Of 93 bipolar subjects, 91 completed the 6-month assessment, and at that time 85.7% still met full criteria for mania or hypomania. Thus, only 14.3% had recovered. One year later the recovery rate was 37% and the relapse rate was 38%. The 2-year follow-up for this group found that 5% were in recovery from mania and 55% of those who had previously recovered had relapsed [63,64].

Only a few studies examined factors that may improve or worsen outcome for young children and adolescents with bipolar disorder. One study assessed the recovery and relapse rates and how they were related to psychosocial factors. Low maternal warmth predicted relapse. The significance of maternal warmth as a predictor is consistent with studies in adults with bipolar disorder. The study also found that living in an intact family was associated with faster recovery. The significance of intact family as a predictor may be unique to childhood mania [64].

DIAGNOSTIC ASSESSMENT

A thorough and extensive evaluation is necessary before diagnosing bipolar disorder in a child or adolescent. Such an evaluation requires a detailed history of both mood and non-mood symptoms and an appraisal of risk factors for bipolar disorder. A comprehensive face-to-face assessment of the child, including a mental status examination, is necessary to rule out pervasive developmental disorders, language and thought disorders, and psychotic symptoms. This assessment may take several hours to complete and could be done by a multidisciplinary team in one day or over several days. A detailed lifeline or timeline including onset, offset and duration of symptoms, stressful life events and history of treatment is helpful in establishing diagnosis. The diagnostic accuracy for bipolar illness in children and adolescents improves when DSM criteria are applied [65].

Several structured and semi-structured interviews may also be used to help assess mania in children. Structured interviews include the Diagnostic Interview for Children and Adolescents, Revised (DICA–R) [66], the Diagnostic Interview Schedule for Children (DISC) [67] and the Children's Interview for Psychiatric Syndromes (ChIPS) [68]. Semi-structured interviews include the Schedule for Affective Disorders and Schizophrenia for School Age Children (KSADS) [69], the Washington University Kiddie and Young Adult Schedule for Affective Disorders and Schizophrenia, Lifetime and Present Episode Version for DSM-IV (WASH-U-KSADS) [70,71] and the Interview Schedule for Children (ISC) [72]. When using standardized assessment instruments, a comprehensive evaluation by a well-trained clinician with extensive experience in diagnosing children and adolescents with psychiatric disorders should be performed to improve diagnostic accuracy.

Clinical rating scales may be helpful in tracking the severity and course of target symptoms of mania. Such rating scales for bipolar disorder used to be underdeveloped and understudied, but at the present time several investigators are looking into the usefulness of various scales. Strober *et al.* [36] used the Beigel–Murphy Scale [73] in assessing severity of mania in adolescents and reported the instrument to be helpful. Fristad *et al.* [74] modified the Mania Rating Scale [75] for use in pre-pubertal manic children. A preliminary study found that it was helpful in differentiating manic children from hyperactive children [76]. The Child Behavior Checklist (CBCL) has been reported to distinguish children with mania from those with ADHD [70,77]. Such rating scales can be used to supplement clinical evaluation.

The diagnostic work-up should be done in a systematic manner. First and foremost, mania secondary to drug use or general medical conditions should be ruled out. Currently, there are no specific laboratory or biological tests that can diagnose bipolar disorder in children and adolescents. Hence, diagnosis is established by considering all data from history, family history and mental status examination. Once the diagnosis has been established, a baseline laboratory assessment that includes a complete blood count with differential, thyroid function tests (including T3, free T4 and TSH), electrolytes, blood urea nitrogen, creatinine, creatinine clearance, liver function tests and electrocardiogram should be performed. These tests are necessary because there are medical conditions that can present with manic symptoms and often children with bipolar disorder require treatment with psychotropic medications.

Medical conditions which may present with manic symptoms include infectious diseases (encephalitis, influenza, syphilis, AIDS), endocrine disorders (hyperthyroidism), tumours, and neurological conditions (temporal lobe epilepsy, multiple sclerosis, Wilson's disease, closed or open head injury). Manic symptoms may be induced by medications (steroids, isoniazid, sympathomimetics) and alcohol or drug abuse.

MANAGEMENT OF BIPOLAR DISORDER IN THE YOUTH

Management of bipolar disorder is complicated and needs to be individually tailored to the needs of the individual child and family. A treatment plan should take into account the fact that the child's symptoms will vary with developmental and environmental changes. Also, symptoms may vary due to the fluctuating nature of the disorder. Therefore, successful treatment plans for bipolarity in children require flexibility and openness by the treating clinician.

Conceptualizing the child's treatment and needs as moving targets is a good way to plan the treatment of this complicated illness. Generally, management of a bipolar child requires pharmacological treatment of manic symptoms and other comorbid psychiatric symptoms. Also, management of suicidal and other emergency behaviours, management of school functioning, management of family stress and caregiver burden, and mental health treatment of other family members is necessary. Hospitalization of the child may be needed during a full-blown manic episode to ensure patient and family safety. Suicidal threats and gestures need to be taken seriously. The family should develop a crisis plan with the members of the treatment team so that in an emergency the parents know how to access the appropriate services efficiently. In acute manic state, clinicians must avoid getting into any arguments or questions regarding the delusional system of the child. After recovery, clinicians should not remind the child of his or her foolish or embarrassing behaviour. It is critical that parents are aware of their child's mood symptoms, sleep habits and pattern of cycling so that they can make environmental and behavioural interventions and abort the development of a full-blown episode.

In addition, parents should be aware of the possible educational impairment associated with bipolar disorder. Bipolar children and adolescents are at risk for learning disabilities [48]. Therefore, psychoeducational testing is important in the comprehensive treatment plan once the child's mood is stable. A bipolar child can be unfocused, unmotivated and lethargic because of mood symptoms, and impulsive, inattentive, anxious or disabled because of comorbid conditions. Prescribed medication may also result in cognitive dullness, fatigue and poor handwriting. Unfortunately, some of these side effects may not completely go away despite careful medication monitoring, dosage reduction and changes in time of administration. Both clinicians and parents should be aware of the long-term implications of this illness pertaining to schooling and career planning. A bipolar child generally falls under the educational label of serious emotional disturbance (SED). According to the 1999 report by the US Department of Education, SED children are four times more likely to drop out of high school than their peers [78].

Pharmacological Treatment

Mania in children is not easily modified without medication. Unfortunately, there are very few treatment options that are evidence based. In general, current pharmaceutical treatment of children and adolescents with bipolar disorder is based on clinical trials in bipolar adults [79,80]. It is common clinical practice to have patients continue on medications for a period of time following remission. However, the optimal length of maintenance treatment remains unclear, and available guidelines are based on limited consensus rather than controlled trial outcomes. There are only limited studies of mood stabilizers and antidepressants in children and adolescents [81]. Also, given the high rates of comorbid conditions, children with paediatric mania may require combinations of medications to adequately manage symptoms [82,83].

There is a risk of inducing a manic episode with the use of antidepressants in children with undiagnosed bipolar disorder. Careful monitoring should be undertaken when prescribing antidepressants to any child with a family history of mood disorders or other risk factors for bipolar disorder, such as depression involving a rapid onset, psychomotor retardation and/or psychotic features [83–85].

Lithium

Lithium is the oldest and most studied mood stabilizer in adults. It is approved by the US Food and Drug Administration (FDA) for treatment of bipolar disorder in adolescents who are 12 years of age or older, but not in pre-pubertal children.

Varanka *et al.* [86] reported on ten hospitalized pre-pubertal manic children with bipolar I disorder. Lithium was used according to dosing guidelines provided by Weller *et al.* [87]. These children tolerated lithium well and reached therapeutic blood levels in a very short period of time. Response rate was comparable to adults. Other open trials also report response rates similar to adults [88].

To date, there is only a single published double-blind randomized controlled trial of lithium in adolescents. This was a prospective placebo-controlled investigation of lithium in adolescents with bipolar disorder and comorbid substance abuse ($n = 25$). In this study, the adolescents' diagnosis of bipolar disorder preceded their substance abuse by several years. After 6 weeks of treatment, subjects treated with lithium showed a statistically significant decrease in positive urine toxicology screens and a significant improvement in GAF (46% in the lithium-treated group versus 8% in the placebo group). This study demonstrated the efficacy of lithium for the treatment of substance use disorders in bipolar adolescents, but did not report on the effect of lithium on the bipolar disorder in these adolescents [89].

Strober *et al.* [90] conducted a naturalistic prospective follow-up study of 37 hospitalized bipolar adolescents treated successfully with lithium. Those who discontinued lithium treatment (against medical advice) were three times more likely to relapse than those who continued lithium.

The largest systematic treatment trial to date was a recent study conducted by Kafantaris *et al.* [91]. This study examined the initial response to lithium treatment and potential predictors of non-response in a sample of 100 acutely manic bipolar I adolescents: 63 met response criteria and 26 achieved remission of manic symptoms at the week 4 assessment. Prominent depressive features, age at first mood episode, severity of mania and comorbidity with ADHD did not distinguish responders from non-responders. When treated with adjunctive antipsychotic medication, subjects with psychotic features at baseline responded as well as subjects without psychosis. In this study, lithium appeared effective for acute stabilization of bipolar symptoms. However, more double-blind, placebo-controlled trials in adolescents with acute mania are needed.

In younger bipolar children, two small placebo crossover studies found lithium superior to placebo [92,93]. Other studies suggest that lithium is relatively well tolerated in children. Side effects have been systematically reported in children as young as 3 years of age [94]. Common lithium side effects in children include weight gain, nausea, diarrhoea, tremor, enuresis, fatigue, ataxia, leukocytosis and malaise. Less commonly seen side effects are renal, ocular, thyroid, neurological, dermatological and cardiovascular. Changes in growth, diabetes and hair loss have also been reported [95,96]. Younger children may experience more side effects than older children [97].

Valproate

Several single case reports and small open series suggest that valproate is an effective mood stabilizer in adolescents [98–100]. Strober [101] examined the clinical course of juvenile bipolar illness treated with valproate compared with a historical control group treated with lithium. Valproate was superior to lithium for the mixed form of mania but was not more efficacious in classic mania.

Common side effects of valproate include sedation, nausea, vomiting, appetite/weight gain and tremor [95]. Lethal cases of hepatic toxicity appear to occur almost exclusively in relatively young children, especially those younger than 2 years who are on multiple medications [102,103].

Valproate has been reported to induce a metabolic syndrome (especially in younger women), characterized by obesity, hyperinsulinemia, lipid abnormalities, polycystic ovaries and hyperandrogenism. In a cohort of Finnish women taking valproate for seizures, 80% of the women who started taking valproate before the age of 20 years had polycystic ovaries compared with 43% of all women taking valproate [104]. Replacing valproate with lamotrigine reduced the severity of this metabolic syndrome in 16 women, which seems to suggest a partial reversibility [105]. Whether this finding generalizes to a psychiatric population is not yet clear, since the study only included women with epilepsy.

Forty patients, aged 7–19 years, with a manic, hypomanic or mixed episode were enrolled in an open-label study of divalproex (2–8 weeks), followed by a double-blind, placebo-controlled period (8 weeks). A total of 22 patients showed at least 51% improvement in Mania Rating Scale (MRS) scores during the open-label period. However, 23 subjects discontinued the study during the open-label period. The reasons were noncompliance, ineffectiveness and intolerability. Thirteen subjects completed the 8-week trial. Of 13 subjects who completed the study, 8 showed marked improvement on the MRS, 4 showed moderate improvement and 1 showed some improvement. The most common adverse events were headache, nausea, vomiting, diarrhoea and somnolence. Too few subjects participated in the double-blind period for statistical analysis [106].

Carbamazepine

Carbamazepine has demonstrated efficacy in adult bipolar disorder. However, there are no controlled studies and only a few anecdotal reports on this drug in children [107]. Garfinkel *et al.* [108] reported on a series of 19 treatment-resistant bipolar adolescents (11 with acute mania and 8 with mixed state) who had an excellent response to a combination of lithium and carbamazepine. Oxcarbazepine has lately become quite popular due to the fact that it does not suppress the bone marrow and does not require blood monitoring. This drug is currently being studied in the USA.

Combination Treatments

Since many youths with bipolar disorder do not respond to valproate or lithium monotherapy, an open-label study was conducted to examine the effectiveness of a combination of valproate and lithium therapy in youths diagnosed with bipolar disorder [109]. Ninety patients (66 males, 24 females) meeting DSM-IV criteria for bipolar I or II disorder, aged 5–17 years, were treated prospectively for up to 20 weeks with valproate and lithium. Significant improvement in all outcome measures was observed by week 8, as well as at the end of study. The combination appeared to be well tolerated.

Bipolar children and adolescents often have comorbid disorders that also complicate their treatment [110]. Data has just started accumulating on combinations of mood stabilizers with stimulants, antidepressants and atypical antipsychotics.

Other Mood Stabilizers

No data on lamotrigine and gabapentin are currently available in bipolar youth. The authors have found lamotrigine to be helpful in depressed bipolar teenagers, especially those with self-cutting behaviours during their mood episodes.

In a chart review study of 26 children and adolescents with DSM-IV bipolar disorder, a significant improvement on the Clinical Global Assessment Scale (CGAS) was found after a treatment of average duration 4.4 months with an average dose of 104 mg/day of topiramate. No serious adverse events were reported [111].

Antipsychotics

Atypical antipsychotics have been recently studied in the treatment of mania in adults. There are some data to support their use in children with bipolar disorder.

Frazier *et al.* [112] used risperidone in 28 youth (mean 10.4 years old) with bipolar disorder (25 mixed and 3 hypomanic). These children received a mean dose of 1.7 mg over an average period of 6.1 months. The authors concluded that 82% of the children showed improvement in both their manic and aggressive symptoms, 69% had improvement in psychotic symptoms, but only 8% showed improvement in ADHD symptoms.

DelBello *et al.* [113] studied 30 manic or mixed bipolar I adolescents (12–18 years) who received an initial valproate dose of 20 mg/kg and were randomly assigned to 6 weeks of combination therapy with quetiapine, titrated to 450 mg/day ($n = 15$), or placebo ($n = 15$). The valproate+quetiapine group demonstrated a significantly greater reduction in Young Mania Rating Scale (YMRS) scores from baseline to endpoint than the valproate+placebo group. Sedation, rated as mild or moderate, was significantly more common in the valproate+quetiapine group. Although the valproate+quetiapine association was generally well tolerated, there was a greater drop-out rate in that group.

Kafantaris *et al.* [114] gave an adjunctive antipsychotic medication in combination with lithium. If the psychosis resolved, the antipsychotic medication dose was gradually tapered and discontinued after 4 weeks of therapeutic lithium levels. Each subject was then given a trial of maintenance lithium monotherapy for up to 4 weeks. Improvement was noticed in 64% of the sample with psychotic features after 4 weeks of combination treatment. However, few maintained their response after discontinuation of the antipsychotic medication. Successful discontinuation of antipsychotic medication was associated with current episode being the first episode, shorter duration of psychosis, and the presence of thought disorder at baseline. The authors concluded that adjunctive antipsychotic medication needs to be maintained for longer than 4 weeks in the vast majority of adolescents with psychotic mania, even though the manic and psychotic symptoms have resolved and lithium is maintained.

Electroconvulsive Therapy

Electroconvulsive therapy (ECT) is rarely used in children and adolescents. The recent literature on the use of ECT to treat mood disorders in children and adolescents only consists of case reports and case series [115]. When used appropriately, this therapy is safe and can change the life of a treatment-resistant child or adolescent. In the USA, for a child or adolescent to receive ECT, two child and adolescent psychiatrists other than the treating psychiatrist should agree that treatment is indicated.

Psychotherapy

A literature search by Fristad *et al.* [116], conducted in 2002, found that at present there are no psychosocial treatments empirically validated or otherwise for children with bipolar disorder. Preliminary data from the child group therapy programme, which was developed as part of multifamily psychoeducational groups (MFPGs), is promising [117].

Early-onset bipolar disorder produces a host of issues for all family members of the affected individual. These issues need to be addressed immediately and consistently in order to maximize the psychological well-being of all involved. Parents must become specialized caregivers to children affected by the disorder. Central to family-based interventions for bipolar disorder is the family's access to a clinician who is well versed in the manifestations of this disorder and who has the flexibility to adapt to the vicissitudes of this illness. Treatment plans must be tailored individually to the family's needs. Holder and Anderson have outlined coping strategies for families in which one or more members are experiencing a serious mental illness [118].

Recently MFPGs have gained popularity and there is reasonable evidence in support of their usefulness [119]. Over time, families participating in these groups showed an attitude shift toward more positive thinking about educational and mental health care systems [120].

Support Groups

Caregivers of children with bipolar disorder often suffer from emotional, physical and financial stress. A primary source of emotional stress is that of watching their child suffer from rejection by peers, school failure, rage attacks, suicide attempts and of coping with the total unpredictability of their child's behaviour. Families can become homebound out of dread of other public episodes of rages and obscenities in the ill child. A raging child is a risk for the physical safety of other family members; he or she may damage property or run away into the street impulsively. Therefore, the caregivers of these children often live in a state of hypervigilance. Another source of emotional stress for these caregivers is navigating uncharted territories, i.e. new systems with their own language and rules. For example, many children with bipolar disorder require special education services or get involved in the juvenile justice system. This can leave the caregiver confused, misunderstood and overwhelmed. Similarly, caregivers report negative experiences when dealing with mental health professionals [121].

As a result of stress associated with their role, caregivers may experience physical problems like sleep disturbances, headaches and exhaustion. Unfortunately financial strain is a given for these families. Insurance coverage is rarely comprehensive, and medications and intensive treatment modalities are expensive. It is estimated that 11% of children with special health care needs do not have any insurance [122]. In addition to the above-mentioned sources of stress, these families suffer isolation because of stigmatization, which may lead to almost total social exclusion from family gatherings, church and community events.

Participation in a support group can alleviate caregiver burden [123,124]. Also, members of parent support groups report more utilization of information and services than non-members [125]. In today's mental health environment, peer-led self-help or mutual help support groups complement the care provided by mental health professionals. More than 70% of Americans suffering from a diagnosable behavioural or mental health disorder will never receive specialized mental health care and instead will rely on these types of groups [126].

Internet Resources

Online support groups have been extremely useful in providing social support to parents who feel isolated [127]. Similar to in-person support groups, members of computer-mediated support groups receive information, advice, emotional support and contact with people in similar situations [128]. One positive outcome of the Internet groups was the creation of the Child and Adolescent Bipolar Foundation (CABF) in 1999 from the parent online support groups in the 1990s. The CABF website (www.bpkids.org) provides users with scientific information about diagnosis, symptoms and treatment of early onset bipolar disorder. Other aspects related to lives of bipolar disorder sufferers are also addressed. Other relevant websites are those of the Depression and Bipolar Support Alliance (DBSA) (www.ndmda.org), the National Alliance for the Mentally Ill (NAMI) (www.nami.org) and the National Institute of Mental Health (NIMH) (www.nimh.nih.gov).

CONCLUSIONS

Almost every aspect of paediatric bipolar disorder requires more study. Many adolescents and children with bipolar disorder do not respond to current first-line pharmacological treatments. Therefore, studies with novel agents should be extended to this population. Given the poor response in many cases to available treatment, in the face of either lack of efficacy or delayed onset of efficacy of single agents, physicians will continue to use combination therapies. Therefore, the resultant drug–drug interactions also need systematic study.

Factors associated with poor and better outcomes are not clear. The role of temperamental dysregulation in the aetiology of child and adolescent bipolar disorder needs further study. Similarly, the relationship and overlap between borderline personality disorders and bipolar disorder needs further investigation in this age group. Developmentally sensitive measures of comorbidity and specific measures for charting different mood episodes and length of mood episodes are needed. For example, the YMRS scores are higher in younger children and higher in boys [129], for reasons that are not clear. Further research will help clinicians and researchers better understand bipolar disorder in children and adolescents. This in turn will result in more accurate diagnosis and more effective treatment.

REFERENCES

1. Anthony J., Scott P. (1960). Manic depressive psychosis in childhood. *J. Child Psychol. Psychiatry*, **1**, 52–72.
2. Kessler R.C., Walters E.E. (1998). Epidemiology of DSM-III-R major depression and minor depression among adolescents and young adults in the National Comorbidity Survey. *Depress. Anxiety*, **7**, 3–14.
3. Lewinsohn P.M., Klein D.N., Seeley J.R. (1995). Bipolar disorders in a community sample of older adolescents: prevalence, phenomenology, comorbidity, and course. *J. Am. Acad. Child Adolesc. Psychiatry*, **34**, 454–463.
4. Luby J. (2003). Depressed preschoolers with bipolar family history: a group at high risk for later switching to mania. *J. Child Adolesc. Psychopharmacol.*, **13**, 187–197.
5. Weller R.A., Weller E.B., Tucker S.G., Fristad M.A. (1986). Mania in prepubertal children: has it been underdiagnosed? *J. Affect. Disord.*, **11**, 151–154.
6. Nottelmann E.D., Jensen P.S. (1995). Bipolar affective disorder in children and adolescents. *J. Am. Acad. Child Adolesc. Psychiatry*, **34**, 705–708.
7. Souery D., Mendlewicz J. (2003). New advances in the understanding and treatment of bipolar disorder. *Int. J. Neuropsychopharmacol.*, **6**, 123–125.
8. Tramontina S., Schmitz M., Polanczyk G., Rohde L.A. (2003). Juvenile bipolar disorder in Brazil: clinical and treatment finding. *Biol. Psychiatry*, **53**, 1043–1049.
9. Srinath S., Janardhan Reddy Y.C., Girimaji S.R., Seshadri S.P., Sabbkrishna D.K. (1998). A prospective study of bipolar disorder in children and adolescents from India. *Acta Psychiatr. Scand.*, **98**, 437–442.
10. Carlson G.A., Strober M. (1978). Manic-depressive illness in early adolescence. A study of clinical and diagnostic characteristics in six cases. *J. Am. Acad. Child Adolesc. Psychiatry*, **17**, 138–153.
11. Gammon G.D., John K., Rothblum E.D., Mullen K., Tischler G.L., Weissman M.M. (1983). Use of a structured diagnostic interview to identify bipolar

disorder in adolescent inpatients: frequency and manifestation of the disorder. *Am. J. Psychiatry*, **140**, 543–547.
12. Suppes T., Leverich G., Keck P., Nolen W.A., Denicoff K.D., Altshuler L.L., McElroy S.L., Rush A.J., Kupka R., Frye M.A., *et al.* (2001). The Stanley Foundation Bipolar Treatment Outcome Network, 2: Demographics and illness characteristics of the first 261 patients. *J. Affect. Disord.*, **67**, 45–59.
13. Hirschfeld R.M.A., Lewis L., Vornick L.A. (2003). Perceptions and impact of bipolar disorder: how far have we really come? Results of the National Depressive and Manic–Depressive Association 2000 survey on bipolar disorder. *J. Clin. Psychiatry*, **64**, 161–174.
14. Boerlin H.L., Gitlin M.J., Zoellner L.A., Hammen C.L. (1998). Bipolar depression and antidepressant-induced mania: a naturalistic study. *J. Clin. Psychiatry*, **59**, 374–379.
15. Howland R. (1996). Induction of mania with serotonin reuptake inhibitors. *J. Clin. Psychopharmacol.*, **16**, 425–427.
16. Bowden C.L. (2002). Update on bipolar disorder: epidemiology, etiology, diagnosis, and prognosis. *Medscape Psychiatry Ment. Health*, **2**(6).
17. Weller E.B., Calvert S.M., Weller R.A. (2003). Bipolar disorder in children and adolescents: diagnosis and treatment. *Curr. Opin. Psychiatry*, **16**, 383–388.
18. Safer D.J. (1997). Changing patterns of psychotropic medications prescribed by child psychiatrists in the 1990s. *J. Child Adolesc. Psychopharmacol.*, **7**, 267–274.
19. Kaplan S.L., Busner J. (1997). Prescribing practices of inpatient child psychiatrists under three auspices of care. *J. Child Adolesc. Psychopharmacol.*, **7**, 275–286.
20. Carlson G.A., Kashani J.H. (1988). Manic symptoms in a non-referred adolescent population. *J. Affect. Disord.*, **15**, 219–226.
21. Klein D.N., Dupue R.A., Slater J.F. (1986). Inventory identification of cyclothymia: IX. Validation in offspring of bipolar I patients. *Arch. Gen. Psychiatry*, **43**, 441–445.
22. Lewinsohn P.M., Klein D.N., Seeling J.R. (2000). Bipolar disorder during adolescence and young adulthood in a community sample. *Bipolar Disord.*, **2**, 281–293.
23. Weissman M.M., Leaf P.J., Tischler G.L., Blazer D.G., Karno M., Bruce M.L., Florio L.P. (1988). Affective disorders in five US communities. *Psychol. Med.*, **18**, 141–153.
24. Smith A.L., Weissman M.M. (1992). Epidemiology. In: Paykel E.S. (ed.) *Handbook of Affective Disorders*. Guilford Press, New York, pp. 111–129.
25. Ballenger J.C., Reus V.I., Post R.M. (1982). The atypical clinical picture of adolescent mania. *Am. J. Psychiatry*, **139**, 602–606.
26. Carlson G.A., Strober M. (1979). Affective disorders in adolescence. *Psychiatr. Clin. North Am.*, **2**, 511–526.
27. Hsu L.K.G., Starzynski J.M. (1986). Mania in adolescence. *J. Clin. Psychiatry*, **47**, 596–599.
28. Strober M., Carlson G.A. (1982). Bipolar illness in adolescents with major depression: clinical, genetic, and psychopharmacologic predictors in a three- to four-year prospective follow-up investigation. *Arch. Gen. Psychiatry*, **39**, 549–555.
29. Weinberg W.A., Brumback R.A. (1976). Mania in childhood: case studies and literature review. *Am. J. Dis. Child.*, **130**, 380–385.
30. White J.H., O'Shanick G. (1976). Juvenile manic-depressive illness. *Am. J. Psychiatry*, **134**, 1035–1036.

31. Varanka T.M., Weller R.A., Weller E.B., Fristad M.A. (1988). Lithium treatment of manic episodes with psychotic features in pre-pubertal children. *Am. J. Psychiatry*, **145**, 1557–1559.
32. Cantwell D.P., Carlson G.A. (eds) (1983). *Affective Disorders in Childhood and Adolescence*. Spectrum, New York.
33. Carlson G.A. (1984). Classification issues of bipolar disorders in childhood. *Psychiatr. Dev.*, **2**, 273–285.
34. Feinstein S.C., Wolpert E.A. (1973). Juvenile manic–depressive illness: clinical and therapeutic considers. *J. Am. Acad. Child Adolesc. Psychiatry*, **12**, 123–136.
35. McGlashan T. (1988). Adolescent versus adult onset of mania. *Am. J. Psychiatry*, **145**, 221–223.
36. Strober M., Morrell W., Burroughs J., Lampert C., Danforth H., Freeman R. (1988). A family study of bipolar I disorder in adolescence. Early onset of symptoms linked to increased familial loading and lithium resistance. *J. Affect. Disord.*, **15**, 255–268.
37. Geller B., Luby J. (1997). Child and adolescent bipolar disorder: a review of the past 10 years. *J. Am. Acad. Child Adolesc. Psychiatry*, **36**, 1168–1176.
38. Geller B., Sun K., Zimerman B., Luby J., Frazier J., Williams M. (1995). Complex and rapid-cycling in bipolar children and adolescents: a preliminary study. *J. Affect. Disord.*, **34**, 259–268.
39. Weckerly J. (2002). Pediatric bipolar mood disorder: review. *J. Dev. Behav. Pediatr.*, **23**, 42–56.
40. Leibenluft E., Charney D.S., Towbin K.E., Bhangoo R.K., Pine D.S. (2003). Defining clinical phenotypes of juvenile mania. *Am. J. Psychiatry*, **160**, 430–437.
41. Wehr T.A., Sack D.A., Rosenthal N.E. (1987). Sleep reduction as a final common pathway in the genesis of mania. *Am. J. Psychiatry*, **144**, 542.
42. Geller B., Williams M., Zimerman B., Frazier J., Beringer L., Warner K.L. (1998). Prepubertal and early adolescent bipolarity differentiate from ADHD by manic symptoms, grandiose delusions, ultra-rapid or ultradian cycling. *J. Affect. Disord.*, **51**, 81–91.
43. Hazell P.L., Carr V., Lewin T.J., Sly K. (2003). Manic symptoms in young males with ADHD predict functioning but not diagnosis after 6 years. *J. Am. Acad. Child Adolesc. Psychiatry*, **42**, 552–560.
44. Chang K.D., Steiner H., Ketter T.A. (2000). Psychiatric phenomenology of child and adolescent bipolar offspring. *J. Am. Acad. Child Adolesc. Psychiatry*, **39**, 453–460.
45. Biederman J., Faraone S.V., Chu M.P., Wozniak J. (1999). Further evidence of a bidirectional overlap between juvenile mania and conduct disorder in children. *J. Am. Acad. Child Adolesc. Psychiatry*, **8**, 8–7.
46. Akiskal H.S. (1995). Developmental pathways to bipolarity: are juvenile-onset depressions pre-bipolar? *J. Am. Acad. Child Adolesc. Psychiatry*, **34**, 754–763.
47. Biederman J., Mick E., Faraone S.V., Spencer T., Wilens T.E., Wozniak J. (2000). Pediatric mania: a developmental subtype of bipolar disorder? *Biol. Psychiatry*, **48**, 458–466.
48. Wozniak J., Biederman J., Kiely K., Ablon J.S., Faraone S.V., Mundy E., Mennin D. (1995). Mania-like symptoms suggestive of childhood-onset bipolar disorder in clinically referred children. *J. Am. Acad. Child Adolesc. Psychiatry*, **34**, 867–876.
49. Anonymous (2001). National Institute of Mental Health research roundtable on prepubertal bipolar disorder. *J. Am. Acad. Child Adolesc. Psychiatry*, **40**, 871–878.

50. Faraone S.V., Biederman J., Wozniak J., Mundy E., Mennin D., O'Donnell D. (1997). Is comorbidity with ADHD a marker for juvenile-onset mania? *J. Am. Acad. Child Adolesc. Psychiatry*, **6**, 1046–1055.
51. Wilens T.E., Biederman J., Millstein R.B., Wozniak J., Hahesy A.L., Spencer T.J. (1999). Risk for substance use disorders in youths with child- and adolescent-onset bipolar disorder. *J. Am. Acad. Child Adolesc. Psychiatry*, **38**, 680–685.
52. Carlson G.A. (2003). Differences in phenomenology related to age of onset in bipolar disorder. Presented at the American Academy of Child and Adolescent Psychiatry Meeting, Miami, 14–19 October.
53. Horowitz H.A. (1975). The use of lithium in the treatment of the drug-induced psychotic reaction. *Dis. Nerv. Syst.*, **36**, 159–163.
54. Horowitz H.A. (1977). Lithium and the treatment of adolescent manic depressive illness. *Dis. Nerv. Syst.*, **38**, 480–483.
55. Borchardt C.M., Bernstein G.A. (1995). Comorbid disorders in hospitalized bipolar adolescents compared with unipolar depressed adolescents. *Child Psychiatry Hum. Dev.*, **26**, 11–18.
56. West S., McElroy S., Strakowski S., Keck P., McConville B. (1995). Attention deficit hyperactivity disorder in adolescent mania. *Am. J. Psychiatry*, **152**, 271–274.
57. Davis R.E. (1979). Manic–depressive variant syndrome of childhood: a preliminary report. *Am. J. Psychiatry*, **136**, 702–706.
58. Geller B. (1997). Controlled study of prepubertal bipolar disorders. Presented at the NIMH Workshop on Prepubertal Bipolar Disorder, Washington, DC, 10–11 March.
59. Geller B., Bolhofner K., Craney J.L., Williams M., DelBello M.P., Gundersen K. (2000). Psychosocial functioning in a prepubertal and early adolescent bipolar disorder phenotype. *J. Am. Acad. Child Adolesc. Psychiatry*, **39**, 1543–1548.
60. Strober M., Schmidt-Lackner S., Freeman R., Bower S., Lampert C., DeAntonio M. (1995). Recovery and relapse in adolescents with bipolar affective illness: a five-year naturalistic, prospective follow-up. *J. Am. Acad. Child Adolesc. Psychiatry*, **34**, 724–731.
61. Carlson G.A., Bromet E.J., Sievers S. (2000). Phenomenology and outcome of subjects with early- and adult-onset psychotic mania. *Am. J. Psychiatry*, **157**, 213–219.
62. Geller B., Zimerman B., Williams M., Bolhofner K., Craney J.L., DelBello M.P., Soutullo C.A. (2000). Six-month stability and outcome of a prepubertal and early adolescent bipolar disorder phenotype. *J. Child Adolesc. Psychopharmacol.*, **10**, 165–173.
63. Geller B., Craney J.L., Bolhofner K., DelBello M.P., Williams M., Zimerman B. (2001). One-year recovery and relapse rates of children with a prepubertal and early adolescent bipolar disorder phenotype. *Am. J. Psychiatry*, **158**, 303–305.
64. Geller B., Craney J.L., Bolhofner K., Nickelsburg M.J., Williams M., Zimerman B. (2002). Two-year prospective follow-up of children with a prepubertal and early adolescent bipolar disorder phenotype. *Am. J. Psychiatry*, **159**, 927–933.
65. Carlson G.A., Fennig S., Bromet E.J. (1994). The confusion between bipolar disorder and schizophrenia in youth: where does it stand in the 1990s? *J. Am. Acad. Child Adolesc. Psychiatry*, **33**, 453–460.
66. Reich W., Weiner Z. Diagnostic Interview for Children and Adolescents (DICA-R-C), DSM III-R version. Unpublished manuscript.

67. Costello E.J., Edelbrock C.S., Costello A.J. (1985). Validity of the NIMH Diagnostic Interview Schedule for Children: a comparison between psychiatric and pediatric referrals. *J. Abnorm. Child Psychol.*, **13**, 579–595.
68. Weller E.B., Weller R.A., Fristad M.A., Rooney M.T., Schecter J. (2000). Children's Interview for Psychiatric Syndromes (ChIPS). *J. Am. Acad. Child Adolesc. Psychiatry*, **39**, 76–84.
69. Chambers W.J., Puig-Antich J., Hirsch M., Paez P., Ambrosini P.J., Tabrizi M.A., Davies M. (1985). The assessment of affective disorders in children and adolescents by semistructured interview. *Arch. Gen. Psychiatry*, **42**, 696–702.
70. Geller B., Warner K., Williams M., Zimerman B. (1998). Prepubertal and early adolescent bipolarity differentiate from ADHD: assessment and validity using the WASH-U-KSADS, CBCL, and TRF. *J. Affect. Disord.*, **51**, 93–100.
71. Geller B., Zimerman B., Williams M., Bolhofner K., Craney J.L., DelBello M.P., Soutullo C. (2001). Reliability of the Washington University in St. Louis Kiddie Schedule for Affective Disorders and Schizophrenia (WASH-U-KSADS) mania and rapid cycling sections. *J. Am. Acad. Child Adolesc. Psychiatry*, **40**, 450–455.
72. Kovacs M.L. (1978). The Interview Schedule for Children. *Psychopharmacol. Bull.*, **21**, 991–994.
73. Beigel A., Murphy D.L., Bunney W.E. Jr (1971). The manic-state rating scale. *Arch. Gen. Psychiatry*, **25**, 256–262.
74. Fristad M.A. Weller E.B., Weller R.A. (1992). The Mania Rating Scale: can it be used in children? A preliminary report. *J. Am. Acad. Child Adolesc. Psychiatry*, **31**, 252–257.
75. Fristad M.A., Weller R.A., Weller E.B. (1995). The Mania Rating Scale (MRS): further reliability and validity studies with children. *Ann. Clin. Psychiatry*, **7**, 127–132.
76. Young R.C., Biggs J.T., Zeigler V.E., Meyer D.A. (1978). A rating scale for mania: reliability, validity and sensitivity. *Br. J. Psychiatry*, **133**, 429–435.
77. Beiderman J., Wozniac J., Kiely K., Ablon S., Faraone S., Mick E., Mundy E., Kraus I. (1995). CBCL scales discriminate prepubertal children with structured interview-derived diagnosis of mania from those with ADHD. *J. Am. Acad. Child Adolesc. Psychiatry*, **34**, 464–471.
78. US Department of Education (1999). *21st Annual Report to Congress on the Implementation of Individuals with Disabilities Education Act*. US Department of Education, Washington, DC.
79. McClellan J., Werry J. (1997). Practice parameters for the assessment and treatment of children and adolescents with bipolar disorder. *J. Am. Acad. Child Adolesc. Psychiatry*, **36** (Suppl. 10), 157S–176S.
80. Kafantaris V. (1995). Treatment of bipolar disorder in children and adolescents. *J. Am. Acad. Child Adolesc. Psychiatry*, **34**, 732–741.
81. Emslie G.J., Mayes T.L. (2001). Mood disorders in children and adolescents: pharmacological treatment. *Biol. Psychiatry*, **49**, 1082–1090.
82. Spencer T.J., Biederman J., Wozniak J., Faraone S.V., Wilens T.E., Mick E. (2001). Parsing pediatric bipolar disorder from its associated comorbidity with the disruptive behavior disorders. *Biol. Psychiatry*, **49**, 1062–1070.
83. Biederman J., Mick E., Prince J., Bostic J.Q., Wilens T.E., Spencer T., Wozniak J., Faraone S.V. (1999). Systematic chart review of the pharmacological treatment of comorbid attention deficit disorder in youth with bipolar disorder. *J. Child Adolesc. Psychopharmacol.*, **9**, 247–256.

84. Altshuler L.L., Post R.M., Leverich G.S., Mikalauskas K., Rosoff A., Ackerman L. (1995). Antidepressant-induced mania and cycle acceleration: a controversy revisited. *Am. J. Psychiatry*, **152**, 1130–1138.
85. Boerlin H., Gitlin M., Zoellner L. (1998). Bipolar depression and antidepressant-induced mania: a naturalistic study. *J. Clin. Psychiatry*, **59**, 374–379.
86. Varanka T.M., Weller R.A., Weller E.B., Fristad M.A. (1988). Lithium treatment of manic episodes with psychotic features in prepubertal children. *Am. J. Psychiatry*, **145**, 1557–1559.
87. Weller E.B., Weller R.A., Fristad M.A. (1986). Lithium dosage guide for prepubertal children: a preliminary report. *J. Am. Acad. Child Psychiatry*, **25**, 92–95.
88. DeLong G.R., Aldershof A.L. (1987). Long-term experience with lithium treatment in childhood: correlation with clinical diagnosis. *J. Am. Acad. Child Adolesc. Psychiatry*, **26**, 389–394.
89. Geller B., Cooper T.B., Sun K., Zimerman B., Frazier J., Williams M., Heath J. (1998). Double blind and placebo controlled study of lithium for adolescent bipolar disorders with secondary substance dependency. *J. Am. Acad. Child Adolesc. Psychiatry*, **37**, 171–178.
90. Strober M., Morrell W., Lampert C., Burroughs J. (1990). Relapse following discontinuation of lithium maintenance therapy in adolescents with bipolar I illness: a naturalistic study. *Am. J. Psychiatry*, **147**, 457–461.
91. Kafantaris V., Coletti D.J., Dicker R., Padula G., Kane J.M. (2003). Lithium treatment of acute mania in adolescents: a large open trial. *J. Am. Acad. Child Psychiatry*, **42**, 1038–1045.
92. DeLong G.R., Nieman G.W. (1983). Lithium-induced behavior changes in children with symptoms suggesting manic–depressive illness. *Psychopharmacol. Bull.*, **19**, 258–265.
93. McKnew D.H., Cytryn L., Buchsbaum M.S., Hamovit J., Lamour M., Rapoport J.L., Gershon E.S. (1981). Lithium in children of lithium-responding parents. *Psychiatry Res.*, **4**, 171–180.
94. Hagino O.R., Weller E.B., Weller R.A., Washing D., Fristad M.A., Kontras S.B. (1995). Untoward effects of lithium treatment in children aged four through six years. *J. Am. Acad. Child Adolesc. Psychiatry*, **34**, 1584–1590.
95. Rosenberg D.R., Holttum J., Gershon S. (1994). *Textbook of Pharmacotherapy for Child and Adolescent Psychiatric Disorders*. Brunner/Mazel, New York.
96. Campbell M., Silva R.R., Kafantaris V., Locascio J.J., Gonzalez N.M., Lee D., Lynch N.S. (1991). Predictors of side effects associated with lithium administration in children. *Psychopharmacol. Bull.*, **27**, 373–380.
97. Whittier M.C., West S.A., Galli V.B., Raute N.J. (1995). Valproic acid for dysphoric mania in a mentally retarded adolescent. *J. Clin. Psychiatry*, **56**, 590–591.
98. Papatheodorou G., Kutcher S.P., Katic M., Szalai J.P. (1995). The efficacy and safety of divalproex sodium in the treatment of acute mania in adolescents and young adults: an open clinical trial. *J. Clin. Psychopharmacol.*, **15**, 110–116.
99. Whittier M.C., West S.A., Galli V.B., Raute N.J. (1995). Valproic acid for dysphoric mania in a mentally retarded adolescent. *J. Clin. Psychiatry*, **56**, 590–591.
100. West S.A., Keck P.E.J., McElroy S.L. (1995). Oral loading doses in the valproate treatment of adolescents with mixed bipolar disorder. *J. Child Adolesc. Psychopharmacol.*, **5**, 225–231.

101. Strober M. (1997). The naturalistic prospective course of juvenile bipolar illness. Presented at the Second International Conference on Bipolar Disorder, Pittsburgh, PA, 20 June.
102. Silberstein S.D., Wilmore L.J. (1996). Divalproex sodium: migraine treatment and monitoring. *Headache*, **36**, 239–242.
103. Bryant A.E. III, Dreifuss F.E. (1996). Valproic acid hepatic fatalities, III: US experience since 1986. *Neurology*, **46**, 465–469.
104. Isojarvi J.I., Laatikainen T.J., Pakarinen A.J., Juntunen K.T., Myllyla V.V. (1993). Polycystic ovaries and hyperandrogenism in women taking valproate for epilepsy. *N. Engl. J. Med.*, **329**, 1383–1388.
105. Isojarvi J.I.T., Ratrya J., Myllyla W., Knip M., Koivunen R., Pakarinen A.J., Tekay A., Tapanainen J.S. (1998). Valproate, lamotrigine, and insulin-mediated risks in women with epilepsy. *Ann. Neurol.*, **43**, 446–451.
106. Wagner K.D., Weller E.B., Carlson G.A., Sachs G., Biederman J., Frazier J.A., Wozniak P., Tracy K., Weller R.A., Bowden C. (2002). An open-label trial of divalproex in children and adolescents with bipolar disorder. *J. Am. Acad. Child Psychiatry*, **41**, 1224–1230.
107. Kowatch R.A., Suppes T., Carmody T.J., Bucci J.P., Hume J.H., Kromelis M., Emslie G.J., Weinberg W.A., Rush A.J. (2000). Effect size of lithium, divalproex sodium, and carbamazepine in children and adolescents with bipolar disorder. *J. Am. Acad. Child Psychiatry*, **39**, 713–720.
108. Garfinkel M., Garfinkel L., Himmelhoch J., McHugh T. (1985). Lithium carbonate and carbamazepine: an effective treatment for adolescent manic or mixed bipolar patients. Presented at the Annual Meeting of the American Academy of Child and Adolescent Psychiatry, San Antonio, TX, 23–27 October.
109. Findling R.L., McNamara N.K., Gracious B.L., Youngstrom, E.A., Stansbrey R.J., Reed M.D., Demeter C.A., Branicky L.A., Fisher K.E., Calabrese J.R. (2003). Combination lithium and divalproex sodium in pediatric bipolarity. *J. Am. Acad. Child Psychiatry*, **42**, 895–901.
110. Kowatch R.A., Sethuraman G., Hume J.H., Kromelis M., Weinberg W.A. (2003). Combination pharmacotherapy in children and adolescents with bipolar disorder. *Biol. Psychiatry*, **53**, 978–984.
111. DelBello M.P., Kowatch R.A., Warner J., Schwiers M.L., Rappaport K.B., Daniels J.P., Foster K.D., Strakowski S.M. (2002). Adjunctive topiramate treatment for pediatric bipolar disorder: a retrospective chart review. *J. Child Adolesc. Psychopharmacol.*, **12**, 323–330.
112. Frazier J.A., Meyer M.C., Biederman J., Woznik J., Wilens T.E., Spencer T.J., Kim G.S., Shapiro S. (1999). Risperidone treatment for juvenile bipolar disorder: a retrospective chart review. *J. Am. Acad. Child Psychiatry*, **38**, 960–965.
113. DelBello M.P., Schwiers M.L., Rosenberg H.L., Strakowski S.M. (2002). A double-blind, randomized, placebo-controlled study of quetiapine as adjunctive treatment for adolescent mania. *J. Am. Acad. Child Psychiatry*, **41**, 1216–1223.
114. Kafantaris V., Coletti D.J., Dicker R., Padula G., Kane J.M. (2001). Adjunctive antipsychotic treatment of adolescents with bipolar psychosis. *J. Am. Acad. Child Adolesc. Psychiatry*, **40**, 1448–1456.
115. Bertagnoli M.W., Borchardt C.M. (1990). A review of ECT for children and adolescents. *J. Am. Acad. Child Adolesc. Psychiatry*, **29**, 302–307.

116. Fristad M.A., Goldberg-Arnold J.S., Gavazzi S.M. (2002). Multifamily psychoeducational groups (MFPG) for families of children with bipolar disorder. *Bipolar Disord.*, **4**, 254–262.
117. Fristad M.A., Goldberg-Arnold J.S. (2003). Psychotherapy for children with bipolar disorder. In: Geller B., DelBello M.P. (eds) *Bipolar Disorder in Childhood and Early Adolescence*. Guilford Press, New York, pp. 358–393.
118. Holder D.A., Anderson B.M. (1990). Psychoeducational family intervention for depressed patients and their families. In: Keitner B.I. (ed.) *Depression and Families: Impact and Treatment*. American Psychiatric Press, Washington, DC, pp. 157–184.
119. Fristad M.A., Gavazzi S.M., Soldano K.W. (1998). Multifamily Psychoeducational groups for childhood mood disorders: a program description and preliminary efficacy data. *Contemp. Fam. Ther.*, **20**, 385–402.
120. Goldberg-Arnold J.S., Fristad M.A., Gavazzi S.M. (1999). Family psychoeducation: giving caregivers what they want and need. *Fam. Relations*, **48**, 411–417.
121. Lefley H.P. (1997). The consumer recovery vision: will it alleviate family burden? *Am. J. Orthopsychiatry*, **67**, 210–219.
122. Newacheck P.W., Strickland B., Shonkoff J.P., Perrin J.M. (1998). An epidemiological profile of children with special health care needs. *Pediatrics*, **102**, 117–123.
123. Cook J.A., Heller T., Pickett-Schenk S.A. (1999). The effect of support group participation on caregiver burden among parents of adult offspring with severe mental illness. *Fam. Relations*, **48**, 405–410.
124. Koroloff N.M., Friesen B.J. (1991). Support groups for parents of children with emotional disorders: a comparison of members and non members. *Community Ment. Health J.*, **27**, 265–279.
125. Norcross, J.C. (2000). Here comes the self-help revolution in mental health. *Psychotherapy*, **37**, 370–377.
126. Sisson D.P., Fristad M.A. (2001). A survey of stress and support for parents of children with early onset bipolar disorder. *Bipolar Disord.*, **3** (Suppl. 1), 58.
127. Bacon E.S., Condon E.H., Fernsler J.I. (2000). Young widows' experience with an Internet self-help group. *J. Psychosoc. Nurs.*, **38**, 24–33.
128. Salem D.A., Bogar G.A., Reid C. (1997). Mutual help goes on-line. *J. Community Psychol.*, **25**, 189–207.
129. Youngstrom E.A., Danielson C.K., Findling R.L., Gracious B.L., Calabrese J.R. (2002). Factor structure of the Young Mania Rating Scale for use with youths ages 5 to 17 years. *J. Clin. Child Adolesc. Psychol.*, **31**, 567–572.

CHAPTER

5

Detecting the Risk for Affective Spectrum Disorders in the Children of Bipolar Parents

Gabriele Masi*, Hagop S. Akiskal‡ and Kareen Akiskal‡

**Stella Maris Scientific Institute of Child Neurology and Psychiatry, Calambrone (Pisa), Italy*
‡University of California at San Diego, and Veterans Administration Medical Center, La Jolla, CA, USA

INTRODUCTION

Awareness of bipolar spectrum disorders in children is rapidly increasing, and a more precise definition of clinical subtypes and early signs is being accomplished. One indication of this greater awareness is the research to detect prodromal features of early-onset disorders in high-risk populations, such as the offspring of bipolar probands [1]. Retrospective findings from adult bipolar patients show that 59% report the onset of their symptoms before the age of 14, with an average time lapse of 5 years between symptom onset and correct diagnosis and treatment [2]. Offspring studies on children and adolescents of people with mental disorders are useful to improve our knowledge about the factors that may influence the development and the natural history of these diseases, including predictors of psychopathology, factors of resilience or early signs of the disorders [1,3]. Furthermore, these studies can improve our capacities of prevention, early diagnosis and timely interventions. They are of great importance to families where one or both parents are bipolar, because they facilitate the detection of bipolar prodromes. The relevant data can be used by patient and advocacy organizations serving bipolar families [4].

Children and adolescents of parents with bipolar disorder are a cohort of intensively studied patients, and many studies are available in the literature on their psychopathological characteristics [5–24]. It is more than of

Early Detection and Management of Mental Disorders.
Edited by Mario Maj, Juan José López-Ibor, Norman Sartorius, Mitsumoto Sato and Ahmed Okasha.
 ISBN 0-470-01083-5.

historical interest that the first study of the clinical characteristics of the offspring of manic–depressive parents was conducted by one of the authors of this chapter, an adult psychiatrist working in a mood clinic [25]. He did so because bipolar mothers bitterly complained that child psychologists, child psychiatrists and paediatricians neglected the affective symptoms of their children as transitory problems, despite insistence by these mothers that they themselves had experienced the same symptoms; they simply wanted their children to receive the earliest possible care. Most child professionals [9–23] ventured into this arena much later. Overall, these studies demonstrate an elevated prevalence of affective disorders, disruptive behaviour disorders and anxiety disorders in the child and adolescent offspring of affected parents. However, prevalence rates reported in the existing studies vary greatly. A number of methodological issues hamper the comparability across studies, and the interpretation of findings [22]. First of all, there is a large variation in the sample composition: most studies used selected clinical samples of adults with bipolar disorder, including inpatients, outpatients or a mix, with different types of bipolar disorder (type I, type II or both), and different degrees of severity. Furthermore, the comparison samples (usually small and unrepresentative) vary greatly among studies. Several studies did not include comparison groups; in several others only healthy volunteers were considered as a control group. The majority of studies included children of normal parents and/or children of psychiatrically ill, nonbipolar parents, and/or medically ill patients. Diagnostic procedures also varied greatly, as well as the diagnostic system of reference, the number of diagnoses and the informants.

All the studies which compared bipolar offspring to healthy volunteers' offspring show that bipolar offspring present an increased risk for a wide range of mental disorders, including mood disorders (major depressive disorder and bipolar disorder), behavioural disorders (mainly attention-deficit/hyperactivity disorder, ADHD), and anxiety disorders [8–10,14, 16–19], suggesting a lack of phenotypic specificity. Rates of mood disorders in bipolar offspring range from 5 to 67% versus 0–38% in children of healthy volunteers, and rates of other mental disorders range from 5 to 52% versus 0–25% in children of healthy volunteers [3]. Subsyndromal and temperamental characteristics are also described in children without concurrent affective episodes in studies of the offspring of bipolar parents [25,26], as well as atypical cognitive functioning [8,27].

Overall, current results emphasize the clinical importance of the routine and systematic assessment of family histories for judging the likelihood of the development of affective disorders, namely a bipolar disorder, in the child and adolescent offspring and siblings of bipolar patients [28]. Why can early signs of bipolar disorder be expected in children of bipolar patients? Because family, twin and adoption studies strongly support the role of genetic factors in the aetiology of bipolar disorder, even though the complex inheritance pattern is not yet clearly understood [29]. This complex inheritance includes, among others, unstable DNA trinucleotide repeat sequences, which appear to expand in length over successive generations, offering, hypothetically, an explanation for the many deviations from Mendelian inheritance in bipolar disorder. These mutations are considered the basis of a clinical phenomenon, called anticipation, characterized by earlier onset and increasingly severe phenotype in younger generations for certain diseases, including bipolar disorder [30–33]. Genetic anticipation may thus lead to increased detection of bipolar disorder in children and adolescents. This is consistent with studies confirming a secular trend in the age of onset of bipolar disorder, with the average age of onset decreasing in more recently born individuals [34].

Besides genetic factors, environmental stressors are related to having a parent with bipolar disorder, who is unstable due to mood swings, possible hospitalizations, substance abuse and other less severe but more persistent behavioural excesses. Families with a bipolar parent report differences in their environment, in terms of cohesion and organization, conflictuality and dyscontrol [35]. This is not surprising, considering the psychosocial disruptions in bipolar patients. During development, the child born into a family with a bipolar parent is exposed to extremes of moods and related social instabilities, validating his or her own inherited proclivity to mood instability [36].

Finally, it is likely that increased use of antidepressants and/or stimulants in bipolar offspring with depression, anxiety or ADHD may elicit an earlier onset of bipolar disorder [37]. However, not all studies support an increased risk for manic switch in young bipolar patients treated with psychostimulants, at least in the short term [38].

THE RISK FOR MOOD DISORDERS

Studies on the risk for early-onset bipolar disorder in the offspring of bipolar patients are made more difficult by the relative uncertainty of the phenomenology of bipolar disorder in childhood, given the developmental differences of the disorder in prepubertal patients, including atypicality of phenomenology [39], and the high frequency of comorbidity, mainly with ADHD [40]. More recently a new effort was made to develop diagnostic criteria for different phenotypes of juvenile mania [41,42], and to produce methodological guidelines, including inclusion and exclusion criteria, for clinical studies in child and adolescent patients with bipolar disorder [43].

An early study found that the risk of developing an affective disorder for first-degree relatives of bipolar probands was 27% if one parent, and 74% if both parents had a bipolar disorder [44]. A meta-analysis of studies conducted before 1997 showed that bipolar offspring (both children and adults) are at 2.7 times higher risk for developing any psychiatric disorder, and 4 times higher risk for developing a mood disorder, compared to children of parents without psychiatric illness [45]. Cyclothymia has been repeatedly found to be more common in bipolar offspring than in controls [12,28,46]. Subsequent studies confirm that about 50% of children of bipolar parents have at least one psychiatric disorder, and bipolar spectrum disorders (bipolar I, bipolar II and cyclothymia) are reported in 14–50% of these children [20,21,25]. It is debatable whether clinical features of bipolar offspring are different from those of bipolar samples which are mixed for the presence or absence of family history [1].

Depressive disorders are frequently reported in the offspring of bipolar parents and, according to several studies [15,17,25], they are the most frequently reported disorder. For Kashani *et al.* [11], depression is more frequent in bipolar offspring (22%) than in offspring of depressed parents, while Hammen *et al.* [17] and Radke-Yarrow *et al.* [18] found higher rates in children of depressed parents than in children of bipolar parents. Longitudinal studies may be needed to explore the eventual bipolar outcome in this population of depressed offspring, in view of the high rates of subsequent manic episodes in early-onset depression [46]. This risk is reported to be even higher in depressed children with a positive family history of bipolar disorder [47].

Duffy *et al.* [20] explored psychopathological features in the offspring of two groups of bipolar parents, divided on the basis of their response to long-term lithium prophylaxis. The leading hypothesis was that the response to lithium prophylaxis was a clinical marker of a more homogeneous, genetically based subgroup of bipolar disorder. Of the 36 children, 19 (52.8%) met DSM-IV criteria for at least one psychiatric disorder (9/21 in the lithium responders' offspring, 10/15 in the lithium nonresponders' offspring). The children of lithium responder parents tended to manifest psychiatric illnesses clustering in the affective domain, with episodic course and fewer comorbid conditions. On the contrary, children of lithium nonresponders tended to present a wider range of psychopathology, a chronic course and a higher comorbidity. These data were confirmed in an expansion of this study with a larger sample and a prospective, longitudinal design [23]. Parents with classical episodic bipolar disorder characterized by complete remissions and an excellent response to lithium tended to have children with typical, episodic affective disorders, with abrupt onset superimposed on a normal premorbid development, and a good quality of remissions. On the contrary, parents with bipolar disorder characterized by incomplete remissions tended to have children with early problems in social and academic functioning, which continued alongside the mood disorder, which itself followed a chronic course with poor quality of remission. Differences in the course of the disorders between the offspring groups did not appear to be attributable to psychosocial stress. These different bipolar phenotypes have been more recently described in greater detail [41]. Whether these phenotypes have different rates of response to lithium treatment is a matter for further research.

Chang *et al.* [21] described cross-sectional psychopathological features in 60 subjects (mean age 11.1 years) from 37 families with at least one bipolar parent. Of these 60 subjects, 33 (55%) had a DSM-IV axis I disorder: 17 subjects (28%) met lifetime (but mostly also current) diagnostic criteria for ADHD, 9 (15%) for major depressive disorder or dysthymia, 9 (15%) for bipolar disorder or cyclothymia, 6 (10%) for oppositional defiant disorder, 3 (5%) for an anxiety disorder, 2 (3%) for obsessive–compulsive disorder and 2 (3%) for tic disorder. Of the children with a diagnosis of bipolar disorder, 88% had a co-occurring ADHD; 81% of offspring with ADHD and 88% of offspring with bipolar disorder were males. Bipolar parents of offspring with bipolar disorder were more likely to have had an ADHD themselves, and there was a tendency to an earlier onset of their psychiatric symptoms, compared to parents of offspring without axis I disorders.

The finding of an association of parental ADHD+bipolar disorder with bipolar offspring suggests the possibility of a genetic transmission of a distinct, more virulent subtype of bipolar disorder with earlier onset and ADHD features [48]. This may be confirmed by the observation that bipolar parents with childhood ADHD tended to have an earlier age of onset of their bipolar symptoms, compared to those without ADHD. Severity of mood symptoms was separately considered in the unilineal or bilineal risk groups (one or two ill parents). Depressed mood, irritability, lack of mood reactivity, rejection sensitivity, social withdrawal and crying were significantly more severe in the bilineal group, while manic symptoms (grandiosity, euphoric mood, decreased need for sleep) did not significantly differ between the groups. These data suggest that an innate difficulty in mood regulation in the highest risk subjects may represent a prodromal state of bipolar disorder, whereas manic symptoms may represent later signs of a more advanced and crystallized presentation of bipolar disorder. Given the cross-sectional design of the study, it was not possible to define longitudinal risk during subsequent development, as well as the rate of remission of the current disorders (the mean age of this cohort was 11.1 years).

More recently a prospective study of prodromal features for bipolarity has been conducted in psychiatrically well Amish children [24]. The risk for bipolar disorder was 38% among children with a bipolar parent, compared with 17% in the control sample. The risk in the control sample was mostly (15 out of 18 children) accounted for by children of psychiatrically well parents who were siblings of a bipolar patient. Children with negative family history rarely received even a low risk rating. The clinical features which were most frequent in children with a bipolar parent were mood lability, low energy, anxiety/worry, hyperalertness, sensitivity and somatic complaints. Increased and decreased energy, decreased sleep and anger/temper were noted to occur periodically in more than 50% of the children, and these miniclusters (episodic affective storms) were considered the more typical prodromal manifestation in children at risk for bipolarity. Disruptive behaviours and conduct problems were very rare in the Amish children with a bipolar parent, presumably due to psychosocial and environmental influence.

Todd *et al.* [28,49] explored mental disorders in children and adolescent members of extended families identified through adult bipolar probands. In the first study [49] there was a significant relationship between the risk of an early-onset affective disorder in children and adolescents, and the degree of genetic relatedness to affected adults in the family, while there was no significant correlation between affective disorders and any of the psychosocial measures. Furthermore, there was not an increased risk of developing disruptive behaviour disorders or anxiety disorders. In the subsequent, extended pilot study [28], 12 of the 50 interviewed offspring (24%) received a lifetime diagnosis of an affective disorder, 6 of bipolar disorder, 5 of depressive disorder and 1 of dysthymia. The offspring of a parent with an affective disorder showed a five-fold higher risk of having an affective disorder diagnosis than the offspring with healthy parents, supporting a major role of genetic factors, compared to presumably shared cultural and environmental factors. An increased risk of anxiety disorders, but not of disruptive behaviour disorders, was found in the bipolar offspring.

ADHD AND OTHER DISRUPTIVE BEHAVIOUR DISORDERS

Childhood-onset bipolar disorder is frequently associated with or preceded by oppositional defiant disorder, conduct disorder or, more frequently, ADHD [40,48,50,51]. The reasons for the association between bipolar disorder and ADHD remain unresolved. It is presently unclear whether this association is a true comorbidity, or a consequence of a diagnostic overlap between the two disorders, or if ADHD is a prodromal condition in the course of bipolar disorder, or a complication of bipolar disorder. Several studies support the finding that adolescent-onset bipolar disorder shows less comorbidity with disruptive behaviour disorders than prepubertal-onset bipolar disorder [40,48,52]. More recently, ADHD has been found as an antecedent in 50% of patients with prepubertal bipolar disorder, compared to 8.7% of patients with adolescent-onset bipolar disorder [52], suggesting that ADHD may be an antecedent or an early sign of a very early-onset bipolar disorder.

Wozniak *et al.* [50] interviewed 46 first-degree relatives of 16 children with a diagnosis of mania. High rates of ADHD comorbidity were found both in the proband children and in the relatives. A five-fold elevated risk for bipolar disorder was observed among relatives of children with ADHD and bipolar disorder, compared to children with ADHD alone [48]. Furthermore, ADHD and bipolar disorder co-occurred in the same relatives more frequently than expected by chance.

Offspring studies on bipolar probands show that about a quarter of bipolar offspring meet criteria for ADHD [9,16–21]. High rates of ADHD in bipolar offspring may be related to an eventual early-onset of bipolar disorder in this population. The presence of ADHD with co-occurring mood difficulties in bipolar offspring may indicate an increased risk for bipolar development.

Carlson and Weintraub [19] grouped bipolar offspring, offspring of parents with other mental disorders and healthy controls by the presence or absence of behavioural or attentional problems, and found that these problems predicted the development of mental disorders in late adolescence or young adulthood. However, attentional and behavioural disorders were associated to later development of mood disorders in bipolar offspring, but not in offspring of parents with other disorders and in healthy controls [19].

Chang *et al.* [21] reported on the psychopathological features of 60 bipolar offspring. ADHD was the most frequent diagnosis (27%). Parents with bipolar disorder who reported to have had an ADHD during childhood more frequently had a child with bipolar disorder than bipolar parents without a history of ADHD [21,53]. Therefore, co-occurring ADHD and bipolar disorder in a parent may increase the risk for early-onset bipolar disorder in offspring.

Significantly lower rates of ADHD are reported in the offspring of bipolar patients in several non-US studies. Duffy *et al.* [20] found only one child with ADHD in the 21 offspring of 13 bipolar parents, and one child with ADHD in the 53 offspring of 30 bipolar probands in the expansion of the same study [23]. This finding was supported by the lack of evidence of attentional problems in both affected and nonaffected children, irrespective of the parents' lithium responsiveness [54]. In Wals *et al.*'s study [22], ADHD was a current diagnosis in 4% of the sample, and a lifetime diagnosis in 5% of the sample.

Given the symptomatological overlap, as well as the developmental relationship between ADHD and early-onset bipolar disorder, a comparison between the offspring of parents with ADHD and of bipolar parents with or without ADHD may help to clarify the relationship between bipolar disorder and ADHD [3].

EUROPEAN VIEWS

A recent study [22] was carried out in 140 adolescent offspring, aged 12–21 years, of bipolar parents living in the Netherlands, 41 of whom (29%) met diagnostic criteria for at least one current DSM-IV mental disorder. The most frequent diagnoses were mood disorder (14%, including 3% with a bipolar disorder), anxiety disorder (8%), substance use disorder (6%), ADHD (4%) and disruptive behaviour disorder (4%). A total of 61 subjects (44%) met criteria for at least one lifetime diagnosis, namely mood disorder (27%, including 3% with bipolar disorder), anxiety disorder (11%), substance use disorder (6%), disruptive behaviour disorder (6%) and ADHD (5%). The Child Behavior Checklist (CBCL) [55] was used in these subjects and in controls from the general population, to assess behavioural and emotional problems, according to self-rating as well as parents' and teachers' evaluation. Higher scores were found for 8 of the 11 subscales of the self-administered CBCL (mostly concerning internalizing problems) in the female probands, and for 4 of the 11 subscales (mostly concerning externalizing problems such as aggressive behaviour) in the male probands. According to teachers' evaluation, there was no significant difference between probands and controls. Overall, this study reported lower rates of psychopathology (in terms of DSM-IV diagnoses, as well as in terms of dimensional scores), compared with those found in studies from US populations. These rates were only slightly different from those found in the general Dutch population with a similar procedure by the same research group [56]. Only the prevalence of mood disorders in the probands was considerably higher than that found in the general population. These findings cast doubts on the previously established conclusion that the adolescent offspring of bipolar patients are at great risk for psychopathology in general, and specifically for bipolar disorder. According to the authors, the difference between their results and those of US studies may be in part due to the modalities of sample recruitment, which may have selected less impaired bipolar parents (two-thirds of the sample were recruited from patients' associations and only one-third from outpatient clinics). However, this hypothesis is not supported by their own data, since differences between the two patient subgroups did not reach statistical significance. Another possible selection bias is related to the fact that only a minority of selected parents agreed to participate, so that the most impaired subjects or the families with the most severely impaired offspring may have been excluded from the study. The Dutch authors also hypothesize that a more frequent use of antidepressants and stimulants in the USA may account for higher rates of pharmacological hypomania. Finally, another possibly relevant factor may be the different conceptualization of bipolar disorder in the USA and in Europe.

European and US conceptualizations of mania in prepubertal children have been summarized recently by Harrington and Myatt [57], who express doubt about the validity of the diagnosis of mania, and particularly about the inferences made about the meaning of some symptoms. According to this view, manic states in prepubertal children are extremely rare. However, the experience of one of the authors of this chapter [52,58] is that paediatric, including prepubertal, mania is common in Italy, and exhibits the same range of comorbidities as reported in the USA.

FOLLOW-UP STUDIES

Prospective follow-up studies are rare in the literature on juvenile bipolarity. One of the major problems in detecting bipolar disorder in children is the extent to which depressive states, temperamental moodiness, "atypical" mood swings with explosive moods and behaviour, and/or ultra-rapid cycling represent variants and/or precursors of clinically more recognizable bipolar disorder. This question cannot be resolved by cross-sectional observation. A family history of bipolar disorder may reinforce the bipolar nature of the presenting mood instability, but, in the absence of genetic markers, prospective follow-up is the ultimate clinical "test" available today for supporting a bipolar diagnosis in a child presenting with such instability. This is what one of the authors of this chapter attempted to accomplish in his mood clinic, where adult manic–depressive patients brought their children or younger siblings with what they deemed to be early signs of bipolarity, similar to what they had experienced as children before the illness fully declared itself at a later age.

In this prospective follow-up over 3–4 years [25], carried out in 68 offspring or siblings (age range 6 to 24 years) of adult bipolar patients, 79% of those with a provisional diagnosis of depression had a depressive recurrence, and 37.5% developed a bipolar disorder (type I or II). Eleven subjects with polysubstance abuse without a clinical affective disorder were re-diagnosed as having either a dysthymic or a cyclothymic disorder during the follow-up. Anxiety disorders, substance abuse and/or disruptive behaviour disorder appeared as antecedents to the full-blown mood disorder rather than coexisting as independent comorbid conditions.

Indeed, the Zahn-Waxler *et al.* study [9], which found that offspring of a bipolar parent showed a range of adjustment problems as infants and toddlers, which continued four years later – including some that could be classified as DSM-III psychiatric disorders – represents a further extension of the same perspective, according to which relatively amorphous mood instability in the children of bipolar mothers crystallizes over time into more recognizable affective disorder.

In a Canadian study, LaRoche *et al.* [15] reported that 24% of 37 school-aged offspring from 21 families with a manic–depressive parent received a positive DSM-III diagnosis, largely in the affective illness spectrum. When the presence of affective traits was considered, a lack of evidence for continuity of psychopathology over a 3–7-year follow-up period resulted in most cases. These data support the notion of a broad bipolar spectrum. Along these lines, Hammen *et al.* [17] observed diagnoses from both past lifetime and prospective follow-up assessments in the offspring of unipolar, bipolar and chronically medically ill mothers, and found that the highest psychopathological risk (including that for bipolar disorder) during all evaluations was in the offspring of unipolar women. Indeed, school-aged children of bipolar mothers experienced fewer chronic, recurrent or new-onset psychiatric disorders over 1–3 years, including both affective disorders alone or in combination with behaviour or anxiety disorders. It would appear to us that some of the so-called "unipolar" offspring of mothers may have been bipolar II cases, whose hypomanic episodes were missed in the clinical evaluation procedure with diagnostic interviews in which 4 days of hypomania are needed for such a diagnosis [59].

Duffy *et al.* [23], in their prospective, longitudinal follow-up study described earlier, reported that offspring of lithium responders tended to have an episodic affective disorder, with an abrupt onset, often preceded by sleep and anxiety disorders, and good recovery. On the contrary, offspring of lithium nonresponders showed early-onset academic and behavioural problems, which continued alongside the mood disorder, which showed chronic course and poor remission. This study supports the characterization of two bipolar phenotypes: a classical, narrow form, and a broad form, with subcontinuous course, incomplete remissions and predominately irritable mood and unstable course. These two phenotypes run in the family and may partly be predicted by lithium response.

Further longitudinal research is needed to follow up children with different psychopathologies, in order to describe putative different pathways to bipolarity. The high frequency of anxiety disorders preceding the onset of bipolar disorder, mainly in the classical form, is considered an antecedent of the full-blown mood disorder rather than "true comorbidity", in the context of variable phenotypic expression during development. The high incidence of current and past anxiety disorders in bipolar offspring (including separation anxiety, panic and social phobic disorders) may in part stem from the chaotic environment and attachment difficulties related to the presence of one or two bipolar parents [35], and in part represent an alternative pathway to bipolarity [60,61]. The latter is suggested by current studies in adults whereby panic and related disorders appear to characterize the bipolar II subtype and its unstable course [62–66].

Follow-up studies are warranted to ascertain the possibility that children with subsyndromal features of bipolar disorder (including temperamental disinhibition, high levels of activity and mood dysregulation) may develop a fully expressed bipolar disorder during childhood, adolescence and early adulthood, in order to describe possible vulnerability factors. It would finally be relevant to study temperamental, genetic and environmental characteristics of children of bipolar parents who never develop psychopathology, in order to define possible factors of resilience.

ENVIRONMENTAL FACTORS

Even if the familial transmission of bipolar disorder has been well established, the concordance rate between identical twins does not approach 100%, suggesting a combined role of genetic predisposition and environmental factors [67]. A bipolar parent with recurrent episodes is often dysfunctional, neglectful or absent, and this chronic or recurrent situation can influence the child's development [35,36]. Negative family interactions, including higher expressed emotions, have been proved to be predictive of relapse in bipolar adolescents and adults [68], but studies considering the family environment in the presence of a bipolar parent, and its effect on offspring, are rare. Conrad and Hammen [69] evaluated the offspring of bipolar mothers and found that a better outcome was associated with social competence and a healthy father. Marital discord, parental divorce, a second parent with psychopathology, and chronicity of illness were predictors of psychopathology in children of bipolar parents [6,13,16,70]. Inoff-Germain *et al.* [70] found that mothers with bipolar disorder had more negative reactions towards their children than mothers with unipolar depression and healthy mothers, supporting the hypothesis that parenting may be a critical element for the psychopathological outcome. Furthermore, socioeconomic status was found to be related to the presence of psychopathology in the offspring [16,18].

Chang *et al.* [35] have specifically explored family environment in families with one bipolar parent, assessed by the Family Environment Scale (FES) [71]. Data show, according to parents' ratings, lower scores on the cohesion and organization scales, and higher scores on the conflict scale, compared to population means. Scores did not differ between families with one or two affected parents, as well as between bipolar offspring with or without an axis I DSM-IV diagnosis. This finding suggests the lack of a specific relationship between negative family environment and the development of psychopathology in the offspring.

TEMPERAMENT AND BIPOLAR VULNERABILITY

Temperamental features can be predictors of later psychopathology [72,73], and a difficult temperament (irregular biological rhythms, irritability, inflexibility) has been suggested to be a premorbid feature in children with bipolar disorder [74,75].

One of the authors of this chapter [76,77] described three temperamental profiles potentially predisposing to adolescent or adult-onset bipolar disorder: the hyperthymic, cyclothymic and irritable types. These are characterized by excesses along the lines of exuberant, overconfident, overenergetic, impulsive, overtalkative, extraverted, meddlesome, uninhibited, stimulus seeking and mood labile traits. In an 11-year prospective study, high self-ratings of mood lability and energetic activity predicted bipolar II switching in depressed patients [46]. Kochman *et al.* [78], using a new scale for cyclothymic-sensitive temperament, showed the same outcome in adolescent major depressions.

Studies of offspring at risk for bipolar disorder have found mood and behavioural difficulties suggestive of an affective dysregulation. A study considering seven 2-year-old sons of bipolar mothers found significant aggressive behaviours during laboratory observations, compared to control offspring of nonaffected mothers [79]. Chang *et al.* [26] addressed this topic in a sample of 53 children and adolescents of bipolar parents, 27 of whom (52%) received a psychiatric diagnosis (28% ADHD, 15.1% anxiety disorder, 13.2% bipolar disorder and 11.3% depression), and were evaluated with a temperament measure [80]. The bipolar offspring as a whole showed lower scores in the general activity scale and higher scores in the approach and rhythm-sleep scales. Bipolar offspring with psychiatric diagnoses showed higher activity levels than bipolar offspring without diagnoses, and lower scores on flexibility, positive mood and task orientation. Grigoroiu-Serbanescu *et al.* [16] found that bipolar offspring with psychopathology had less emotional stability, less frustration tolerance, and more anxiety and shallowness in relationships and schoolwork than bipolar offspring without psychopathology. All these findings may support the hypothesis that temperamental features such as less emotional stability, intolerance to frustration and irregular biological rhythms may predispose to a variety of psychopathologies.

The foregoing findings are consistent with the temperament construct of behavioural disinhibition [81,82]. This temperamental quality, evident in early childhood, is characterized by a tendency to seek out novelty, approach unfamiliar stimuli, and display disinhibition of speech or action. This temperament can often be associated with higher ratings of school behaviour problems, and may be linked with later disruptive behaviour and comorbid mood disorders, especially in high-risk populations such as bipolar offspring. These findings are also consistent with previous data from a study on a nonclinical cohort of high school students, which showed a correlation between decreased flexibility/increased distractibility and presence of depression, substance abuse and delinquency [83].

In an interactional model, a combination of genetic vulnerability with environmental stressors, deficient coping strategies and maladaptive patterns of behaviour may lead to development of full-blown bipolar disorder [84]. We have formulated a pathogenetic model of bipolarity in which temperament plays a pivotal role in mediating between putative "mood genes" and clinical phenotypes [61].

PREDICTORS OF PSYCHOPATHOLOGY

The majority of bipolar offspring will not develop bipolar disorder. It is therefore crucial to detect, from an early age, predictors of bipolar development in this high-risk population [1]. Early detection of a prodromal state may allow timely and specific interventions and prevention of a poorer outcome.

Research on prodromal signs in this population did not give definite results. Carlson and Weintraub [19] found that attentional and behavioural problems during childhood were not more frequent in the offspring of bipolar parents than in the offspring at risk for other, non-bipolar, psychiatric disorders. However, a unique relationship between childhood problems and young adulthood mood disorders was found only in the bipolar risk group. Fergus *et al.* [85], based on parental retrospective report, suggested that the earlier of these childhood problems clustered around irritability/dyscontrol, i.e. temper tantrums, poor frustration tolerance, impulsivity and agressivity.

Preschool children with depression and a family history of bipolar disorder show higher rates of restlessness or motor agitation, compared to depressed children without family history of bipolar disorder [86]. Follow-up studies are needed to investigate rates of later switching to mania.

Subsyndromal bipolar disorder has been described in 6% of adolescents in the community, but a longitudinal assessment showed that none of the adolescents with subsyndromal mania met criteria for full-blown bipolar disorder type I in their early 20s [87]. In the study on Amish children [24], the presence of episodic miniclusters of increased and decreased energy, decreased sleep and anger/temper were considered the more typical prodromal manifestation in children at higher risk for bipolarity. The nature and the natural history of these subsyndromal forms, both subcontinuous and episodic, deserve further research.

It has been hypothesized that bipolar offspring show deficits consistent with the syndrome of nonverbal learning disabilities (NLD) [8]. A recent test of this hypothesis showed that children at risk for bipolar disorder have a significantly higher verbal IQ than performance IQ, as well as psychomotor deficits, but academic deficiencies in mechanical arithmetic relative to reading and spelling abilities, typical of NLD, were not demonstrated [27]. Whether these cognitive abnormalities are predictive of the development of bipolar disorder is still unclear, even though they are similar to those found in adults with bipolar disorder [88].

Duffy *et al.* [54] explored whether some significant symptoms of inattention were present among the 53 offspring of 30 bipolar patients, with ($n = 24$) or without ($n = 29$) psychopathologies (mostly in the mood and/or anxiety domain). A lack of evidence of premorbid ADHD and an absence of current attentional problems was found with an objective measure (a cancellation test), even though with a subjective measure (a self-administered ADHD rating scale) a significant difference was found between the well and psychiatrically ill, as well as between those with and those without an affective disorder. This led to the hypothesis that attentional difficulties may reflect the activity of the underlying mental disorder rather than a real attentional problem, and caution against a possible overdiagnosis of ADHD in the presence of another Axis I disorder.

A dimensional approach can help to define behavioural and emotional profiles in children and adolescents of bipolar parents, capturing earlier manifestations of the disorder even before a categorical diagnosis. One example of this approach is the CBCL [55], a format reporting the behavioural and emotional problems of children (4–18 years) as described by parents. Dienes *et al.* [89] reported higher scores on all the CBCL scales in bipolar offspring. Within these offspring, subjects with a diagnosable mental disorder (bipolar disorder, ADHD, depression and/or anxiety) scored significantly higher than those without a clinical disorder on numerous CBCL subscales. The offspring with bipolar disorder were more pervasively disturbed than the rest of the clinical portion of the sample, even though several scales did not distinguish the bipolar disorder and ADHD groups. Furthermore, ADHD and depressed/anxious children did not differ as well at the CBCL. These findings led to the suggestion that a prodromal-subclinical bipolar disorder in ADHD and depressed/anxious children of bipolar parents (as well as in nonclinical bipolar offspring) may have determined higher scores at the CBCL, compared to non-bipolar offspring.

Kochman *et al.* [78] demonstrated that, among adolescents with major depression, trait cyclothymia with extreme lability was a predictor of suicide attempts in a 2-year prospective follow-up, as well as of the development of bipolar disorder. Such data underscore the immense public health importance of the foregoing treatment efforts.

NEUROBIOLOGICAL ASPECTS

The longitudinal study of a high-risk population such as bipolar offspring may help to reveal possible markers of disease which distinguish subjects who will eventually develop bipolar disorder (or other psychopathologies) from subjects who will not. Even though it may be difficult to ascertain whether these markers predispose to the disorder, or if they are the first signs of the disorder, the identification of these markers could allow earlier diagnoses and timely interventions [1]. Unfortunately, relevant findings to date are extremely scarce.

A magnetic resonance imaging (MRI) analysis of offspring of bipolar patients showed that they had increased hippocampal volumes, compared to healthy volunteer offspring [90]. Longitudinal data to determine whether this hippocampal abnormality is related to a bipolar outcome are still not available.

Another study using magnetic resonance spectroscopy (MRS) found that bipolar offspring with bipolar disorder had decreased *N*-acetyl-aspartate (NAA) to creatine (Cr) ratios in the right dorsolateral prefrontal cortex (DLPFC), while bipolar offspring with mood and disruptive behavioural disorder but not bipolar disorder had unchanged NAA/Cr ratios in the same cerebral region [91]. Information about the NAA before the onset of bipolar disorder and before the onset of pharmacological treatment was not available. The NAA/Cr ratio tends to decrease as illness duration increases [91].

TREATMENT IMPLICATIONS

Early detection of prodromal symptoms or signs in high-risk populations offers a window of opportunity for preventive and therapeutic interventions (psychotherapy as well as pharmacotherapy), and allows avoidance of treatments (antidepressants, stimulants) which may worsen the clinical course of the disorder [37].

Psychoeducational as well as psychotherapeutic interventions on children and their parents (either affected or not) can help them to manage life experiences or family stressors. On the pharmacological side, lithium did not result to be superior to placebo in the treatment of 30 prepubertal children with depression and a positive family history of mood disorders (40% with a parent with bipolar disorder, 40% with a more distant bipolar familiality and 20% with family history of major depression only) [92]. Divalproex has been openly studied in bipolar offspring with mood or behavioural disorders and mild affective symptoms, but without a full-blown bipolar disorder [93]: of the 23 subjects who completed the study, 18 (78%) were considered responders according to the Clinical Global Impression (CGI) improvement score (very much or much improved). The majority of responders improved within the first 4 weeks of treatment. These preliminary findings suggest a possible preventive pharmacological intervention in a high-risk population not yet with a fully developed bipolar disorder.

Methodological issues of an ongoing 8-week, randomized, placebo-controlled study with antikindling agents in 60 bipolar offspring with either cyclothymia or bipolar disorder not otherwise specified have been reported [94], but results are still not available. Donovan *et al.* [95] did report in a small double blind study that explosive and labile moods in adolescence falling short of clear-cut criteria for bipolarity responded to valproate.

CONCLUSIONS

In the offspring of bipolar patients, a broad spectrum of psychopathology can be observed:

1. Childhood depression is at high risk for bipolar transformation.
2. Childhood anxiety disorders may represent precursors of bipolar I disorder, or alternative clinical expression of bipolar II disorder.
3. ADHD, especially when the parent has a combined ADHD–bipolar disorder diagnosis, is a marker for early-onset bipolar disorder.
4. "Classical" episodic euphoric mania is rare in prepubertal children, unless the parent has a lithium-responding bipolar disorder.
5. Most children diagnosed as bipolar manifest stormy, ultra-rapid-cycling course. Loaded family history for bipolar disorder represents a family marker for this early-onset severe phenotype of bipolar disorder.
6. Temperamental excesses along mood-labile and overconfident lines are often precursors of bipolarity in children.

7. Cyclothymia may predict major depression with suicidality in teens, many of whom have bipolar disorder.
8. Environmental factors represent nonspecific parameters in the precipitation and aggravation of the course of bipolar disorders in children and adolescents.
9. The early detection of prodromal symptoms or signs in this high-risk population offers a window of opportunity for preventive and therapeutic interventions, which may be improved by further longitudinal studies exploring premorbid cognitive and physiological endophenotypes and structural/functional brain abnormalities.

REFERENCES

1. Chang K., Steiner H., Dienes K., Adleman N., Ketter T. (2003). Bipolar offspring: a window into bipolar disorder evolution. *Biol. Psychiatry*, **53**, 945–951.
2. Lish J.D., Dime-Meenan S., Whybrow P.C., Price R.A., Hirschfeld R.M. (1994). The National Depressive and Manic-Depressive Association (DMDA) survey of bipolar members. *J. Affect. Disord.*, **31**, 281–294.
3. Del Bello M.P., Geller B. (2001). Review of studies of child and adolescent offspring of bipolar parents. *Bipolar Disord.*, **3**, 325–334.
4. Akiskal K., Akiskal H.S. (2003). Préface. In: Kochman F., Menard JA (eds) *Les Troubles Bipolaires*. Sanofi-Synthélabo, Paris, pp. 2–3.
5. O'Connell R.A., Mayo J.A., O'Brien J.D., Misrshedaie P. (1979). Children of bipolar manic depressives. In: Mendlewicz J, Shopsin B (eds) *The Genetics of Affective Disorder*. Spectrum, New York, pp. 61–87.
6. Kuyler P.L., Rosenthal L., Igel G., Dunner D.L., Fieve R.R. (1980). Psychopathology among children of manic–depressive patients. *Biol. Psychiatry*, **15**, 589–597.
7. LaRoche C., Cheifetz P.N., Lester E.P. (1981). Antecedents of bipolar affective disorders in children. *Am. J. Psychiatry*, **138**, 986–988.
8. Decina P., Kestembaum C.J., Farber S., Kron L., Gargan M., Sackeim H.A., Fieve R.R. (1983). Clinical and psychological assessment of children of bipolar probands. *Am. J. Psychiatry*, **140**, 548–553.
9. Zahn-Waxler C., Mayfield A., Radke-Yarrow M., McKnew D.H., Cytryn L., Davenport Y.B. (1988). A follow-up investigation of offspring of parents with bipolar disorder. *Am. J. Psychiatry*, **145**, 506–509.
10. Gershon E.S., McKnew D., Cytryn L., Hamovit J., Schreiber J., Hibbs E., Pellegrini D. (1985). Diagnoses in school age children of bipolar affective disorder patients and normal controls. *J. Affect. Disord.*, **8**, 283–291.
11. Kashani J.H., Burk J.P., Horwitz B., Reid J.C. (1985). Differential effects of subtype of parental major affective disorder on children. *Psychiatry Res.*, **15**, 195–204.
12. Klein D.N., Depue R.A., Slater J.F. (1985). Cyclothymia in the adolescent offspring of parents with bipolar affective disorder. *J. Abnorm. Psychol.*, **94**, 115–127.

13. LaRoche C., Cheifetz P.N., Lester E., Schibuk L., DiTommaso E., Engelsmann F. (1985). Psychopathology in the offspring of parents with bipolar affective disorders. *Can. J. Psychiatry*, **30**, 337–343.
14. Hammen C., Gordon D., Burge D., Adrian C., Jaenicke C., Hiroto D. (1987). Maternal affective disorders, illness, and stress: risk for children's psychopathology. *Am. J. Psychiatry*, **144**, 736–741.
15. LaRoche C., Sheiner R., Lester E., Benierakis C., Marrache M., Engelsmann F., Cheifetz P. (1987). Children of parents with manic–depressive illness: a follow-up study. *Can. J. Psychiatry*, **32**, 563–569.
16. Grigoroiu-Serbanescu M., Christodorescu D., Jipescu I., Totoescu A., Marinescu E., Ardelean V. (1989). Psychopathology in children aged 10–17 of bipolar parents: psychopathology rate and correlates of the severity of the psychopathology. *J. Affect. Disord.*, **16**, 167–179.
17. Hammen C., Burge D., Burney E., Adrian C. (1990). Longitudinal study of diagnoses in children of women with unipolar and bipolar affective disorder. *Arch. Gen. Psychiatry*, **47**, 1112–1117.
18. Radke-Yarrow M., Nottelman E., Martinez P., Fox M.B., Belmont B. (1992). Young children of affectively ill parents: a longitudinal study of psychosocial development. *J. Am. Acad. Child Adolesc. Psychiatry*, **31**, 68–77.
19. Carlson G.A., Weintraub S. (1993). Childhood behavior problems and bipolar disorder – relationship or coincidence? *J. Affect. Disord.*, **28**, 143–153.
20. Duffy A., Alda M., Kutcher S., Fusee C., Grof P. (1998). Psychiatric symptoms and syndromes among adolescent children of parents with lithium-responsive or lithium-nonresponsive bipolar disorder. *Am. J. Psychiatry*, **155**, 431–433.
21. Chang K.D., Steiner H., Ketter T.A. (2000). Psychiatric phenomenology of child and adolescent bipolar offspring. *J. Am. Acad. Child Adolesc. Psychiatry*, **39**, 453–460.
22. Wals M., Hillegers M.H., Reichart C.G., Ormel J., Nolen W.A., Verhulst F.C. (2001). Prevalence of psychopathology in children of a bipolar parent. *J. Am. Acad. Child Adolesc. Psychiatry*, **40**, 1094–1102.
23. Duffy A., Alda M., Kutcher S., Cavazzoni P., Robertson C., Grof E., Grof P. (2002). A prospective study of the offspring of bipolar parents responsive and nonresponsive to lithium treatment. *J. Clin. Psychiatry*, **63**, 1171–1178.
24. Egeland J.A., Shaw J.A., Endicott J., Pauls D.L., Allen C.R., Hostetter A.M., Sussex J.N. (2003). Prospective study of prodromal features for bipolarity in well Amish children. *J. Am. Acad. Child Adolesc. Psychiatry*, **42**, 786–796.
25. Akiskal H.S., Downs J., Jordan P., Watson S., Daugherty D., Pruitt D.B. (1985). Affective disorders in referred children and younger siblings of manic–depressives. Mode of onset and prospective course. *Arch. Gen. Psychiatry*, **42**, 996–1003.
26. Chang K.D., Blasey C., Ketter T.A., Steiner H. (2004). Temperament characteristics of child and adolescent bipolar offspring. *J. Affect. Disord.*, **77**, 11–20.
27. McDonough-Ryan P., DelBello M., Shear P.K., Ris D.M., Soutullo C., Strakowski S.M. (2002). Academic and cognitive abilities in children of parents with bipolar disorder: a test of the nonverbal learning disability model. *J. Clin. Exp. Neuropsychol.*, **24**, 280–285.
28. Todd R.D., Reich W., Petti T.A., Joshi P., DePaulo J.R. Jr, Nurnberger J. Jr, Reich T. (1996). Psychiatric diagnoses in the child and adolescent members of extended families identified through adult bipolar affective disorder probands. *J. Am. Acad. Child Adolesc. Psychiatry*, **35**, 664–671.

29. Tsuang M.T., Faraone S.V. (1990). *The Genetics of Mood Disorders*. The Johns Hopkins University Press, Baltimore, MD.
30. Ross C.A., McInnis M.G., Margolis R.L., Shi-Hua L. (1993). Genes with triplet repeats: candidate mediators of neuropsychiatric disorders. *Trends Neurosci.*, **16**, 254–260.
31. Alda M., Grof P., Ravindran L., Cavazzoni P., Duffy A., Grof E., Zvolsky P., Wilson J. (2000). Anticipation in bipolar affective disorder: is age at onset a valid criterion? *Am. J. Med. Genet.*, **96**, 804–807.
32. McInnis M.G., McMahon F.J., Chase G.A., Simpson S.G., Ross C.A., DePaulo J.R. Jr (1993). Anticipation in bipolar affective disorder. *Am. J. Hum. Genet.*, **53**, 385–390.
33. Goossens D., Del Favero J., Van Broeckhoven C. (2001). Trinucleotide repeat expansions: do they contribute to bipolar disorder? *Brain Res. Bull.*, **56**, 243–257.
34. Rice J., Reich T., Andreasen N.C., Endicott J., Van Eerdewegh M., Fishman R., Hirschfeld R.M., Klerman G.L. (1987). The familial transmission of bipolar illness. *Arch. Gen. Psychiatry*, **44**, 441–447.
35. Chang K.D., Blasey C., Katter T.A., Steiner H. (2001). Family environment of children and adolescents with bipolar parents. *Bipolar Disord.*, **2**, 68–72.
36. Akiskal H.S. (1996). The temperamental foundations of mood disorders. In: Mundt C.H., Freeman H.L. (eds) *Interpersonal Factors in the Origin and Course of Affective Disorders*. Gaskell, London, pp. 3–30.
37. Soutullo C.A., DelBello M.P., Ochsner J.E., McElroy S.L., Taylor S.A., Strakowski S.M., Keck P.E. Jr. (2002). Severity of bipolarity in hospitalized manic adolescents with history of stimulant or antidepressant treatment. *J. Affect. Disord.*, **70**, 323–327.
38. Galanter C.A., Carlson G.A., Jensen P.S, Greenhill L.L., Davies M., Li W., Chuang S.Z., Elliott G.R., Arnold L.E., March J.S., *et al.* (2003). Response to methylphenidate in children with attention deficit hyperactivity disorder and manic symptoms in the multimodal treatment study of children with attention deficit hyperactivity disorder titration trial. *J. Child Adolesc. Psychopharmacol.*, **13**, 123–136.
39. Biederman J. (1995). Developmental subtypes of juvenile bipolar disorder. *Harv. Rev. Psychiatry*, **3**, 227–230.
40. Faraone S.V., Biederman J., Wozniak J., Mundy E., Mennin D., O'Donnell D. (1997). Is comorbidity with ADHD a marker for juvenile-onset mania? *J. Am. Acad. Child Adolesc. Psychiatry*, **36**, 1046–1055.
41. Liebenluft E., Charney D.S., Towbin K.E., Bhangoo R.K., Pine D.S. (2003). Defining clinical phenotypes of juvenile mania. *Am. J. Psychiatry*, **160**, 430–437.
42. Cragney J.L., Geller B. (2003). A prepubertal and early adolescent bipolar disorder I phenotype: review of phenomenology and longitudinal course. *Bipolar Disord.*, **5**, 243–256.
43. Carlson G.A., Jensen P.S., Findling R.L., Meyer R.E., Calabrese J., DelBello M.P., Emslie G., Flynn L., Goodwin F., Hellander M., *et al.* (2003). Methodological issues and controversies in clinical trials with child and adolescent patients with bipolar disorder: report of a consensus conference. *J. Child Adolesc. Psychopharmacol.*, **13**, 13–27.
44. Gershon E.S., Hamovit J., Guroff J.J., Guroff J.J., Dibble E., Leckman J.F., Sceery W., Targum S.D., Nurnberger J.I. Jr, Goldin L.R., *et al.* (1982). A family study of schizoaffective, bipolar I, bipolar II, unipolar, and normal control probands. *Arch. Gen. Psychiatry*, **39**, 1157–1167.

45. Lapalme M., Hodgins S., Laroche C. (1997). Children of parents with bipolar disorder: a meta-analysis of risk for mental disorders. *Can. J. Psychiatry*, **42**, 623–631.
46. Akiskal H.S., Maser J.D., Zeller P., Endicott J., Coryell W., Keller M., Warshaw M., Clayton P., Goodwin F. (1995). Switching from "unipolar" to bipolar II: an 11-year prospective study of clinical and temperamental predictors in 559 patients. *Arch. Gen. Psychiatry*, **52**, 114–123.
47. Geller B., Fox L.W., Clark K.A. (1994). Rate and predictors of prepubertal bipolarity during follow-up of 6- to 12-year-old depressed children. *J. Am. Acad. Child Adolesc. Psychiatry*, **33**, 461–468.
48. Faraone S.V., Biederman J., Mennin D., Wozniak J., Spencer T. (1997). Attention-deficit hyperactivity disorder with bipolar disorder: a familial sybtype? *J. Am. Acad. Child Adolesc. Psychiatry*, **36**, 1168–1176.
49. Todd R.D., Reich W., Reich T. (1994). Prevalence of affective disorder in the child and adolescent offspring of a single kindred: a pilot study. *J. Am. Acad. Child Adolesc. Psychiatry*, **33**, 198–207.
50. Wozniak J., Biederman J., Mundy E., Mennin D., Faraone S.V. (1995). A pilot family study of childhood-onset mania. *J. Am. Acad. Child Adolesc. Psychiatry*, **34**, 1577–1583.
51. Kovacs M., Pollock M. (1995). Bipolar disorder and comorbid conduct disorder in childhood and adolescence. *J. Am. Acad. Child Adolesc. Psychiatry*, **34**, 715–723.
52. Masi G., Toni C., Perugi G., Travierso M.C., Millepiedi S., Mucci M., Akiskal H.S. (2003). Externalizing disorders in consecutively referred children and adolescents with bipolar disorder. *Compr. Psychiatry*, **44**, 184–189.
53. Sachs G.S., Baldassano C.F., Truman C.J., Guille C. (2000). Comorbidity of attention deficit – hyperactivity disorder with early- and late-onset bipolar disorder. *Am. J. Psychiatry*, **157**, 466–468.
54. Duffy A., Grof P., Kutcher S., Robertson C., Alda M. (2001). Measures of attention and hyperactivity symptoms in a high-risk sample of children of bipolar parents. *J. Affect. Disord.*, **67**, 159–165.
55. Achenbach T.M. (1991). *Manual for the Child Behavior Checklist/4–18 and 1991 Profile*. University of Vermont Department of Psychiatry, Burlington, VT.
56. Verhulst F.C., van der Ende J., Ferdinand R.F., Kasius M.C. (1997). The prevalence of DSM-III-R diagnoses in a national sample of Dutch adolescents. *Arch. Gen. Psychiatry*, **54**, 329–336.
57. Harrington R., Myatt T. (2003). Is preadolescent mania the same condition as adult mania? A British perspective. *Biol. Psychiatry*, **53**, 961–969.
58. Masi G., Toni C., Perugi G., Mucci M., Millepiedi S., Akiskal H.S. (2001). Anxiety disorders in consecutively referred children and adolescents with bipolar disorder: a neglected comorbidity. *Can. J. Psychiatry*, **46**, 797–802.
59. Benazzi F., Akiskal H.S. (2003). Refining the evaluation of bipolar II: beyond the strict SCID-CV guidelines for hypomania. *J. Affect. Disord.*, **73**, 33–38.
60. Akiskal H.S. (1995). Developmental pathways to bipolarity: are juvenile-onset depressions prebipolar? *J. Am. Acad. Child Adolesc. Psychiatry*, **34**, 754–763.
61. Masi G., Perugi G., Toni C., Millepiedi S., Mucci M., Bertini N., Akiskal H.S. Obsessive–compulsive bipolar comorbidity: focus on children and adolescents. *J. Affect. Disord.*, 78, **175.**
62. Savino M., Perugi G., Simonini E., Soriani A., Cassano G.B., Akiskal H.S. (1993). Affective comorbidity in panic disorder: is there a bipolar connection? *J. Affect. Disord.*, **28**, 155–163.

63. Chen Y.W., Dilsaver S.C. (1995). Comorbidity of panic disorder in bipolar illness: evidence from the Epidemiologic Catchment Area Survey. *Am. J. Psychiatry*, **152**, 280–282.
64. MacKinnon D.F., Xu J., McMahon F.J., Simpson S.G., Stine O.C., McInnis M.G., DePaulo J.R. (1998). Bipolar disorder and panic disorder in families: an analysis of chromosome 18 data. *Am. J. Psychiatry*, **155**, 829–831.
65. Perugi G., Akiskal H.S., Ramacciotti S., Nassini S., Toni C., Milanfranchi A., Musetti L. (1999). Depressive comorbidity of panic, social phobic and obsessive–compulsive disorders: is there a bipolar II connection? *J. Psychiatr. Res.*, **33**, 53–61.
66. MacKinnon D.F., Zandi P.P., Gershon E.S., Nurnberger J.I. Jr., DePaulo J.R. Jr (2003). Association of rapid mood switching with panic disorder and familial panic risk in familial bipolar disorder. *Am. J. Psychiatry*, **160**, 1696–1698.
67. Bertelsen A., Harvald B., Hauge M. (1977). A Danish twin study of manic–depressive disorders. *Br. J. Psychiatry*, **130**, 330–351.
68. Miklowitz D.J., Goldstein M.J., Nuechterlein K.H., Snyder K.S., Mintz J. (1988). Family factors and the course of bipolar affective disorder. *Arch. Gen. Psychiatry*, **45**, 225–231.
69. Conrad M., Hammen C. (1993). Protective and resource factors in high and low-risk children: a comparison of children with unipolar, bipolar, medically ill, and normal mothers. *Dev. Psychopathol.*, **5**, 593–607.
70. Inoff-Germain G., Nottelman E.D., Radke-Yarrow M. (1992). Evaluative communications between affective ill and well mothers and their children. *J. Abnorm. Child Psychol.*, **20**, 189–212.
71. Moos R. (1974). *Family Environment Scale*. Consulting Psychologist Press, Palo Alto, CA.
72. Biederman J., Rosenbaum J.F., Hirshfeld D.R., Faraone S.V., Bolduc E.A., Gersten M., Meminger S.R., Kagan J., Snidman N., Reznick J.S. (1990). Psychiatric correlates of behavioral inhibition in young children of parents with and without psychiatric disorders. *Arch. Gen. Psychiatry*, **47**, 21–26.
73. Hirschfeld-Becker D.R., Biederman J., Faraone S.V., Violette H., Wrightsman J., Rosenbaum J.F. (2002). Temperamental correlates of disruptive behavior disorders in young children: preliminary findings. *Biol. Psychiatry*, **51**, 563–574.
74. Chess S., Thomas A. (1985). Temperamental differences: a critical concept in child health care. *Pediatr. Nurs.*, **11**, 167–171.
75. Carlson G.A. (1995). Identifying prepubertal mania. *J. Am. Acad. Child Adolesc. Psychiatry*, **34**, 750–753.
76. Akiskal H.S., Khani M.K., Scott-Strauss A. (1979). Cyclothymic temperamental disorders. *Psychiatr. Clin. North Am.*, **2**, 527–554.
77. Akiskal H.S., Mallya G. (1987). Criteria for the "soft" bipolar spectrum: treatment implications. *Psychopharmacol. Bull.*, **23**, 68–73.
78. Kochman F.J., Hantouche E.G., Ferrari P., Lancrenon S., Bayart D., Akiskal H.S. (in press). Cyclothymic temperament as a prospective predictor of bipolarity and suicidality in children and adolescents with major depressive disorder. *J. Affect. Disord.*
79. Zahn-Waxler C., Cummings E.M., McKnew D.H., Radke-Yarrow M. (1984). Altruism, aggression, and social interactions in young children with a manic–depressive parent. *Child Dev.*, **55**, 112–122.
80. Windle M., Lerner R.M. (1986). Reassessing the dimensions of temperament individuality across the life span: the Revised Dimensions of Temperament Survey (DOTS-R). *J. Adolesc. Res.*, **1**, 213–230.

81. Kagan J., Reznick J.S., Snidman N. (1988). Biological bases of childhood shyness. *Science*, **240**, 167–171.
82. Hirshfeld-Becker D.R., Biederman J., Calltharp S., Rosenbaum E.D., Faraone S.V., Rosenbaum J.F. (2003). Behavioral inhibition and disinibition as hypothesized precursor of psychopathology. *Biol. Psychiatry*, **53**, 985–999.
83 Windle M. (1991). The difficult temperament in adolescence: associations with substance use, family support, and problem behaviors. *J. Clin. Psychol.*, **47**, 310–315.
84. Post R.M. (1992). Transduction of psychosocial stress into the neurobiology of recurrent affective disorder. *Am. J. Psychiatry*, **149**, 999–1010.
85. Fergus E.L., Miller R.B., Luckenbaugh D.A., Leverich G.S., Findling R.L., Speer A.M., Post R.M. (2003). Is there progression from irritability/dyscontrol to major depressive and manic symptoms? A retrospective community survey of parents of bipolar children. *J. Affect. Disord.*, **77**, 71–78.
86. Luby J.L., Mrakotsky C. (2003). Depressed preschoolers with bipolar family history: a group at high risk for later switching to mania. *J. Child Adolesc. Psychopharmacol.*, **13**, 187–197.
87. Lewinshon P.M., Klein D.N., Seley J. (2000). Bipolar disorder during adolescence and young adulthood in a community sample. *Bipolar Disord.*, **2**, 281–293.
88. Martinez-Aran A., Vieta E., Colom F., Reinares M., Benabarre A., Gasto C., Salamero M. (2000). Cognitive dysfunctions in bipolar disorder: evidence of neuropsychological disturbances. *Psychother. Psychosom.*, **60**, 2–18.
89. Dienes K.A., Chang K.D., Blasey C.M., Adleman N.E., Steiner H. (2002). Characterization of children of bipolar parents by parent report CBCL. *J. Psychiatr. Res.*, **36**, 337–345.
90. DelBello M.P., Soutullo C.A., Ryan P., Graman S.M., Zimmerman M.E., Getz G.E., Lake K.A., Strakowski S.M. (2000). MRI analysis of children at risk for bipolar disorder. *Biol. Psychiatry*, **47** (Suppl.), 13S.
91. Chang K.D., Adleman N., Dienes K., Naama B.-G., Reiss A., Ketter T.A. (2003). Decreased *N*-acetylaspartate in children with familial bipolar disorder. *Biol. Psychiatry*, **53**, 1059–1065.
92. Geller B., Cooper T.B., Zimmerman B., Frazier J., Williams M., Heath J., Warner K. (1998). Lithium for prepubertal depressed children with family history predictors of future bipolarity: a double-blind, placebo-controlled study. *J. Affect. Disord.*, **51**, 165–175.
93. Chang K.D., Dienes K., Blasey C., Adleman N., Ketter T., Steiner H. (2003). Divalproex monotherapy in the treatment of bipolar offspring with mood and behavioral disorders and at least mild affective symptoms. *J. Clin. Psychiatry*, **64**, 936–942.
94. Findling R.L., Gracious B.L., McNamara M.K., Calabrese J.R. (2000). The rationale, design, and progress of two maintenance treatment studies in pediatric bipolarity. *Acta Neuropsychiatrica*, **12**, 136–138.
95. Donovan SJ, Stewart JW, Nunes EV, Quitkin FM, Parides M, Daniel W, Susser E, Klein DF. (2000). Divalproex treatment for youth with explosive temper and mood lability: a double-blind, placebo-controlled crossover design. *Am. J. Psychiatry*, **157**, 818–820.

CHAPTER

6

The "Difficult" Child: Main Underlying Syndromes and Differential Diagnosis

Sam Tyano and Iris Manor

Geha Psychiatric Hospital, Petach-Tikvah, Israel

INTRODUCTION

Of the referrals to child outpatient mental health clinics, the highest percentage is represented by children who are defined as "difficult" and are described more specifically as exhibiting various behavioural problems.

"Difficult" children are those who are not easy to live with. They are the opposite of "easy" children; that is, they create difficulties for the environment in which they live, are a nuisance and draw a lot of attention. Under this label we can find children who are sad, maladjusted, impulsive, post-traumatic, psychotic and so forth. All of them present difficulties to those around them, yet they are totally different from one another.

The common denominator of all these children is a behaviour which is unpleasant, strident to the environment, and creates provocation and friction. Most of them are violent. A large number of them will start off as children with certain difficulties, will develop into annoying and/or infuriating children, and will end up as violent children. Some of them will be diagnosed as psychopaths, a diagnosis that does not exist in current main classifications, but includes those who are emotionally "burnt out" and derive pleasure from violence. Others will be mistakenly diagnosed as psychopaths, since their smooth, unemotional surface conceals depression and anxiety. Other children will be diagnosed under other headings, if they even manage to get that far, and do not remain in the "garbage can" of the generalization "violent children", which in many people's opinion does not necessitate further attention.

Early Detection and Management of Mental Disorders.
Edited by Mario Maj, Juan José López-Ibor, Norman Sartorius, Mitsumoto Sato and Ahmed Okasha.
 ISBN 0-470-01083-5.

A "difficult" child is sometimes one who experiences himself or herself as difficult. A large number of children experience themselves as a heavy burden and are extremely critical of their own behaviour and functioning. Several of these children develop "self-fulfilling prophecies" since, with time, they indeed become hard to handle as a result of the depression and behaviour disorders they develop.

The most sensitive question is distinguishing between the "easy" and the "difficult" child. When does the child's behaviour lose the quality of "easiness"? Every child has occasional outbursts and sometimes hits others, but continuity of difficult behaviour turns the child into a "difficult" one. As opposed to the normal child, who presents outbursts from time to time, the "difficult" child presents these behaviours over time, and even if not continually, at least most of the time.

Another element is that of surprise or, alternatively, suddenness. The "easy" child is likely to have outbursts, lose concentration and be hyperactive and violent in certain circumstances, for example in the event of tiredness, severe emotional stress, etc. On the contrary, the "difficult" child is subject to surprising, unexpected outbursts without any apparent provocation. Thus, when this behaviour appears, it shocks others and angers them by the very fact of its being unexpected.

The third element is the setting: the same behaviours that cause the child to be "difficult" are liable to appear in any setting. It is impossible to expect these problems to be confined to the school or any other oppressive external framework; they will appear in a large variety of frameworks.

Of course, perceiving the child as "difficult" depends not only on the child's behaviour, but also on the parents' patience and tolerance of this behaviour. A child's behaviour may be perceived by one family as normal, and by another family as "difficult", disturbing and even threatening.

In our estimation, for all practical purposes, the boundary between "easy" and "difficult" is the tolerance line. Any time the child's behaviour becomes oppressive and causes suffering to the environment and to himself or herself, he or she is a "difficult" child. Oppression constitutes a necessary, if not sufficient, factor in diagnosing a child as "difficult". The factors that make the child "difficult" will be significant not only for the diagnosis itself, but for the treatment, which will focus on changing these factors, whether they are "child factors" or "family factors".

On the emotional level, the "difficult" child arouses frustration and feelings of indignity and anger, and places the adult who is struggling with him or her in a position of insufficient knowledge, lack of control and doubt. Thus, the "difficult" child stimulates a vicious circle perpetuating difficulty and distress. Accordingly, when we deal with the "difficult" child, we are dealing with a complex child–environment model, which continues to develop over time, and in which interaction soon becomes the central focus.

In this chapter we will discuss those syndromes which are most frequently behind the profile of the "difficult" child and their differential diagnosis. We will devote space and attention to these syndromes according to their relative frequency, with the exception of organic disorders which, due to space constraints, will only be covered in the framework of differential diagnosis.

ASSESSMENT OF THE "DIFFICULT" CHILD

The classical presenting picture of the "difficult" child is that of a parent or a teacher rushing a child with deviant behavioural symptoms to the psychiatrist, while the child himself/herself is usually unaware or denying any existing problem.

The first step in the assessment of the "difficult" child is history taking. This includes detailed medical, developmental and psychiatric history not only of the patient, but of the family as well. All sources of information must be used – the child, his/her parents, teachers, etc. – in order to create a picture as clear as possible of the child's inner and outer world. As part of this history, there are several structured and semistructured interviews dealing with the history of the child. One of the most well known is the Kiddie Schedule for Affective Disorders and Schizophrenia (K-SADS) [1]. This is a semistructured interview that examines many details, with room for clarifications regarding major symptoms of several disorders in the framework of the differential diagnoses mentioned in this chapter.

The next step would be a clinical examination, which should allow the evaluation of possible comorbidities, acute situations, central personality characteristics, strengths and weaknesses and the child's self-perception as an individual and as part of the community. Clinical examination can be structured, semistructured or unstructured. Neurological and physical examinations are a must in this phase of assessment, mostly to rule out organic diagnoses.

At this point, the clinician must assess the gathered data and check if diagnostic criteria of any of the disorders dealt with in this chapter are met. If not, follow-up may still be warranted according to the circumstances and clinical picture. If diagnostic criteria for any disorder are met, the use of rating scales, neuropsychological tests and neuroimaging tools is indicated.

Rating scales, also sometimes called behavioural checklists, allow quantitative ratings of the adult's evaluation of the child's behaviour and are used as a cornerstone in the clinical evaluation of the child. Their drawback is their subjectivity, as well as the adult's limited knowledge of the child's acts and thoughts. Accordingly, they constitute an essential but insufficient evaluation tool.

Rating scales demand judgement of the child's behaviour in binary terms (yes/no) or in quantitative degree of severity. They are very easy to administer and encompass many functional areas, from internalizing conditions such as depression and introversion to externalizing conditions such as violence or delinquency. Prominent examples of such scales are the Child Behavior Checklist (CBCL) and the Revised Child Behavior Checklist (RCBP) [2].

Widely used scales to assess attention-deficit/hyperactivity disorder (ADHD) include the Conners Rating Scale [3] and the Swanson, Nolan and Pelham Questionnaire (SNAP-IV) [4]. The Eyberg Child Behavior Inventory [5] is used to evaluate conduct disorder (CD) and oppositional defiant disorder (ODD). Common scales for the assessment of post-traumatic stress disorder (PTSD) are the Children's PTSD Inventory (CPTSDI) [6], the Trauma Symptom Checklist for Children (TSCC) [7], the Angie/Andy Cartoon Trauma Scale (ACTS) [8], the Pediatric Emotional Distress Scale (PEDS) [9], the Clinician-Administered PTSD Scale for Children (CAPS-C) [10], the Adolescent Dissociative Experience Scale (ADES) [11], the Children's Perceptual Alteration Scale (CPAS) [12] and the Child Dissociative Checklist (CDC) [13]. The most frequently used rating scale for mood disorders is the Childhood Depression Rating Scale – Revised (CDRS-R) [14], which is a modified version of the Hamilton Depression Rating Scale.

Neuropsychological assessment is necessary when there is a suspicion of a brain disorder, or there is already evidence of brain damage and a need to estimate the nature and the extent of the influence of the damage on cognition, personality and behaviour of the injured individual, or it is impossible to evaluate the situation using the conventional tools of the clinical interview or a regular psychological test. There are a number of comprehensive batteries of neuropsychological tests for children. The purpose of all of them is to assess various functions, such as short-term, medium and long-term memory, motor, visual and spatial perception, orientation, language, cognition, constructing and creating concepts, problem solving and more, by means of various performance tasks.

The continuous performance tests assess the child's ability to cope with a relatively monotonous and boring task over time. This method is considered one of the most reliable ways of differentiating between children suffering from ADHD and normal children. There are a number of subtypes of this test: the Conners' Continuous Performance Test [15], the Test of Variables of Attention (TOVA) [16], and others.

ATTENTION DEFICIT/HYPERACTIVITY DISORDER (ADHD)

ADHD is conceptualized as a disorder affecting several life spheres, including learning and social behaviour. However, in light of its prevalence and characteristics, Koschack *et al.* [17] and others consider it a trait, and present it as a differentiated style rather than a dysfunction.

A comparison between the ICD-10 and the DSM-IV demonstrates the different ways this disorder is perceived and the difficulties involved in understanding it. According to the DSM-IV, ADHD belongs to a group of behavioural disorders, also including ODD and CD. According to this system, children fulfilling the criteria for both ADHD and CD are a separate group with different aetiological, clinical and prognostic characteristics. On the other hand, the ICD-10 identifies the group of hyperkinetic disorders, subdivided into a "disorder of activity and attention" and a "hyperkinetic conduct disorder". The ICD-10 makes no mention of pure attention deficit disorder, and the basic requirement for the diagnosis of hyperkinetic disorders is a combination of attention deficit and hyperactivity. This difference from the DSM-IV is significant, because the ICD-10 system actually ignores 30% of the children who suffer from attention difficulties, i.e. 2–3% of all children in the general population. From the American point of view, this means ignoring the difficulties and distress of many children while, from the European point of view, an inappropriate attitude towards those children is prevented. It is clear that this divergence is due to different ideological points of view regarding the appropriate way to define disorders in children.

Epidemiology

From a review of the relevant literature published during the past four years, it seems that the prevalence of ADHD ranges between 7% and 16% [18–22]. This large range of percentages is probably the result of having examined different ages as well having employed different diagnostic tools. Moreover, the possibility of underdiagnosis or overdiagnosis should also be considered. A research study conducted in Israel [23] with adolescents who were at the initial stages of examinations prior to military service (thus, a healthy population sample) found a prevalence of ADHD of 4.9%. Thus, we are discussing a disorder that is prevalent among a population which is defined as healthy.

In clinical studies, the diagnosis of ADHD is more frequent among males than females, with a ratio of 9:1, compared to only 4:1 in epidemiological studies. Part of the gap between boys and girls may be explained by the fact that the disorder is much more easily identified in boys, due to their marked hyperactivity, i.e. the gap is in part the result of selective referral of boys to clinics. Nevertheless, the fact that a difference between boys and girls was also evident in epidemiological studies indicates that boys have an intrinsic greater tendency to develop ADHD.

ADHD is prevalent among all social strata, with no relationship to social or economic status. In clinical studies there is indeed a higher prevalence of patients from lower socioeconomic status, but this is probably due to the more frequent referral of these patients to public clinics, which can be more easily monitored.

Contrary to what was believed in the past, ADHD does not disappear in adolescence. The most frequent diagnostic age is the elementary school, when the disorder becomes evident due to educational and social requirements. Another wave of referrals is at junior high school age, when there is an increase in the number of adolescents who are diagnosed as having a pure attention deficit disorder, detected as a result of increasingly complex school requirements. The accepted estimate to date is that two-thirds of ADHD children continue to suffer from it in adulthood, although the hyperactivity component fades somewhat, whereas in a third of subjects the disorder partially or totally fades [24,25].

Clinical Picture

Early Childhood

The three components that constitute the basis for the diagnosis of ADHD, both at school age and earlier, are inattention, impulsiveness and hyperactivity. Nevertheless, levels of activity and attention in infancy are totally different from those at the kindergarten or school stage. In most cases, a suspicion of ADHD is not raised before the age of 2 years. When a 1-year-old baby is very active, does not sleep very much during the day, wakes up frequently at night, does not have regular biological rhythms and does not play on his/her own, the tendency is to diagnose a difficult character, in other words, a variation within the norm, and not ADHD, which is a deviation from the norm. When there is in addition a disturbance in senso-motor regulation, a diagnosis of regulation disorder will usually be made [26].

In a longitudinal research study from birth until the age of 7 years, Palfrey *et al.* [27] found that only 3% of parents of infants up to the age of 14 months expressed concern regarding inattention or hyperactivity problems in their children, compared to 13% of parents of children aged 14 to 29 months. Forty percent of children showed varied levels of ADHD up to kindergarten age, while only 5% continued to suffer from it later on.

The diagnosis should include physical, emotional, cognitive/developmental and family examinations. Blackman [28] suggests the following criteria for distinguishing between troublesome behaviours and ADHD in early childhood: (a) a cluster of hyperactivity, impulsiveness and/or distraction that is higher in intensity and frequency than what would be expected at the child's age and developmental stage; (b) the symptoms are prolonged for over 12 months; (c) the symptoms should be evident in different situations and in the presence of people who are not the child's parents; and (d) there is a decline in social and familial functioning as a result of these symptoms.

Elementary School Children

Understanding the situation at this age is based on what we call the "pearl model" [29]. A pearl evolves as a result of a grain of some substance penetrating into an oyster, while layers are built up around it as a result of interaction between the irritant and the body of the oyster. The perception nowadays is that ADHD is fundamentally organic, i.e. it results from a minor change in the brain's structure and its functioning. Due to continuous interactions of the child with him/herself and the outside world, layers of psychological and social characteristics are formed around the organic grain, that eventually shape a clinical picture.

The "classical" child with ADHD is one who got through the early developmental years with no difficulty. Parents frequently describe him or her as an easy child, at times a bit naughty, but certainly not beyond the normal range for his or her age. An intelligent child will frequently be described as concentrating well when the child has an initial interest in the subject at hand and determines the rate of progress. Typical examples of this are television, computers and Lego, in all three of which the problem of mobilizing and sustaining attention is circumvented, since they provide changing stimuli that are intrinsically interesting to the child and two of them include a defined scenario, which in itself enables attention to be mobilized.

The first period in which difficulties begin to be reported for these children is when academic demands begin. As attention, memory and organizing abilities gain in importance, difficulties begin to surface. In accordance with this, the peak period for diagnosing ADHD is during elementary school, especially in the lower grades. The most common case is of a child who arrives apparently with no former problem or difficulties (apparently – since a retrospective analysis reveals that slight difficulties and attention problems were evident but were ignored), and suddenly finds himself or herself in a situation in which he or she starts to have difficulties and to fail.

The Educational Aspect

The educational aspect mainly involves frustration and underachievement that may not always be apparent on the surface. When we are dealing with overt underachievement, the frustration is greater, but the difficulty is easier to detect, so that a referral may be made for diagnosis and treatment. On the other hand, covert underachievement may remain undetected, or may only be detected at a much later stage, when there has already been irreparable damage to motivation and learning habits. The major protective factors are high IQ, motivation, strong family support and the earliest possible diagnosis and treatment. Among the major risk factors are other learning disabilities, concealment, denying that there is difficulty and comorbidity in the child or in the family.

The Social Aspect

With entry into elementary school, the sudden shock and decline in learning proficiency is frequently accompanied by a parallel decline in social functioning. It is possible to divide ADHD children into two types. The first group of children has good social skills and abilities that serve as a protective factor. These children use their social acumen as a compensation and disguise for their learning difficulties. The self-esteem of these children is less damaged and their inner perceptions are much better. Despite this, it is not uncommon in conversation for them to express hurt and anger regarding matters connected with learning. They also consider themselves stupid, or at least "unfit for learning", and this is an ever-present weak spot in their lives and performance. The other, more problematic group includes those children who have both social and learning difficulties.

To sum up, the basic problem, which is organic in nature, is accompanied by social difficulties that are no less problematic, perhaps even more so, academically speaking. This is due to the fact that finding a solution to social problems is more time-consuming and complex, and dependent on how fixated the ADHD child is on his or her low social or academic status.

OPPOSITIONAL DEFIANT DISORDER (ODD) AND CONDUCT DISORDER (CD)

ODD is characterized by disobedient, rebellious and negative behaviour. There is a gradual appearance of quarrels with adults, and outbreaks of rage, anger and resentment, which range from slight to annoying. The child transgresses rules and laws of authority figures, behaves rebelliously towards them and provokes their anger. He or she tends to blame others for his/her mistakes and behaviour.

It is extremely rare that ODD does not appear at home, but it does definitely happen that its expression in other frameworks is minor. Generally the start of the clinical expression is at home, and at a later stage it spreads to educational and social frameworks outside the home. In this case, the child is likely to suffer from relatively lower academic achievement than his/her ability warrants and social isolation. Then, damage to self-esteem, mood disorders and substance abuse are liable to appear.

Especially worrisome is the evolution of the disorder to CD. In this case, symptoms will appear that pose a threat to others' rights: bullying, arson, abuse of humans and animals, sexual assault, theft and more. Obviously, the individual clinical expression of the symptoms will be in accordance with the child's age and developmental stage.

The age of onset of ODD is early childhood, whereas the age of onset of CD is early adolescence, although it is possible to diagnose it as early as at age 8. There are researchers who see a developmental progression between the two disorders, but this issue remains open to research. The age of onset seems to be earlier in children who also suffer from ADHD [30].

The average prevalence reported in current available studies is 6% of all boys and 11% of all girls for ODD, and 7–8% of boys and 3–4% of girls for CD [31]. Other researchers report an even higher prevalence for ODD, fluctuating between 5% and 25% [32].

According to a survey conducted by Burke *et al.* [33], ODD is a relatively benign disorder, but it increases the risk for CD. The frequency of the development of ODD to CD in girls is not clear, since girls tend to develop CD without a history of ODD. It is also not clear if the less serious characteristics of CD in girls, such as lying, develop into more serious ones, such as theft.

POST-TRAUMATIC STRESS DISORDER (PTSD)

PTSD is an emotional and behavioural syndrome following a traumatic event in the family or outside it. In the family setting, it is the result of traumas such as physical or sexual abuse, or the loss of a parent. Outside the family, it is connected with traffic accidents, natural disasters, war or terror. In childhood PTSD, the person's subjective experience of the event is at least as important as any objective characteristics of the trauma [34].

As opposed to what was thought in the past, there is evidence now that children are more likely to develop PTSD than adolescents and adults [35,36]. This tends to be more true of girls than boys, although this finding is still questionable [37,38]. Accordingly, this is a diagnosis that requires attention and should be ruled out in every case of a "difficult" child who is referred for evaluation.

The DSM–IV category of PTSD mainly concerns adults. Scheeringa *et al.* [39] developed a set of alternative criteria, in which re-experiencing is expressed by reiterative games, recollection of the event, nightmares, flashbacks and distress at discovering elements that recall the event. Numbing is expressed by limited play activities and social introversion, limited affect and loss of developmental skills that had already appeared. Arousal is expressed as nightmares, insomnia, waking up frequently, loss of concentration, hypervigilance and exaggerated startle response. In addition, there is a unique subgroup of symptoms, including new aggressiveness, renewed appearance of separation anxiety, fear of going to the bathroom alone, fear of the dark or any apparently baseless suddenly appearing fear.

There are no studies to date estimating prevalence of PTSD in children. Yule's survey [40] presents a number of reports from recent years, according to which the incidence rate in children who underwent a traffic accident is around 20%, while it is about 10–12% in children who were hospitalized as a result of "common childhood mishaps". Children who develop PTSD as a result of injury may be the same children who suffer from ADHD or ODD, since children from these populations tend to be more involved in accidents and various injuries.

PTSD in children includes three groups of symptoms: recurrent experience of the trauma, avoidance traits (such as emotional withdrawal, refusal to deal with the trauma, etc.) and arousal symptoms (such as insomnia, irritability, concentration difficulties and heightened startle response) [41]. The third group of symptoms is the one that makes these children "difficult".

In the initial stage, the child generally reacts to the trauma with separation anxiety, and in more severe cases with regression (e.g. bedwetting at night). Regression can at times be to very early stages of childhood. A 10-year-old child who arrived at our clinic about 6 years ago, whose classmates introduced a pencil into his sexual organ, regressed to a developmental stage of 2 years old for a period of a year and only regained speech 4 years after the trauma. Difficulties with falling asleep and waking up in the middle of the night appear. A lower stimulus threshold is present, as well as expressions of unexpected aggression. The most important element in the diagnosis is the change that takes place in the child's behaviour. This change, when compared with previous behaviour, must bring the clinician to suspect a traumatic event.

MOOD DISORDERS

Mood disorders in children and adolescents are often severe and liable to cause significant morbidity and mortality [42,43]. For several years childhood depression was underdiagnosed, but today we are better able to identify and diagnose it in early childhood. Mania is undergoing the same process today. In certain cases, what was defined as ADHD or behaviour disorder turns out to be a "covert mania". In follow-up studies of ADHD and disruptive behaviours, a high frequency of mood disorders (including bipolar disorder) has been observed, which were diagnosed at a later stage in the child's life. Therefore, the greater our ability to refine the clinical criteria of mania in children and develop suitable scales, the better will we be able to identify maniform conditions at a younger age and differentiate them from ADHD and behaviour disorders. However, bipolar disorder, ADHD, disruptive behaviours and drug abuse are also likely to co-occur in the same subjects [44]. These subjects are also more likely to undergo traumas and fulfil criteria for PTSD.

Estimates regarding the prevalence of major depression in children and adolescents range between 4% [45] and 25% [46]. Mania is a much rarer disorder: less than 1% of children and adolescents suffer from manic symptoms. The appearance of depression or mania is more frequent in adolescents than in children. In children, the prevalence of major depression is equal in males and females, whereas in adolescence this ratio changes to 2:1 in favour of girls. The prevalence of bipolar disorder is identical for both sexes at all ages.

Major Depression

According to the DSM-IV, the criteria for diagnosing childhood and adolescent depression are identical to those for adults, apart from the fact that irritability can appear instead of sadness. In addition, the depressed child tends to exhibit anxiety symptoms (for example, abandonment anxiety), somatic complaints and behavioural modifications to a greater extent than adults. This clinical profile, even though it is not specific, must cause the clinician to suspect depression.

The age of the depressed child and his/her mental level play a central role in the clinical profile of the disorder. Most children do not demonstrate affective verbal expressions before the age of 7. They express depression by means of nonverbal communication, such as facial expressions or bodily stance, whose exact interpretation by the clinician demands considerable experience and sensitivity. At school age, not only does the child's ability to verbally describe his/her mood improve, but teachers' parameters are added as well as the child's functional level in school as a means of evaluating his/her condition. In adolescence, depression becomes gradually more similar to adult depression.

In treating the child who is suffering from ADHD, it is important to remember that psychostimulants are liable to arouse a clinical depression which was previously covert. Depressive symptoms also play a prominent role in the clinic for children with CD/ODD. On the other hand, a behaviour disorder may lead the child to recurrent social failures that in turn lead to damage of self-worth and subsequently to depression. Accordingly, depression is one of the main phenomena that must be examined and discounted in children exhibiting any kind of behaviour disorder. This demand is especially vital in light of the empathic failure that these children create, due to which internalizing disorders are not examined or diagnosed sufficiently [47].

PTSD is also characterized by a high prevalence of depressive symptoms. Many children who exhibit clinical depression conceal a history of acute or chronic trauma. In addition, these children are liable to be "many-layered": i.e. depression may be the most prominent clinical feature, and only a more in-depth evaluation will make it possible to locate the old trauma and other characteristics of PTSD, which are hiding beneath the behavioural turmoil. This combination of PTSD and depression is one of the most challenging and difficult to decipher conditions among those included under the heading of "the difficult child".

Bipolar Disorder

Children generally tend to exhibit mixed states, with short periods of strong lability of mood and irritability [48]. This causes diagnostic difficulties and creates situations of underdiagnosis. In adolescents, the clinical presentation is very similar to that of adults: elated mood or irritability, pressured speech, excessive sexuality, delusions of grandeur and lack of sleep.

A psychotic profile can accompany depression or mania, and this is an indication of seriousness and a risk factor for recurrence.

Epidemiological studies show that children and adolescents suffering from bipolar disorder almost always develop additional disorders [49]. These generally include CD, ODD and ADHD, as well as substance abuse and anxiety disorders. Several researchers are convinced that bipolar disorder appearing at a young age represents a more difficult and persistent form of the illness [50]. Suicidal ideation and attempts are at least as frequent in bipolar adolescents as in adults.

A striking characteristic is the familial connection between ADHD, bipolar disorder and behavioural disorders, and the branching out at later stages of one diagnosis (bipolar disorder) from the earlier diagnoses (ADHD or behavioural disorder). This indicates the importance of bipolar disorder in relation to the "difficult" child, who is generally diagnosed initially as suffering from ADHD or behavioural disorder or from a combination of the two.

Outcome

At least 50% of children and adolescents suffering from major depression, and 90% of those suffering from bipolar disorder, will continue to suffer from it in adulthood. Pine *et al.* [51] showed that depressive symptoms in adolescence (even without the existence of major depression) strongly predict a major depressive episode in adulthood. Little is known of the longitudinal outcome of childhood-onset mania. Geller *et al.* [48] checked the outcome of 89 children with mania and found poor outcome: low recovery rates and high relapse rates compared with adults. They could not rule out the hypothesis that childhood mania responds less well to mood stabilizers. Moreover, prepubertal onset is associated with rapid cycling and worse prognosis [52]. Early-onset and comorbidity cases are expected to suffer from this disorder in adulthood as well [52].

DIFFERENTIAL DIAGNOSIS

Childhood-onset Psychosis

The clinical picture of childhood-onset psychosis may include a tendency towards isolation and becoming reserved and withdrawn, but also soft neurological signs, delayed language development and attention deficit. These features, which might be characteristic of children who suffer from ADHD, do sometimes cause diagnostic confusion. They raise the question of whether a child who was diagnosed with ADHD and later with schizophrenia suffered from the outset from early signs of the latter disorder.

This question is important, since the traditional treatment for ADHD, i.e. psychostimulants, conflicts with the common treatment for schizophrenia, and there are those who assert that it might even increase the risk of developing the symptoms of the latter disorder. In a recent study, ADHD was diagnosed in 31% of first-degree relatives of schizophrenic patients, much more than should be expected in the general population [53]. In addition, it was found that among these children there were more prominent characteristics of cognitive and perceptive disturbances, as well as neurological signs. Obviously, these findings strengthen the suspicion that these early symptoms can be preliminary signs for the development of schizophrenia.

Children suffering from ODD are also likely to camouflage signs of childhood psychosis. Impaired judgement of reality and cognitive disabilities are liable to appear as promiscuous behaviour, violence and delinquency such as theft or lying, which the child does not perceive as such due to the distorted reality in which he/she lives [54]. Treatment of ODD is indeed closer to treatment of psychotic conditions than treatment of ADHD. However, if the child is actually suffering from psychosis, it constitutes insufficient and incorrect treatment, so that the differential diagnosis is an important one.

Children suffering from PTSD are also likely to be misleading by creating a pseudo-psychotic picture, primarily due to the dissociative characteristics that accompany this disorder. For example, children who have undergone sexual abuse frequently exhibit dissociative, sexual/seductive or anxious behaviours [55,56]. These children are also likely to exhibit visual and auditory hallucinations caused by "flashbacks", irritability and mistrust, detachment and avoidance. These characteristics are liable to suggest the presence of a psychotic condition, especially if the clinician has not considered the possibility of physical or sexual trauma.

Pervasive Developmental Disorders (PDD)

The differentiation between pervasive developmental disorders (PDD) and ADHD may appear obvious. However, many children who have these disorders in various degrees of severity also exhibit symptoms of ADHD and even respond well to psychostimulants. This is especially true of Asperger's syndrome, which is more elusive from a diagnostic point of view than the other syndromes belonging to this group. Since the main characteristics of Asperger's syndrome include severe and persistent disturbances in social interactions and development of limited and repetitive behavioural patterns, interests and activities, these children show a significant clinical impairment in important functional areas such as the social or occupational sphere. An example of the confusion in this area is given by the work of Ghaziuddin *et al.* [57], which describes comorbidities of Asperger's syndrome and shows that the most common comorbidity in these children is that with ADHD.

A study that examined the development of children who were later diagnosed with PDD not otherwise specified (PDD-NOS) compared to children with ADHD found that in early childhood it was very hard to detect any significant differences between the groups [58]. In an examination of the social functioning of children suffering from ADHD, high functioning autism or PDD-NOS [59], the children with autism were characterized by the highest (least normative) scores on social functioning scales; the next highest scores were of children with PDD-NOS, and the lowest were those of ADHD children. On the other hand, on the "acting-out" scale, the highest scores were given to children with ADHD, whereas on the "social insight" scale there was no difference between children with ADHD and those with PDD-NOS.

Another group of researchers [60] compared children with PDD-NOS, ADHD or other mental disorders and healthy controls according to their ability to recognize emotions and theory of mind (ToM). Children with PDD-NOS and with ADHD showed difficulties in emotion recognition and ToM in ways that could not be distinguished from one another. In contrast, children who exhibited behavioural disorders or depression did not show such difficulties and responded like healthy children. A distinction between the two groups of ADHD and PDD-NOS could only be made for second-order functioning in the ToM.

From a therapeutic point of view, it was also found that children suffering from PDD responded as well to stimulants as did children with ADHD [61]. The main observable response was relief from restlessness and excess movement. At the same time, it was found that attention improved as well.

Another important differential diagnosis is that between children with PDD and those suffering from PTSD. Some PTSD characteristics in infancy (overarousal and hypervigilance on the one hand, and detachment, recoiling from people and introversion on the other) are similar to those of PDD. Much further research is needed in this sphere.

Organic Syndromes

In every diagnostic and evaluative process of a child suffering from a mental disorder, it is necessary to take into account the possibility that an organic condition exists that is causing or exacerbating the disorder. A physical examination must be performed, including a full neurological examination and routine blood tests. In every case where there is a suspicion of physical illness, experts from other fields must be consulted and supplementary tests performed, such as imaging procedures. Overlooking a physiological factor and delaying treatment of it is liable to be fatal or lead to irreparable damage, therefore a high suspicion index and a rapid response on the part of the psychiatrist are essential.

Several physical disorders may produce psychiatric symptoms: they include tumours, intoxications, nutritional deficiencies and metabolic disorders. Unusual mental symptoms, positive results in physiological or neurological examinations or laboratory tests, signs of cognitive impairment or a family history of hereditary physical illness must all arouse suspicion and stimulate further investigation.

An additional significant element is the high risk of comorbidity between "difficult child" syndromes and a secondary organic disorder due to physical injury. For example, children suffering from ADHD tend to bruise more easily, suffer from injuries demanding hospitalization and from head injuries and develop organic residua. In a study by DiScala *et al.* [62], the characteristics of injuries suffered by ADHD children were compared to those of children not suffering from this disorder. It was found that children suffering from ADHD are more likely to be injured as pedestrians or cyclists and to suffer from self-inflicted injuries. In addition, they are more likely to suffer from multiple physical injuries, head injuries and more severe injuries. The time they spent in hospital was longer, and they were referred to the intensive care unit more frequently. In this study, 53% of the cases resulted in long-term injury or disability, as opposed to 48% in non-ADHD children. As a result, they were also referred more often to rehabilitation wards. Another study [63], conducted in children who suffered closed head injuries, showed a high prevalence of ADHD prior to the injury. In addition, many children developed ADHD after the injury.

The possible development of a vicious circle, in which ADHD or behaviour disorder will expose the child to physical injury, and the physical injury will lead to a deterioration of behaviour, should be considered.

Differential Diagnoses of ADHD in Early Childhood

ADHD in early childhood presents a slightly different and unique differential diagnosis. The conditions to be considered are the following:

1. A deviation from the norm (difficult temperament), involving difficulty in regulation, much crying, difficulty in calming down, hyperactivity, etc.
2. Children who have been given no clear limits.
3. Behavioural disorder or rebellious opposition disorder. Rarer at these ages, although they exist.
4. Deviations in IQ (talented/retarded).

5. Spasms of petit mal type. This condition causes staring into space and dissociation. It appears mostly at ages 5–6 years, but might appear even earlier. The disease is relatively easy to diagnose, since a characteristic pattern can be detected on electroencephalogram.
6. Chronic inflammation of the middle ear, antihistaminic medications.
7. Undiagnosed sight and hearing problems.
8. Other physical and/or chronic conditions, such as hyperthyroidism, hypothyroidism and severe anaemia.
9. Genetic syndromes: fragile X syndrome, William's syndrome, neuro-developmental pervasive disorder.
10. PDD.
11. Psychosis.
12. Infancy affective disorders, including anxiety disorder, infantile depression and mixed disorder of emotional expressiveness. In these children, the inappropriateness of affect stands out more than attention difficulties, although these certainly exist.
13. Child–parent attachment disorder with self-endangerment [64]. In this case, the tendency for self-endangerment, aggressiveness and impulsiveness displayed by the small child are aimed at capturing the attention of an unavailable or incapable parent, and for this reason they will appear mainly when the child is interacting with the parent. In severe and prolonged cases, these behaviours will appear in the presence of any adult whom the child sees as a potential psychological parent.
14. Regulatory disorders, motorically disorganized/impulsive type: although the concept of regulatory disorders in affect, attention and processing sensory information is well known to clinicians, much work is still needed in order to determine the validity of these diagnoses.
15. PTSD of infancy. Irritability and attention difficulties are very common in young children who have experienced trauma, yet the origins of PTSD and ADHD are entirely different, so in most cases it is easy to distinguish between the two. At the same time, in complex cases where the young child is chronically exposed to difficult experiences, diagnosis is harder.

PROGNOSIS

The prognosis of the "difficult" child is extremely variable. Two "difficult" children exhibiting a similar clinical picture and sometimes sharing the same diagnosis can develop in two opposite directions: one will grow up to be a mentally healthy adult, free from the symptoms from which he suffered in childhood; the other will exhibit increasingly more symptoms, suffer from one or more disorders as described in this chapter, develop comorbid disorders, such as substance abuse, and later decline rapidly into a situation of significant social dysfunction.

The prognosis depends on several factors, including the diagnosis, the severity of the symptoms, the age of onset of the difficulties, the child's other characteristics (traits, tendencies, IQ, etc.), the interaction of the child with his/her family and the legitimization given him/her to function at different levels, the environmental demands, the support systems, the nature of individual and family coping, the nature of treatment and the response to it. Concerning pharmacological treatment, several factors are to be considered: the existence of an effective pharmacological treatment; the specific effectiveness for the individual child; whether the parents are prepared to give medication to their children. This last question may sound rather strange, but in many parts of the world there is a widespread apprehension regarding pharmacological treatment, accompanied by stigma and ignorance, so that even if there is an effective, available medication, parents refuse to administer it.

AN INTEGRATIVE–DYNAMIC MODEL OF THE DIFFICULT CHILD

Our understanding of the "difficult" child is based on our perception of three major components: (a) the integration among personality components, (b) the interaction between the child and the environment and (c) the dynamic of these processes.

The development of the "difficult" child is based on an organic nucleus that is in constant interaction with other characteristics of the person carrying it. In addition, and important to the same degree, is the interaction that develops between the child and his/her environment, starting with his/her parents and ending with large social systems. These interactions determine the development of the difficult child's characteristics, and in fact constitute a central factor in formulating the diagnosis, whether it is ADHD, ODD/CD or PTSD. Not surprisingly, in light of the complexity of these processes, it may be expected that there will be multiple diagnoses. In fact, these diagnoses are only descriptive; that is, they describe symptoms, and their developmental process is common in more fundamental ways. In addition, since frequently there is a common aetiological source, the same child is likely to be diagnosed differently at different stages in his/her development. Here dynamism, the third component of the model, enters the picture.

In our view, alongside the integration of the three axes, there is an additional important component in understanding the "difficult" child: the time continuum. The subject of time is raised often in matters such as the time when the symptoms appeared and the developmental process of the disorder, since development is dynamic by definition. Furthermore, continuity is referred to, for example in the area of ADHD. One of the criteria of DSM-IV deals with the importance of the presence of at least some of the symptoms before the age of 7. This continuity is crucial for understanding the integrative nature of the disorder and its having a primary organic source, but it also sheds additional light on the process. Since development is dynamic, the child progressively changes from one point in time to another. This stems from two reasons.

First, the biological clock acts differently in different situations, so that different syndromes and disorders, including innate ones, appear at different points in time and modify existent interactions. Over and above these changes, there are also environmental changes, which are synchronized with time, for example, school entry, passing from one grade to another and accompanying changes in academic requirements, entry into social frameworks, such as youth groups, etc. These changes may seem artificial (not built-in), but since they are environmental, and the environment has a tremendous impact on phenomenological development, they are no less important than innate organic factors. These changes are time-dependent, and their existence exacerbates or discourages further development of the "difficult child" phenomenon as well as determining its final form.

Second, the same disorders existing at a certain age are likely to appear totally different at another point in time, again due to changes in the interactions they create between the child and the environment. Therapy constitutes an additional factor, which creates different interactions, biological, as well as psychological and social. In this part of the continuity factor it is possible to include the concept of risk factors and protective factors, or alternatively the currently more acceptable concept of resilience. This phenomenon is much broader than the factors themselves, but stems from the continuous interaction among them, which is dynamic and has an existence of its own.

It is interesting to compare the time motif in the development of the "difficult child" with the time motif in normative development. In childhood, there exist two opposing concepts of time: "maternal time" and "paternal time". Paternal time deals with external, real time, and is in many senses unavoidable; it reflects the laws of reality that are a combination of natural and man-made laws. The child grows, he or she secretes hormones, learning requirements change according to age, while social demands change as well. On the other hand, maternal time reflects the child's internal experience, and his ability to experience change and cope with it. Abnormal development means that these two times gradually separate, so that the child cannot experience from within the changes and demands that are perceived as imposed from without, leading to a disconnection and "freezing" of time in various pathological ways. While working with children, we frequently observe how parents encountering different organic difficulties of their child, as well as various systems that deal with the child, attempt to cope with the child's difficulties by means of the time continuum, in other words, by stopping the progress of time and its demands, so that it will be in accord with the child's development. A typical example of this is keeping a child in the kindergarten for another year, although he is supposed to advance to first grade. The explanation given by the parents and the system is "to allow the child to mature", but this explanation is problematic, since maturity means the creation of renewed harmony among the different developmental axes. Thus, harmony should be achieved by closing gaps, by treating organic difficulties and by processing traumas, not by artificially intervening in the time clock. This intervention in systemic frameworks is an illusion, since it creates the impression that it is possible to stop time. This is a dangerous illusion in itself, but it is even more dangerous when it encourages one to ignore a constant ongoing time-dependent dynamic process. This is liable to be the ultimate factor in the development of the "difficult child". This is due to the fact that the child who has suffered until now from ADHD or an untreated traumatic syndrome will gradually become a child whose environment cannot support him or her, and who gets no enjoyment out of his or her development.

A significant principle stems from recognizing the time element and its importance: that of equilibrium. The child's functioning is based on equilibrium, which constitutes the different protective and risk factors that make up the child's different characteristics and the interaction among them. The importance of time lies both in the existence of a constantly fluid process and of key points that mark changes within this process. That is, in the same way that it is impossible to bathe twice in the same river, it is impossible to diagnose the same child twice. The change that occurs is ongoing, continuous and inevitable. In other words, both the integration and the interaction that make up the personality model are in constant motion, while factors are added to the equation and subtracted from it at all times. However, as was stated above, we have here dynamic and not static equilibrium. It follows from this that risk factors are those in which equilibrium is upset, which is likely to happen at any time, but especially at key points. For example, a risk factor is when a child with ADHD enters first grade and is expected to do things that were not demanded of him in the past. Naturally, additional factors enter into the set of "considerations":

intelligence, strengths, additional traits, the existence of an additional diagnosis, the fact of the child's diagnosis before he enters school, whether he is being treated, etc. In a situation in which equilibrium is upset, symptoms appear, so this is the time when it is possible to make a diagnosis and begin preventive treatment (according to DSM-IV, it is impossible to offer treatment until distress is evident). On the other hand, at this stage the symptoms are liable to begin developing at a rapid rate, so that early preventive treatment must be immediate.

On the other hand, the fact of dynamism provides an advantage and protection, since in the same way as equilibrium may be upset, so can it be righted when there is continual change. Diagnosis, the beginning of treatment or changes in it, different living conditions and so forth are all likely to facilitate a return of equilibrium. This is an additional reason for the importance of early diagnosis and treatment: when equilibrium is righted, the phenomenon of the "difficult child" will recede.

A necessary conclusion from what was stated above is that in opposition to different psychiatric or psychological diagnoses, the "difficult child" phenomenon is itself time-dependent, and is definitely likely to be temporary. The same child who was "difficult" yesterday is likely to be an "easy" or "normal" child (or any other opposing judgmental expression) tomorrow, according to the place at which his equilibrium system is located in the field of motion.

CONCLUSIONS

The "difficult" child is a behavioural term, which expresses the attitude of adults towards the child's adjustment difficulties to his/her environment on the one hand and the manner in which the child expresses his/her distress on the other. Since frequently what is presented is a symptom, this behaviour encompasses a range of professional diagnoses. We discussed in this chapter the most prevalent diagnoses that come to expression in this way. In order to facilitate understanding, we divided these disorders, but it is important to mention that not only does comorbidity exist among them, but more than half the children suffering from one of them is suffering from an additional psychiatric disorder.

Behaviour disorder is the most prevalent presenting symptom in children referred to outpatient clinics. Prompt diagnosis in these cases is especially crucial due to its preventative aspect. With the tools at our disposal today, we can prevent the development of the disorder in adolescence or adulthood. In other cases we can help the child arrive at a satisfactory integration into his/her immediate environment in order to develop with the maximum utilization of the creative and intellectual potential at his or her disposal. It is necessary to begin this diagnosis as early as infancy, so as to warn the environment regarding the existence of a disorder and help the family arrive at a new equilibrium. This will allow the child to find his or her place in the family dynamic and later in the social environment.

An understanding of the "difficult" child is based on the bio-psycho-social model at all its levels. At the aetiological level, it affords a broad understanding of the syndrome's development, starting from the genetic and up to the environmental–cultural level. At the clinical level, it allows deployment of the clinic. This begins with understanding neurotransmitter levels and the way brain waves function and ends with the impact on the environment of the child's behaviour and his or her interactions with it that reflect on all aspects of life. At the therapeutic level, this model demands combined treatment, which touches a totality of symptomatic characteristics and affords parallel and decisive attention to the child's various difficulties.

We suggest a model based on the integration and interaction between all the various characteristics, both external and internal, of the child's world, in addition to the time-perception component, which is significant in understanding the development rate of this syndrome as well as its recession and situational circumstances. In other words, we suggest a model in which a dynamic syndrome is presented, which is likely to worsen or improve at different times and in different circumstances according to the child's situation. This dynamic model of increased severity or improvement emphasizes both the importance of early preventive therapy, which advances improvement of the syndrome, and its situational nature as reflected in its social and cultural aspects.

The "difficult" child in one situation will be an easy and convenient child in another. Understanding this dynamic imparts to the syndrome the dimension of a trait, as well as emphasizing and strengthening the importance of a total therapeutic approach.

An internal difficulty in the child's normative development can be expressed in deviant behaviour. This behaviour, a temporary external reaction, must be examined in order to help the child, but will not necessarily lead to his or her diagnosis, i.e. to the existence of psychopathology. In conclusion, we suggest here an approach which views the "difficult" child as a child who suffers from biological, emotional or social disharmony. This child, under specific and individual stress factors, including temperament, internal and external demands, and interaction with the environment will develop the "difficult child syndrome". The syndrome is onion-like, hence it needs a careful and patient evaluation in order to be fully understood.

REFERENCES

1. Chambers W.J., Puig-Antich J., Hirsch M., Paez P., Ambrosini P.J., Tabrizi M.A., Davies M. (1985). The assessment of affective disorders in children and adolescents by semistructured interview. Test–retest reliability of the Schedule for Affective Disorders and Schizophrenia for school-age children, present episode version. *Arch. Gen. Psychiatry*, **42**, 696–702.
2. Achenbach T.M. (1991). *Manual for the Child Behavior Checklist 14–18 and 1991 Profile*. University of Vermont, Department of Psychiatry, Burlington, VT.
3. Conners C.K. (1997). *The Conners' Rating Scales (revised). Technical Manual*. Multi-Health Systems, Toronto.
4. Swanson J.M., Kraemer H.C., Hinshaw S.P., Arnold L.E., Conners C.K., Abikoff H.B., Clevenger W., Davies M., Elliott G.R., Greenhill L.L. *et al.* (2001). Clinical relevance of the primary findings of the MTA: success rates based on severity of ADHD and ODD symptoms at the end of treatment. *J. Am. Acad. Child Adolesc. Psychiatry*, **40**, 168–179.
5. Eyberg S.M., Robinson E.A. (1983). Conduct problem behavior: standardization of a behavioral rating scale with adolescents. *J. Clin. Child Psychol.*, **12**, 347–354.
6. Saigh P.A. (1989). The development and validation of the Children's Post-traumatic Stress Disorder Inventory. *Int. J. Spec. Education*, **4**, 75–84.
7. Sadowski C.M., Friedrich W.N. (2000). Psychometric properties of the Trauma Symptom Checklist for Children (TSCC) with psychiatrically hospitalized adolescents. *Child Maltreat.*, **5**, 364–372.
8. Praver F., Pelcovitz D., DiGiuseppe R. (1996). *Angie/Andy Cartoon Trauma Scales*. Multi-Health Systems, North Tonawanda.
9. Saylor C.F., Swenson C.C., Reynolds S.S., Taylor M. (1999). The Pediatric Emotional Distress Scale: a brief screening measure for young children exposed to traumatic events. *J. Clin. Child Psychol.*, **28**, 70–81.
10. Nader K., Blake D., Kriegler J., Pynoos R. (1994). *Clinician Administered PTSD Scale for Children (CAPS-C), Current and Lifetime Diagnosis Version, and Instruction Manual*. UCLA Neuropsychiatric Institute and National Center for PTSD, Los Angeles, CA.
11. Armstrong J.G., Putnam F.W., Carlson E.B., Libero D.Z., Smith S.R. (1997). Development and validation of a measure of adolescent dissociation: the Adolescent Dissociative Experiences Scale. *J. Nerv. Ment. Dis.*, **185**, 491–497.
12. Evers-Szostak M., Sanders S. (1992). The Children's Perceptual Alteration Scale (CPAS): a measure of children's dissociation. *Dissociation*, **5**, 91–97.
13. Putnam F.W., Helmers K., Trickett P.K. (1993). Development, reliability, and validity of a child dissociation scale. *Child Abuse Negl.*, **17**, 731–741.
14. Poznanski E.O., Freeman L.N., Mokros H.B. (1985). Children's Depression Rating Scale-Revised (September 1984). *Psychopharmacol. Bull.*, **21**, 979–990.
15. Conners C.K. (1995). *Conners' Continuous Performance Test*. Multi-Health Systems, Toronto.
16. Greenberg L.M., Kindschi C.L. (1996). T*est of Variables of Attention Clinical Guide*. Universal Attention Disorders, St. Paul, MN.
17. Koschack J., Kunert H.J., Derichs G., Weniger G., Irle E. (2003). Impaired and enhanced attentional function in children with attention deficit/hyperactivity disorder. *Psychol. Med.*, **33**, 481–489.
18. Rowland A.S., Umbach D.M., Catoe K.E., Stallone L., Long S., Rabiner D., Naftel A.J., Panke D., Faulk R., Sandler D.P. (2001). Studying the epidemiology

of attention-deficit hyperactivity disorder: screening method and pilot results. *Can. J. Psychiatry*, **46**, 931–940.

19. Barbaresi W.J., Katusic S.K., Colligan R.C., Pankratz V.S., Weaver A.L., Weber K.J., Mrazek D.A., Jacobsen S.J. (2002). How common is attention-deficit/hyperactivity disorder? Incidence in a population-based birth cohort in Rochester, Minn. *Arch. Pediatr. Adolesc. Med.*, **156**, 217–224.
20. Benjasuwantep B., Ruangdaraganon N., Visudhiphan P. (2002). Prevalence and clinical characteristics of attention deficit hyperactivity disorder among primary school students in Bangkok. *J. Med. Assoc. Thai.*, **85** (Suppl. 4), S1232–1240.
21. Montiel-Nava C., Pena J.A., Lopez M., Salas M., Zurga J.R., Montiel-Barbero I., Pirela D., Cardozo J.J. (2002). Estimations of the prevalence of attention deficit hyperactivity disorder in Marabino children. *Rev. Neurol.*, **35**, 1019–1024.
22. Pineda D.A., Lopera F., Palacio J.D., Ramirez D., Henao G.C. (2003). Prevalence estimations of attention-deficit/hyperactivity disorder: differential diagnoses and comorbidities in a Colombian sample. *Int. J. Neurosci.*, **113**, 49–71.
23. Zohar A.H., Ratzoni G., Pauls D.L., Apter A., Bleich A., Kron S., Rappaport M., Weizman A., Cohen D.J. (1992). An epidemiological study of obsessive–compulsive disorder and related disorders in Israeli adolescents. *J. Am. Acad. Child Adolesc. Psychiatry*, **31**, 1057–1061.
24. Adler, L.A., Chua, H.C. (2002). Management of ADHD in adults. *J. Clin. Psychiatry*, **63** (Suppl. 12), 29–35.
25. Pary R., Lewis S., Matuschka P.R., Rudzinskiy P., Safi M., Lippmann S. (2002). Attention deficit disorder in adults. *Ann. Clin. Psychiatry*, **14**, 105–111.
26. Greenspan S., Weider S. (1993). Regulatory disorders. In: Zeanah C.H. Jr (ed.) *Handbook of Infant Mental Health*. Guilford Press, New York, pp. 280–290.
27. Palfrey J.S., Levine M.D., Walker D.K., Sullivan M. (1985). The emergence of attention deficits in early childhood: a prospective study. *Dev. Behav. Ped.*, **6**, 339–348.
28. Blackman J.A. (1999). Attention deficit/hyperactivity disorder in preschoolers: does it exist and should we treat it? *Pediatr. Clin. North Am.*, **46**, 1011–1025.
29. Manor I., Tyano S. (2001). ADHD in elementary school age. In: Manor I., Tyano S. (eds) *To Live with ADHD*. Dyonon, Tel Aviv, pp. 89–111.
30. Biederman J., Faraone S.V., Milberger S., Jetton J.G., Chen L., Mick E., Greene R.W., Russell R.L. (1996). Is childhood oppositional defiant disorder a precursor to adolescent conduct disorder? Findings from a four year follow up of children with ADHD. *J. Am. Acad. Child Adolesc. Psychiatry*, **35**, 1193–1204.
31. Loeber R., Stouthamer-Loeber M., Farrington D.P., Lahey B.B., Keenan K., White H.R. (2002). Three longitudinal studies of children's development in Pittsburgh: the Developmental Trends Study, the Pittsburgh Youth Study, and the Pittsburgh Girls Study. *Crim. Behav. Ment. Health*, **12**, 1–23.
32. Malmquist C.P. (1991). Conduct disorder. Conceptual and diagnostic issues. In: Wiener J.M. (ed.) *Textbook of Childhood and Adolescent Psychiatry*. American Associated Press, Washington, DC, pp. 279–287.
33. Burke J.D., Loeber R., Birmaher B. (2002). Oppositional defiant disorder and conduct disorder: a review of the past 10 years, part II. *J. Am. Acad. Child Adolesc. Psychiatry*, **41**, 1275–1293.
34. Foy D.W, Madvig B.T, Pynoos R.S., Camillieri A.J. (1996). Etiologic factors in the development of post traumatic stress disorder in children and adolescents. *J. School Psychol.*, **34**, 133–145.

35. Fletcher K.E. (1996). Childhood posttraumatic stress disorder. In: Mash E.J., Barkley R.A. (eds) *Child Psychopathology*. Guilford Press, New York, pp. 242–276.
36. Yule W. (1992). Post traumatic stress disorder in child survivors of shipping disasters: the sinking of the "Jupiter". *Psychother. Psychosom.*, **57**, 200–205.
37. Shannon M.P., Lonigan C.J., Finch A.J., Taylor C.M. (1994). Children exposed to disaster: epidemiology of post traumatic symptoms and symptom profiles. *J. Am. Acad. Child. Adolesc. Psychiatry*, **28**, 225–229.
38. Vila G., Witrowski P., Tondini M.C., Perez-Diaz F., Mouren Simeoni M.C., Jouvent R. (2001). A study of posttraumatic disorders in children who experienced an industrial disaster in the Briey region. *Eur. Child Adolesc. Psychiatry*, **10**, 10–18.
39. Scheeringa M.S., Zeanah C.H., Drell M.J., Larrieu J.A. (1995). Two approaches to the diagnosis of posttraumatic stress disorder in infancy and early childhood. *J. Am. Acad. Child Adolesc. Psychiatry*, **34**, 191–200.
40. Yule W. (2001). Posttraumatic stress disorder in the general population and in children. *J. Clin. Psychiatry*, **62** (Suppl. 17), 23–28.
41. Salmon K., Bryant R.A. (2002). Posttraumatic stress disorder in children. The influence of developmental factors. *Clin. Psychol. Rev.*, **22**, 163–188.
42. Brent D.A. (1987). Correlates of the medical lethality of suicide attempts in children and adolescents. *J. Am. Acad. Child Adolesc. Psychiatry*, **26**, 87–91.
43. Fleming G.E., Offord D.R. (1990). Epidemiology of childhood depressive disorders: a critical review. *J. Am. Acad. Child Adolesc. Psychiatry*, **29**, 571–580.
44. Biederman J., Mick E., Wozniak J., Monuteaux M.C., Galdo M., Faraone S.V. (2003). Can a subtype of conduct disorder linked to bipolar disorder be identified? Integration of findings from the Massachusetts General Hospital Pediatric Psychopharmacology Research Program. *Biol. Psychiatry*, **53**, 952–960.
45. Whitaker A., Johnson J., Shaffer D., Rapport J.L. (1990). Uncommon troubles in young people: prevalence estimates of selected psychiatric disorders in a nonrefered population. *Arch. Gen. Psychiatry*, **47**, 487–496.
46. Lewinsohn P.M., Rohde P., Seeley J.R. (1998). Major depressive disorder in older adolescents: prevalence, risk factors and clinical implications. *Clin. Psychol. Rev.*, **18**, 765–794.
47. Lewis D.O., Yeager C.A. (2002). Conduct disorder. In: Lewis M. (ed.) *Child and Adolescent Psychiatry – A Comprehensive Textbook*, 3rd edn. Lippincott Williams & Wilkins, Philadelphia, PA, pp. 670–681.
48. Geller B., Craney J.L., Bolhofner K., Nickelsburg M.J., Williams M., Zimerman B. (2002). Two-year prospective follow-up of children with a prepubertal and early adolescent bipolar disorder phenotype. *Am. J. Psychiatry*, **159**, 927–933.
49. Lewinsohn P.M., Klein D.N., Seeley J.R. (1995). Bipolar disorders in a community sample of older adolescents: prevalence, phenomenology, comorbidity and course. *J. Am. Acad. Child Adolesc. Psychiatry*, **34**, 454–463.
50. Bellivier F., Golmard J.L., Rietschel M., Henry C., Leboyer M. (2003). Age at onset in bipolar I affective disorder: further evidence for three subgroups. *Am. J. Psychiatry*, **160**, rz999–1001.
51. Pine D.S., Cohen E., Cohen P., Brook J. (1999). Adolescent depressive symptoms as predictors of adult depression: moodiness or mood disorder? *Am. J. Psychiatry*, **156**, 133–135.
52. Kessler R.C., Avenevoli S., Ries K., Merikanges R. (2001). Mood disorders in children and adolescents: an epidemiologic perspective. *Biol. Psychiatry*, **49**, 1002–1014.

53. Keshavan M.S., Sujata M., Mehra A., Montrose D.M., Sweeney J.A. (2003). Psychosis proneness and ADHD in young relatives of schizophrenia patients. *Schizophr. Res.*, **59**, 85–92.
54. Volkmar F.R., Tsatsanis K.D. (2002). Childhood schizophrenia. In: Lewis M. (ed.) *Child and Adolescent Psychiatry – A Comprehensive Textbook*, 3rd edn. Lippincott Williams & Wilkins, Philadelphia, PA, pp. 745–754.
55. Wekerle C., Wolfe D.A. (1996). Child maltreatment. In: Mash E.J., Barkleye R.A. (eds) *Child Psychopathology*. Guilford Press, New York, pp. 492–537.
56. Wolfe V.V. (1998). Child sexual abuse. In: Mash E.J., Barkleye R.A. (eds) *Treatment of Childhood Disorders*, 2nd edn. Guilford Press, New York, pp. 545–597.
57. Ghaziuddin M., Weidmer-Mikhail E., Ghaziuddin N. (1998). Comorbidity of Asperger syndrome: a preliminary report. *J. Intellect. Disabil. Res.*, **42**, 279–283.
58. Roeyers H., Keymeulen H., Buysse A. (1998). Differentiating attention-deficit/hyperactivity disorder from pervasive developmental disorder not otherwise specified. *J. Learn. Disabil.*, **31**, 565–571.
59. Luteijn E., Luteijn F., Jackson S., Volkmar F., Minderaa R. (2000). The children's Social Behavior Questionnaire for milder variants of PDD problems: evaluation of the psychometric characteristics. *J. Autism Dev. Disord.*, **30**, 317–330.
60. Buitelaar J.K., Kooij J.J. (2000). Attention deficit hyperactivity disorder (ADHD): etiology, diagnosis and treatment. *Ned. Tijdschr. Geneeskd.*, **144**, 1716–1723.
61. Aman M.G., Langworthy K.S. (2000). Pharmacotherapy for hyperactivity in children with autism and other pervasive developmental disorders. *J. Autism Dev. Disord.*, **30**, 451–459.
62. DiScala C., Lescohier I., Barthel M., Li G. (1998). Injuries to children with attention deficit hyperactivity disorder. *Pediatrics*, **102**, 1415–1421.
63. Gerring J.P., Brady K.D., Chen A., Vasa R., Grados M., Bandeen-Roche K.J., Bryan R.N., Denckla M.B. (1998). Premorbid prevalence of ADHD and development of secondary ADHD after closed head injury. *J. Am. Acad. Child Adolesc. Psychiatry*, **37**, 647–654.
64. Zeanah C.H., Boris N.W. (2000). Disturbances and disorders of attachment in early childhood. In: Zeanah C.H. Jr (ed.) *Handbook of Infant Mental Health*. Guilford Press, New York, pp. 353–368.

CHAPTER

7

Precursors, Prodromes and Early Detection of Eating Disorders

Regina C. Casper

Stanford University Medical School, Stanford, CA, USA

INTRODUCTION

Anorexia nervosa (AN) and bulimia nervosa (BN) pose significant health problems for female adolescents and young adult women. The unique combination of psychological issues and physical impairment and an often prolonged course disrupt psychological and physical growth at a crucial developmental period, with sometimes lasting effects on long-term health.

AN typically has its onset in adolescence and rarely in childhood. The incidence of AN is low, 4.2 cases per 100,000 population [1–5], and point prevalence estimates range between 0.1% and 1% in adolescent female populations and from 0.004% to 0.01% in adolescent males. A higher prevalence compared to the incidence suggests that AN rarely remits spontaneously and does not respond easily to treatment. Affected young people, even if they ultimately recover, may be exposed to many years of suffering. In fact AN is now the third most common chronic condition among adolescent girls in the US, after obesity and asthma [1,6]. The cost of long-term disability to health and welfare services due to chronic AN can be significant [7].

BN is a disorder of late adolescence and young adulthood. Incidence rates for BN are 12.2 per 100,000 population [8]. One-year, lifetime and point prevalence estimates for BN are higher than for AN: they are 1.5%, 2.6–2.8% and 4.2%, respectively, for females, and lifetime prevalence is 0.4% for males [9–12]. In outcome studies of hospitalized and clinic populations, a third of BN patients take a chronic course.

Despite heightened public awareness of the burden of eating disorders, their prevalence has not declined. The major argument of this chapter is that

Early Detection and Management of Mental Disorders.
Edited by Mario Maj, Juan José López-Ibor, Norman Sartorius, Mitsumoto Sato and Ahmed Okasha.
 ISBN 0-470-01083-5.

knowledge about precursors or "forerunners", which may constitute risk factors in the causal chain of events, provides an opportunity to identify vulnerable populations. Furthermore, understanding the precursors and early manifestations of the eating disorders may lead to better informed and more effective preventive measures. Given the complexity of psychiatric disorders, identifying variables that place a population at risk may not only serve as guidance for preventive intervention, which can have tremendous psychological and economic benefits to the individual, to families and to society as a whole, but it may also provide cues to the aetiology of the disorder.

PRECURSORS AS "RISK FACTORS"

Precursors may be risk factors, but not all risk factors are precursors. For the purpose of our discussion here, only correlates shown to precede the disorder will be considered. Kraemer *et al.* [13] described risk factor as "a characteristic, experience or event that, if present, is associated with an increase in the probability (risk) of a particular outcome over the base rate of the outcome in the general unexposed population". According to Kraemer *et al.* [13], risk factors may work together in different ways to produce an outcome: as mediating (explaining why and how another factor affects outcome), moderating (specifying under what conditions another factor will affect outcome), independent (factors that are unrelated in source and time and are co-dominant), overlapping (related factors that occur in the same time frame and have equal weight on the outcome) and proxy (a global factor of which only one component is a risk factor).

In preventive medicine, epidemiological studies have generally served to identify risk factors. Unfortunately, in eating disorders research, population-based studies are scarce, and few have determined the absolute risk, the overall probability of developing the disease in the population at large [14]. In the eating disorders, associations with variables preceding the illness have by and large been determined from clinical studies; for this reason, the term "precursor" is not only descriptively, but also methodologically more accurate than the term "risk factor". One of the drawbacks of using clinical populations is that information from clinical samples, with their generally higher comorbidity than cases drawn from the general population, can complicate interpretations. For example, in the eating disorders, comorbidity might influence aspects of the family's or the individual's functioning, but might have less of an impact on precursors like eating or exercising habits. Moreover, precursors may not be specific: the same precursor may be a risk factor for a depressive or an anxiety disorder. No prospective studies, which would assess the relative risk of premorbid variables to contribute to the particular disorder, have so far been published.

SHARED PRECURSORS FOR AN AND BN

Certain trends in contemporary Western and increasingly Eastern society [15] increase the risk for an essential precursor to occur, namely food restriction or dieting. Foremost among those trends is slimness as a beauty ideal for contemporary women. Thinness as a personal goal, linked to expectations that it will bring social approval and improved self-confidence, presents a challenge to all female adolescents who do not fit the ideal shape. Societal attitudes sensitize these young women to body dissatisfaction, enhancing chances for dietary restriction to bring about body weight loss. An equally important factor is the simplistic belief that everyone can ultimately attain a "perfect" body shape. This challenge to reshape the body is keenly experienced by female adolescents, who accumulate adipose tissue with the growth spurt of puberty. By contrast, male adolescents welcome weight increases and tend to exercise to increase muscle strength.

The emphasis on dietary restriction occurs in a population that has become heavier [16]. In 1983, the norms for body weights listed in the Metropolitan Life Insurance Tables were adjusted upward from the earlier 1964 version. The high prevalence of dieting among female adolescents, between 60% and 80% in the Western hemisphere [17,18], viewed against the low incidence and prevalence of eating disorders, suggest that the relative risk – the magnitude of the association between exposure and disease – is low for AN and somewhat higher for BN. As Bruch [19] aptly commented, "there is an epidemic of dieting, but not an epidemic of eating disorders".

PRECURSORS TO ANOREXIA NERVOSA

Premorbid Body Weight

Few attempts have been made to assess pre-illness body weight in AN. From those few reports, there is no evidence that premorbid body weight deviates from the normal range. Parental reports of pre-illness weights described 12% of AN patients to have been "overweight" from the first year to adolescence [20]. Based on clinical premorbid weight histories, 48% of AN patients were below and 52% were above the 98 percentile of Canadian Standards [21]. In Coners *et al.*'s study [22], recalled overweight was not more common in AN patients than in an age-matched female population.

An accurate calculation of pre-illness body weight would ideally be based on year by year weight deviations derived from records of the patients' paediatric growth curves.

Childhood Activity Level

Davis *et al.* [23] found that half of AN patients compared to a quarter of BN patients reported being more physically active during childhood than the average girl.

Dieting Exposure

Contrary to expectations, exposure to factors favouring dieting does not seem to be a precursor for AN. Fairburn *et al.* [24] showed that AN patients did not differ from healthy controls or from general psychiatric control subjects in their level of exposure to dieting vulnerability domain variables, unlike BN patients. Hence, dieting risk for AN patients, in particular dieting risk related to familial shape and weight concerns, does not appear to be different from the general population.

Individual Psychological Traits and Personality Features

A reliable assessment of pre-illness personality traits is difficult to make without prospective studies. As it is, most personality research has been done retrospectively and some studies have relied on the patient's memory alone, with its subjective bias, instead of obtaining information from independent interviews of parents or other relatives. It is also difficult to judge personality features during the acute stage of the disorder, since the starvation state tends to reinforce rigidity and controlling tendencies [25]. Other manifest features may be a consequence of a comorbid psychiatric disorder: for instance, depressive symptoms affect self-esteem [25]. On the other hand, the overall stability of personality traits into adulthood makes it possible to obtain valid information from patients after full recovery [26,27].

These methodological problems notwithstanding, studies have consistently identified childhood personality traits of high self-expectations and high moral standards along with rigidity as precursors [27].

Research which led to the suggestion to subtype AN based on eating patterns noted early on differences in the patient's childhood personality [20,28]. Restricting AN patients were more often described by their parents as introverted and perfectionistic than binge-eating/purging patients, who tended to be more outgoing as children. Rastam [29] reported a high frequency of premorbid obsessive–compulsive personality disorder in a population-based sample. The existence of traits of obsessionality and social avoidance in AN patients were confirmed by Wentz *et al.* [30] in a follow-up study of the same sample. In two other follow-up studies, women who had recovered from the restricting type of AN and were assessed along normal personality dimensions [31] displayed higher moral standards and rigidity, along with greater emotional, cognitive and behavioural control, than sisters or healthy controls [26], and more obsessive–compulsive personality traits, such as perfectionism, rigidity and preference for order and symmetry [27].

More recently, studies have focused on personality traits reflecting "perfectionism" as a risk factor, albeit different studies have measured different components of perfectionism. Fairburn *et al.* [24] found that negative self-evaluation and perfectionism ("high personal standards") as a childhood characteristic distinguished AN patients from healthy and psychiatric controls. Bulik *et al.* [32] found "concern over mistakes" but not "personal standards" to increase the odds ratio of AN, yet in her study neither characteristic was a predictor for AN. Perfectionism defined in Webster as "a disposition to regard anything short of perfection as unacceptable" tends to coexist with low self-esteem in AN. In a population-based female twin sample, Walters and Kendler [3] found low self-esteem and a higher level of neuroticism to be associated with AN. Low self-esteem also occurred in those without a history of depression. Confirmatory evidence for a poor self-concept comes from three independent studies which described very low (self-critical) self-image scores in adolescents with acute AN by comparison with healthy and depressed adolescents [33–35].

Family Interaction, Environment and Psychopathology

The family characteristics identified by Bruch [19], Selvini-Palazzoli [36] and Minuchin *et al.* [37] – rigidity, overprotectiveness, enmeshment, avoidance of conflict – may be somewhat more common in anorectic families than in families with psychosomatically or psychiatrically ill children, yet overall family dynamics show a great deal of variability. Parental styles and parent–child interactions differ between families of different AN subtypes. Families of restricting AN patients present high levels of cohesion, a calm, orderly, "perfect" environment not different from healthy controls [38], by contrast with families of bulimic AN patients, in which in particular fathers tend towards affective dyscontrol with expressions of hostility [39].

Controlled family studies of AN have described strong familial aggregation in AN families, with intergenerational transmission, but there was no clustering of affective disorders, unless AN coexisted with a depressive disorder [40]. These findings were confirmed in a study of males with AN, which observed a twenty-fold increase of AN in female relatives. Conversely, bulimia nervosa was relatively uncommon among relatives of males with AN [41].

PRODROMES OF ANOREXIA NERVOSA

Significant Weight Loss

Significant weight loss is acknowledged by patients as a critical prodromal risk factor. Patients report the appearance of the anorectic attitude around a weight loss of 15% of their previous weight [42]. A specified amount of weight loss is also a symptom of AN. The loss of weight during the prodromal phase may be induced by dieting but this is not necessarily the case. Other causes of weight loss may be fasting practices [43], or the loss of weight might be the consequence of a physical illness or a depressive disorder. As a symptom of AN, weight loss is typically defended and its seriousness is denied by the patient.

Drive for Activity

Few studies have enquired about the patients' premorbid activity level, but all of them report greater than average physical activity in a majority of patients. Kron *et al.* [44] conducted personal interviews and found that 84% of AN patients tended to be more active premorbidly. Davis *et al.* [23] found on the basis of interviews that AN patients were more physically active than controls from adolescence onwards, as well as prior to the onset of anorexia nervosa: 73% of patients engaged in excessive exercise; 60% were competitive athletes prior to the onset of their disorder; 60% reported that sport or exercise predated dieting. Three-quarters of AN patients claimed that physical activity levels steadily increased during the period when food intake and weight loss decreased the most. Subpopulations in whom exercise is encouraged (athletes) may be at risk for developing anorexia nervosa [45].

Eating Problems in Early Childhood

Food fads and "picky eating" in early childhood have been associated with AN [46,47], whereas pica and family conflicts during meals in early childhood seem to be precursors for BN [48]. Karwautz *et al.* [49] have recently used a discordant patient/sister design and confirmed evidence of poor feeding in childhood for AN.

PRECURSORS FOR BULIMIA NERVOSA

Chronic Caloric Restriction and Dieting

Food deprivation in healthy individuals, which is experienced as a stress by the organism, has been known to increase the risk of binge eating. As described by Keys *et al.* [50], if normal individuals, after having undergone chronic food restriction, regain access to food, they experience food cravings and uncomfortable overeating to the point of eating "immense" meals. Such overeating occasionally leads to compensatory behaviours such as vomiting to relieve the discomfort. Dieting exposure has been identified as a risk factor for BN by Fairburn *et al.* [51].

Premorbid Body Weight

In BN, unlike in AN, individual and familial overweight and critical comments about weight shape and eating habits appear to play a significant role as precursors. A greater proportion of patients reported childhood obesity than either healthy controls or general psychiatric control subjects, and BN patients reported more parental obesity than either control group [51]. The McKnight investigators [52] identified thin body preoccupation and social pressure as predictive for the onset of BN, for the partial syndrome BN and for binge eating disorder. Greater previous weight fluctuations and rates of dieting emerged as predisposing variables in the twin study by Kendler *et al.* [53].

Rumination

Postprandial vomiting and regurgitation are regular features of BN except in cases when excessive exercise is used to burn calories from binge eating. The ability to learn to reverse habitually oesophageal peristalsis or to regurgitate in BN bears a relationship to rumination disorder of infancy. Rumination is a syndrome characterized by effortless repetitive regurgitation of small amounts of food from the stomach. The food is then partially or completely rechewed, reswallowed, or expelled. There is preliminary evidence that rumination might be a precursor from a report by Blinder

[54], who found primary ruminatory behaviour to antedate BN. Fairburn and Cooper [55] and Chial *et al.* [56] reported rumination in BN, but did not comment on the patients' premorbid habits. Rumination as a symptom or a syndrome is an unappreciated condition in adults and underinvestigated in BN [57]. More systematic research might clarify whether the two disorders are related.

Age at Menarche

Menarche occurred at an earlier age in subjects with bulimia compared to psychiatric control subjects [51]. The earlier age at menarche may not be an independent factor, but very likely is weight related. Frisch and McArthur have reported that the amount of body fat is related to onset of menarche [58]. Because BN subjects have higher rates of childhood obesity, they would be expected to experience menarche at an earlier age. A tendency towards overweight and earlier exposure to the bodily changes of puberty would further increase body dissatisfaction and the chances for dieting.

Individual and Personality Traits

Personality characteristics of BN patients by and large appear to fall within the normal range. Kendler *et al.* [11] found no association with avoidant features in BN based on analyses of the Virginia twin registry. The same authors reported similar levels of extraversion in BN and controls. In a clinical study [25], hospitalized BN patients did not differ from normal controls on self-control and risk-taking dimensions; however, in comparison with restricting AN patients, BN patients scored higher on impulsivity and lower on belief in traditional values, suggesting that the personality characteristics of BN patients cover the wide range of normal variation, but they differ compared to restricting AN patients.

Fairburn *et al.* [51] reported negative self-evaluation and perfectionism, the latter assessed as "high personal standards", as risk factors for BN. Factors different from those in AN seem to generate the negative self-evaluation, since BN patients tend to grow up in a family environment fostering critical attitudes.

Family Interaction, Environment and Psychopathology

Studies provide strong evidence for family dysfunction in BN. More conflict expression without resolution and distant fathers have been found to distinguish families with a BN daughter from families of healthy controls and families with restricting AN daughters [59]. Kendler *et al.* [11] reported low levels of paternal care as well as parental substance abuse and parental depression associated with definite and probable cases of BN. In another analysis, Kendler *et al.* [53] reported that familial–environmental influences substantially influenced the liability to BN. Fairburn *et al.* [51] recorded low parental contact, more negative comments from family members about appearance, eating habits and weight, and parental arguments in comparison to psychiatric controls. Rates of parental alcoholism, depression and drug abuse were also increased. A significant problem with Fairburn *et al.*'s risk factor studies in eating disorders [24,51] is that all information concerning the families, including the psychiatric diagnoses, was obtained from the patients and not derived from independent interviews of family members.

PREVENTION AND INTERVENTION PROTOCOLS INCORPORATING INFORMATION ABOUT PRECURSORS

Specific prevention programmes directed at school populations, with the aim to modify unhealthy eating attitudes and weight regulation practices and to reduce the prevalence of dieting, have given generally disappointing results [60,61].

Even a prevention intervention which focused on "three principal components (instruction on the harmful effects of unhealthful weight regulation; promotion of healthful weight regulation through the practice of sound nutrition and dietary principles and regular aerobic physical activity; development of coping skills for resisting the diverse socio-cultural influences linked to thinness and dieting)" effectively improved the knowledge about nutrition, effects of dieting, and causes of body fat, but failed to reduce dieting frequency or eating patterns in high school students [61].

Similarly, a curriculum of ten lessons taught by the classroom teachers for fifth graders – designed to encourage healthy eating, exercise, and body image while discouraging calorie-restrictive dieting, exercising for weight loss and the development of body dissatisfaction – improved the children's information about nutrition, effects of dieting and causes of body fat, but produced no changes in the children's eating patterns, exercise patterns, weight reduction attempts and teasing of fat children [62].

Recently, Wade *et al.* [63] have reported on the outcome of a school-based media literacy programme, an interactive exercise examining the effectiveness of media messages and a self-esteem enhancement programme for reducing three "risk" factors (weight and shape concerns, focus on weight and shape and dietary restraint) in an unselected sample of 8th grade boys and girls. The media intervention produced a reduction in weight concern only, while the self-esteem enhancement programme failed to affect any of the risk measures compared to the control condition.

Whereas the initial prevention trials have focused on providing psycho-educational information about eating disorders, unhealthy eating practices and the consequences of weight fluctuations to all high school students, more recent trials have targeted populations considered at risk.

One of the more sophisticated interactive intervention programmes is described by Stice *et al.* [64], who recruited adolescent girls who expressed body image concerns. The intervention consisted either of help with developing a healthy lifestyle that incorporated a balanced diet and regular exercise, or of a "dissonance" intervention in which participants were asked to help create a body acceptance programme for younger girls. The dissonance intervention programme and the healthy weight control intervention produced reductions in thin ideal internalization, in negative affect and in bulimic pathology, but did not reduce body dissatisfaction or dieting. Of interest is that the effects of the healthy lifestyle programme were more pronounced and longer lasting.

A methodologically different approach, testing whether body image and eating disturbances contribute to the increase in major depression that occurs among girls during adolescence, is directly relevant to intervention efforts. Stice *et al.* [65] analysed data from a 4-year school-based longitudinal study and found that elevated body dissatisfaction, dietary restraint and bulimic symptoms at study entry predicted onset of subsequent depression among initially non-depressed youth when controlling for initial depressive symptoms. This study highlights the importance of mood changes in BN which would need to be taken into consideration in prevention efforts. The study confirms that the body image and eating-related problems in puberty constitute proximate risk factors for depression and contribute to the elevated rates of depressive disorders in adolescent girls.

EARLY DETECTION OF EATING DISORDERS

The value of early detection of a disorder is generally undisputed in medicine. Foremost among the benefits of early detection is the chance for early treatment, enhancing the likelihood for a shorter duration of illness and a full recovery. Commonly, heightened public awareness about medical disorders facilitates early diagnosis; however, so far this has not happened in the eating disorders. Certainly one reason is that the public finds it difficult to distinguish between widespread and perhaps justified dieting efforts that often lead to disordered eating and the restrictive eating habits seen in the eating disorders. Since in the early phase the signs and symptoms of intractable dieting – e.g. refusal to eat, weight loss, sense of loss of control over eating – can overlap with the symptoms in AN or BN, physicians and health care personnel need to be cognizant of the differences in the signs associated with temporary dieting and the symptoms of an eating disorder.

The more accurate the classification and the more concise the diagnostic criteria for a disorder, the easier is its detection. The phenotype of AN has been stable over centuries and can be classified with validity. As stated in ICD-10 [66], "the clinical features of the syndrome are easily recognized, so that the diagnosis is reliable with a high level of agreement between clinicians". Nonetheless, the diagnostic criteria have evolved. Differences between DSM-IV [67] and ICD-10 [66] indicate that clinicians have not always reduced the complex clinical features in the same way into diagnostic categories. To a substantial extent clinical emphasis and not experimental evidence has introduced changes into the diagnostic criteria.

The DSM-IV comprises three syndromes: AN, BN and eating disorder not otherwise specified, whereas the ICD-10 includes, in addition to AN and BN, atypical AN and atypical BN, overeating associated with other psychological disturbances, vomiting associated with other psychological disturbances, other eating disorders, and eating disorders unspecified. There is close agreement on the criteria for the two major syndromes discussed in this chapter. Regarding AN, the principal conceptual difference is the strong emphasis on an attitudinal dimension as a principal criterion in the DSM-IV, namely the individual's "refusal" to maintain a minimally normal body weight as opposed to the assessment of "body weight loss" as the primary criterion in the ICD-10. Another difference is the subdivision into the restricting and binge eating/purging subtypes in the DSM-IV. This subdivision is important, because subtype differences go beyond the clinical manifestations and have implications for treatment and ultimately to pinpoint aetiological differences [25]. The purging and nonpurging types of bulimia nervosa in DSM-IV correspond to BN proper and hyperorexia nervosa in ICD-10.

The early detection of AN is hampered first by factors inherent in the disease process, especially the denial of illness. AN patients typically identify with the weight loss and assert that they are well and that all is normal [68]. This denial of illness not infrequently extends to family members. Second, food restriction and the high value placed on exercise for a healthy body fit cultural norms and may not be recognized as prodromes to AN. BN patients also tend to be secretive about their abnormal eating pattern. Moreover, the demarcation between shape concerns of a dieting person and between eating binges and great variations in intake is imprecise, as feelings of remorse and guilt and a sense of loss of control may follow simple overeating.

Essentially, children, adolescents or young women with AN or BN do not wish to come to the attention of physicians. Comparisons between the numbers of BN patients in epidemiological treatment studies and the prevalence of BN in females aged 16–24 suggest that a minority of individuals with BN seek treatment [69]. For the medical practitioner, the appearance of physical symptoms such as amenorrhoea in AN or parotid gland swelling in BN aids in detecting the disorders [70], albeit not necessarily in the early stages. Clearly, important to consider in the differential diagnosis is the fact that AN occurs primarily in Caucasian women and is virtually non-existent in Afro-American women [69].

The information that classic AN can occur in childhood may not be common knowledge. Bryant-Waugh and Lask [71] reported that few medical practitioners in the UK were familiar with AN in childhood. A mere 31% among paediatricians and only 3% of family practitioners in a geographical area mentioned a possible diagnosis of AN when they were asked to evaluate two case vignettes of childhood AN. More recently Nicholls *et al.* [72] have pointed out that at most 50% of childhood cases fit the diagnostic criteria of the DSM-IV or ICD-10, with the remainder falling into the category eating disorder not otherwise specified. These authors have reported that the criteria developed by their group at Great Ormond Street Hospital, the GOS criteria, diagnosed most children with high inter-rater reliability. Interestingly, the primary GOS criterion for the patient's attitude in AN is not "refusal" but "determined weight loss". The GOS criteria for BN are quite concise: "recurrent binges and purges; sense of lack of control; morbid preoccupation with weight and shape", but they do not specify the minimum frequency of the behaviour.

The first step towards early detection of eating disorders would be to train general practitioners in their diagnosis. Such training effectively doubled the incidence rate in the epidemiological survey of Hoek *et al.* [73] by comparison with the incidence reported by Turnbull *et al.* [8] for AN (8.1 versus 4.2/100,000 population), but not for BN (12.2 versus 11.5/100,000 population).

Screening refers to the performance of a medical evaluation and/or diagnostic test in asymptomatic persons in the hope that early diagnosis may lead to improved outcome. The simplest and shortest screening instrument for AN which gives information about eating concerns and behaviours is the Eating Attitudes Test (EAT 40 or EAT 26) by Garner *et al.* [74]. The score reflects whether an individual is free of concerns, is dieting preoccupied or has abnormal attitudes or behaviours. The instrument has been widely validated. For identifying BN in young women, two simple questions – "Are you satisfied with your eating pattern?" ("no" response) and "Do you ever eat in secret?" ("yes" response) – had a sensitivity of 1.0 and a specificity of 0.9 for BN and hence had a high validity for detecting BN [75].

The screening survey conducted by Rathner and Messner [76] in over 500 schoolgirls confirmed the relevance of using multiple antecedent risk variables for early case detection. Even though the yield of clinical cases was low – a point prevalence of 1.3 % for AN and no cases of BN – all AN cases and subclinical cases were detected in the at-risk groups.

The screening tool developed by the McKnight investigators [52] for disordered eating contains a weight concern scale, the Rosenberg Self-Esteem Scale, and two depression scales. Interestingly, the test–retest reliabilities for the scales were high for the older girls, but low for the elementary school children, suggesting that the younger group might not have understood some questions or concepts. This survey was not designed to detect eating disorders. In fact, it would require a longitudinal study following the same population to examine whether scores on the various scales or changes in scores can predict the onset of disordered eating. Such a large-scale longitudinal study would need to cover the entire period of high risk for the development of eating disorders, for example 8–18 years for AN and 13–25 years for BN, in order to be useful for early identification of eating disorders.

CONCLUSIONS

On the basis of clinical research, a broad range of clinical correlates have been identified as precursors to eating disorders. Their influence on the individual and the disease process operates through environmental, biological and psychological domains. Socioculturally determined precursors are shared between AN and BN, yet others seem to be disease specific. In AN, especially the restricting form, a drive for activity and a personality tending towards cognitive, emotional and behavioural inhibition, rigidity and perfectionism seem to be of importance [27]. The antecedent conditions for BN include a tendency towards familial overweight, a familial tendency towards affective and substance abuse disorders and an environment that increases the risk of dieting, none of which are typically associated with AN.

One of the key questions is whether a particular precursor is a risk factor, given that several studies have used the latter term [24,51,53]. The answer requires well-designed prospective studies. The factor in question and any other factor possibly interacting with it would need to be measured prospectively in the population at risk and in control populations throughout the ages of risk – throughout adolescence for AN and into young adulthood for BN – to prove a main or interactive effect on disease development. Clearly, this type of study has not been done and is unlikely to be done soon, considering the enormity of the task.

Although each precursor alone is unlikely to bring about AN or BN, each in combination with others contributes to a permissive environment in which a genetic or physiological predisposition is more likely to be expressed. In this sense precursor conditions expose dispositions. For example, a persistent negative energy balance induced by dieting appears to enhance a drive for activity in individuals who may be genetically susceptible to AN [77]. Since the energizing effect of increased activity levels counteracts the fatigue brought about by the starvation state, this predisposition would permit the weight loss to proceed to dangerously low levels without causing alarm. In BN, food restriction occurs against a background of a healthy appetite and emotional lability, making dieting a stressful proposition. In this model, then, severe caloric restriction resulting in weight loss would represent a specific antecedent variable for AN and so would disordered restrictive eating for BN.

Some precursor conditions may be preventable; others might be modifiable through treatment. Among the preventable precursors and prodromes, prolonged food restriction or abstinence from food for whichever reason stand out. Cultural expectations are subject to change. For example, fasting for religious reasons now infrequently provides the incentive for chronic food restriction resulting in AN [43]. It is conceivable, even if it seems improbable, as long as food is abundantly available in the Western and increasingly in the Eastern world [15], leading to excess consumption, that women might adopt aesthetic principles favouring a fuller feminine body, obviating the need for dieting.

Quite apart from these sociocultural forces, childhood personality traits of introversion, excessive control, caution, perfectionism and rigidity, which likely follow a pattern of familial transmission, need to be considered as predisposing factors for the development of AN, in particular the restricting type, albeit a certain proportion of patients with the bulimic type of AN seem to share caution, perfectionism and rigidity in childhood, along with greater emotional instability [26]. Even if the transmission of personality traits is believed to be partly genetic [78], the environment, including treatment, can mitigate or reinforce personality trends [79].

If the primary motivation underlying the caloric restriction is not reasonable dieting, but the wish for control over one's life and/or the need for social approval through achieving thinness, it would be more effective to help young girls who feel ineffective and ignored to achieve control over their lives and attain recognition through developing better and more rewarding relationships with people instead of focusing on body weight control. It must be recognized that negative affectivity is a nonspecific risk factor for AN, implicated also in panic attacks and major depression, whereas anxiety sensitivity, so far not described in AN, appears to be a specific factor that increases the risk for serious panic attacks in adolescents [80].

Furthermore, the effect of any of the precursors must be understood in the context of other precursor variables contributing to the development of the disorder. The "risk factor" literature, for instance, provides no information regarding the relative weight or severity of the antecedent condition necessary to increase the likelihood of an eating disorder, yet a certain amount of weight loss seems to be necessary to consolidate the anorectic attitude [42].

How, then, can the knowledge about precursors be applied to prevent eating disorders? Most of the screens differ widely with regard to their objective, their psychometric properties and the validation methodology used. The majority of available screens identify current diagnostic categories of eating disorders; only a few are appropriate for the identification of at-risk behaviours or to predict future eating disorders. The EAT-40 remains an instrument with standardized properties and a high sensitivity [74]. An item-by-item analysis can identify individuals at risk for AN or BN. It is less well known how truthfully survey questions are being answered by individuals with eating disorders. College admission surveys and the students' subsequent health records could provide data to test this question. Since unhealthy eating behaviours have been found to increase the risk for depression, screening surveys and preventive intervention programmes need to incorporate questions about mood disorders symptoms. So far, intervention programmes primarily directed at reducing body dissatisfaction as one of the reasons for dieting have been successful at improving knowledge about good nutrition, the perils of dieting and weight loss, yet they have failed at changing behaviour, such as reducing the dieting frequency or unhealthy eating patterns.

Without knowing more about the aetiological processes, in particular the biological and genetic structure underlying the eating disorders, the mechanisms through which precursors work together remain elusive. The literature on antecedents reviewed here suggests that eating disorders are conditions in which the expression of the genotype – e.g. certain personality dimensions and a drive for activity for AN, and familial tendencies towards overweight, affective disorders and substance abuse disorders for BN – occurs in the presence of a particular environmental exposure, severe or repeated dietary restriction, sanctioned by contemporary Western society.

REFERENCES

1. Kendell R., Hall D., Babigian H. (1973). The epidemiology of anorexia nervosa. *Psychol. Med.*, **3**, 200–203.
2. Hoek H. (1991). The incidence and prevalence of anorexia nervosa and bulimia nervosa in primary care. *Psychol. Med.*, **21**, 455–460.
3. Walters E., Kendler K. (1995). Anorexia nervosa and anorexic-like syndromes in a population-based female twin sample. *Am. J. Psychiatry*, **152**, 64–71.
4. Wakeling A. (1996). Epidemiology of anorexia nervosa. *Psychiatry Res.*, **62**, 3–9.
5. Willi J., Grossman S. (1983). Epidemiology of anorexia nervosa in a defined region of Switzerland. *Am. J. Psychiatry*, **140**, 564–567.
6. Fisher M., Golden N.H., Katzman D.K., Kreipe R.E., Rees J., Schebendach J., Sigman G., Ammerman S., Hoberman H. (1995). Eating disorders in adolescents: a background paper. *J. Adolesc. Health*, **16**, 420–437.
7. Su J., Birmingham C. (2003). Anorexia nervosa: the cost of long-term disability. *Eat. Weight Disord.*, **8**, 76–79.
8. Turnbull S., Ward A., Treasure J., Jick H., Derby L. (1996). The demand for eating disorder care. An epidemiological study using the general practice research database. *Br. J. Psychiatry*, **169**, 705–712.
9. Hoek H., Brook F. (1985). Patterns of care of anorexia nervosa. *J. Psychiatr. Res.*, **19**, 155–160.
10. Bushnell J.A., Wells J.E., Hornblow A.R., Oakley-Browne M.A., Joyce P. (1990). Prevalence of three bulimia syndromes in the general population. *Psychol. Med.*, **20**, 671–680.
11. Kendler K., MacLean C., Neale M., Kessler R., Heath A., Eaves L. (1991). The genetic epidemiology of bulimia nervosa. *Am. J. Psychiatry*, **148**, 1627–1637.
12. Pagsberg A.K., Wang A.R. (1994). Epidemiology of anorexia nervosa and bulimia nervosa in Bornholm County, Denmark, 1970–1989. *Acta Psychiatr. Scand.*, **90**, 259–265.
13. Kraemer H., Stice C., Kazdin A., Offord D., Kupfer D. (2001). How do risk factors work together? Mediators, moderators and independent, overlapping and proxy risk factors. *Am. J. Psychiatry*, **158**, 848–856.
14. Rastam M., Gillberg C., Garton M. (1989). Anorexia nervosa in a Swedish urban region: a population-based study. *Br. J. Psychiatry*, **155**, 642–646.
15. Lee S., Chan Y., Hsu L. (2003). The intermediate term outcome of Chinese patients with anorexia nervosa in Hong Kong. *Am. J. Psychiatry*, **160**, 967–972.
16. Williamson D. (1993). Descriptive epidemiology of body weight and weight change in US adults. *Ann. Intern. Med.*, **119**, 646–649.
17. Nylander I. (1971). The feeling of being fat and dieting in a school population: epidemiologic interview investigation. *Acta Sociomed. Scand.*, **3**, 17–26.
18. Schleimer K. (1983). Dieting in teenage schoolgirls: a longitudinal prospective study. *Acta Paediatr. Scand.*, **312** (Suppl.), 1–54.
19. Bruch H. (1980). Preconditions for the development of anorexia nervosa. *Am. J. Psychoanal.*, **40**, 169–172.
20. Casper R., Eckert E., Halmi K., Goldberg S., Davis J. (1980). Bulimia: its incidence and clinical significance in patients with anorexia nervosa. *Arch. Gen. Psychiatry*, **37**, 1030–1035.
21. Shinder S., Shephard R. (1993). Relationship of premorbid mass and energy intake to increase of body mass during the treatment of anorexia nervosa. *Int. J. Eat. Disord.*, **14**, 65–73.

22. Coners H., Remschmidt H., Hebebrand J. (1999). The relationship between premorbid body weight, weight loss, and weight at referral in adolescent patients with anorexia nervosa. *Int. J. Eat. Disord.*, **26**, 171–178.
23. Davis C., Kennedy S., Ravelski E., Dionne M. (1994). The role of physical activity in the development and maintenance of eating disorders. *Psychol. Med.*, **24**, 957–967.
24. Fairburn C.G., Cooper Z., Doll H.A., Welch S.L. (1999). Risk factors for anorexia nervosa. *Arch. Gen. Psychiatry*, **56**, 468–476.
25. Casper R., Hedeker D., McClough J. (1992). Personality dimensions in eating disorders and their relevance for subtyping. *J. Am. Acad. Child Adolesc. Psychiatry*, **31:**, 830–840.
26. Casper R. (1990). Personality features of women with good outcome from restricting anorexia nervosa. *Psychosom. Med.*, **52**, 156–170.
27. Srinivasagam N., Kaye W., Plotnikov K., Greeno C., Weltzin T., Rao A. (1995). Persistent perfectionism, symmetry, and exactness after long-term recovery from anorexia nervosa. *Am. J. Psychiatry*, **152**, 1630–1634.
28. Strober M. (1980). Personality and symptomatological features in young nonchronic anorexia patients. *J. Psychosom. Res.*, **24**, 353–359.
29. Rastam M. (1992). Anorexia nervosa in 51 Swedish adolescents: premorbid problems and co-morbidity. *J. Am. Acad. Child Adolesc. Psychiatry*, **31**, 819–829.
30. Wentz E., Gillberg C., Gillberg I., Rastam M. (2001). Ten-year follow-up of adolescent onset anorexia nervosa: psychiatric disorders and overall functioning scales. *J. Child Psychol. Psychiatry*, **42**, 613–622.
31. Tellegen A. (1982). *A Multidimensional Personality Questionnaire*. University of Minnesota, Minneapolis, MN.
32. Bulik C.M., Tozzi F., Anderson C., Mazzeo S.E., Aggen S., Sullivan P.F. (2003). The relation between eating disorders and components of perfectionism. *Am. J. Psychiatry*, **160**, 366–368.
33. Casper R., Offer D., Ostrov E. (1981). The self-image of adolescents with acute anorexia nervosa. *J. Pediatrics*, **98**, 656–661.
34. Swift W., Bushnell N., Hanson P., Logeman T. (1986). Self-concept in adolescent anorexics. *J. Am. Acad. Child Adolesc. Psychiatry*, **25**, 826–835.
35. Steinhausen H., Vollrath M. (1993). The self-image of adolescent patients with eating disorders. *Int. J. Eat. Disord.*, **13**, 221–227.
36. Selvini-Palazzoli M. (1970). The families of patients with anorexia nervosa. In: Anthony E., Koupernik, C. (eds). *The Child in His Family*. John Wiley & Sons, New York, pp. 137–145.
37. Minuchin S., Rosman B., Baker L. (1978). *Psychosomatic Families: Anorexia Nervosa in Context*. Harvard University Press, Cambridge, MA.
38. Casper R., Troiani M. (2001). Family functioning in anorexia nervosa differs by subtype. *Int. J. Eat. Disord.*, **30**, 338–342.
39. Strober M., Salkin B., Burroughs J., Morrell W. (1982). Validity of the bulimia-restrictor distinction in anorexia nervosa: parental personality characteristics and family psychiatric morbidity. *J. Nerv. Ment. Dis.*, **170**, 345–351.
40. Strober M., Katz J. (1987). Do eating disorders and affective disorders share a common etiology? A dissenting opinion. *Int. J. Eat. Disord.*, **6**, 171–180.
41. Strober M., Freeman R., Lampert C., Diamond J., Kaye W. (2001). Males with anorexia nervosa: a controlled study of eating disorders in first-degree relatives. *Int. J. Eat. Disord.*, **29**, 263–269.
42. Casper R., Davis J. (1977). On the course of anorexia nervosa. *Am. J. Psychiatry*, **134**, 974–978.

43. Bell R. (1985). *Holy Anorexia*. University of Chicago Press, Chicago, IL.
44. Kron L., Katz J., Gregory G., Weiner H. (1978). Hyperactivity in anorexia nervosa: a fundamental clinical feature. *Compr. Psychiatry*, **19**, 433–440.
45. Yates A., Leehey K., Shisslak C. (1983). Running – an analogue of anorexia? *N. Engl. J. Med.*, **308**, 251–255.
46. Rose J. (1943). Eating inhibitions in children in relation to anorexia nervosa. *Psychosom. Med.*, **5**, 117–124.
47. Jacobs B., Isaacs S. (1986). Pre-pubertal anorexia: a retrospective controlled study. *J. Child Psychol. Psychiatry All. Discipl.*, **27**, 237–250.
48. Marchi M., Cohen P. (1990). Early childhood eating behaviors and adolescent eating disorders. *J. Am. Acad. Child Adolesc. Psychiatry*, **29**, 112–117.
49. Karwautz A., Rabe-Hesketh S., Hu X.Z.J., Sham P., Collier D.A., Treasure J.L. (2001). Individual-specific risk factors for anorexia nervosa: a pilot study using a discordant sister-pair design. *Psychol. Med.*, **31**, 317–329.
50. Keys A., Brozek J., Henschel A., Mickelsen O., Taylor H. (1950). *The Biology of Human Starvation*. University of Minnesota Press, Minneapolis, MN.
51. Fairburn C., Welch S., Doll H., Davies B., O'Connor E. (1997). Risk factors for bulimia nervosa: a community-based case–control study. *Arch. Gen. Psychiatry*, **54**, 509–517.
52. The McKnight Investigators (2003). Risk factors for the onset of eating disorders in adolescent girls: results of the McKnight Longitudinal Study. *Am. J. Psychiatry*, **160**, 248–254.
53. Kendler K., Walters E., Neale M., Kessler R., Heath A., Eaves L. (1995). The structure of the genetic and environmental risk factors for six major psychiatric disorders in women. *Arch. Gen. Psychiatry*, **52**, 374–383.
54. Blinder B. (1983). Bulimia: the binge–purge compulsion. In: Cauwels J. (ed.) *Bulimia*. Doubleday, New York.
55. Fairburn C.G., Cooper P. (1984). Rumination in bulimia nervosa. *Br. Med. J.*, **288**, 826–827.
56. Chial H., Camilleri M., Williams D., Litzinger K., Perrault J. (2003). Rumination syndrome in children and adolescents: diagnosis, treatment, and prognosis. *Pediatrics*, **111**, 158–162.
57. Parry-Jones B. (1994). Mercycism or rumination disorder. A historical investigation and current assessment. *Br. J. Psychiatry*, **165**, 303–314.
58. Frisch R., McArthur J. (1974). Menstrual cycles: fatness as a determinant of minimum weight for height necessary for their maintenance or onset. *Science*, **185**, 949–951.
59. Johnson C., Flach R. (1985). Family characteristics of 105 patients with bulimia. *Am. J. Psychiatry*, **142**, 1321–1324.
60. Paxton S. (1993). A prevention program for disturbed eating and body dissatisfaction in adolescent girls. *Health Educ. Res.*, **8**, 43–51.
61. Killen J.D., Taylor C.B., Hammer L.D., Litt I., Wilson D.M., Rich T., Hayward C., Simmonds B., Kraemer H., Varady A. (1993). An attempt to modify unhealthful eating attitudes and weight regulation practices of young adolescent girls. *Int. J. Eat. Disord.*, **13**, 369–384.
62. Smolak L., Levine M.P., Schermer F. (1998). A controlled evaluation of an elementary school primary prevention program for eating problems. *J. Psychosom. Res.*, **44**, 339–353.
63. Wade T.D., Davidson S., O'Dea J. (2003). A preliminary controlled evaluation of a school-based media literacy program and self-esteem program for reducing eating disorder risk factors. *Int. J. Eat. Disord.*, **33**, 371–383.

64. Stice E., Hayward C., Cameron R., Killen J., Taylor C. (2000). Body-image and eating disturbances predict onset of depression among female adolescents: a longitudinal study. *J. Abnorm. Psychol.*, **109**, 438–444.
65. Stice E., Trost A., Chase A. (2003). Healthy weight control and dissonance-based eating disorder prevention programs: results from a controlled trial. *Int. J. Eat. Disord.*, **33**, 10–21.
66. World Health Organization (1992). *The ICD-10 Classification of Mental and Behavioural Disorders: Clinical Descriptions and Diagnostic Guidelines.* World Health Organization, Geneva.
67. American Psychiatric Association (1994). *Diagnostic and Statistical Manual of Mental Disorders*, 4th edn. American Psychiatric Association, Washington, DC.
68. Lasègue E. (1873). De l'anorexie hystérique. *Archives Générales de Médecine*, **1**, 385–403.
69. Striegel-Moore R., Dohm F., Kraemer H., Taylor C., Daniels S., Crawford P., Schreiber G. (2003). Eating disorders in white and black women. *Am. J. Psychiatry*, **160**, 1326–1331.
70. Casper R. (1998). Recognizing eating disorders in women. *Psychopharmacol. Bull*, **34**, 267–269.
71. Bryant-Waugh R., Lask B. (1990). Can pediatricians and family practitioners recognize anorexia nervosa in children? Presented at the Fourth International Conference on Eating Disorders, New York, 22–26 April.
72. Nicholls D., Chater R., Lask B. (2000). Children into DSM don't go: a comparison of classification systems for eating disorders in childhood and early adolescence. *Int. J. Eat. Disord.*, **28**, 317–324.
73. Hoek H., Bartelds A., Bosveld J., van der Graaf Y., Limpens V.E., Maiwald M., Spaaij C. (1995). Impact of urbanization on detection rates of eating disorders. *Am. J. Psychiatry*, **152**, 1272–1278.
74. Garner D.M., Olmstedt M.P., Bohr Y., Garfinkel P.E. (1982). The Eating Attitudes Test: psychometric features and clinical correlates. *Psychol. Med.*, **12**, 871–878.
75. Freund K.M., Graham S.M., Lesky L.G., Moskowitz M. (1993). Detection of bulimia in a primary care setting. *J. Gen. Intern. Med.*, **8**, 236–242.
76. Rathner G., Messner K. (1993). Detection of eating disorders in a small rural town: an epidemiological study. *Psychol. Med.*, **23**, 175–184.
77. Casper R.C. (1998). Behavioral activation and lack of concern, core symptoms of anorexia nervosa? *Int. J. Eat. Disord.* **24**, 381–393.
78. Arbelle S., Benjamin J., Golin M., Kremer I., Belmaker R., Ebstein R. (2003). Relation of shyness in grade school children to the genotype for the long arm of the serotonin transporter promoter region polymorphism. *Am. J. Psychiatry*, **160**, 671–676.
79. Kagan J., Reznick J., Snidman N. (1987). The physiology and psychology of behavioral inhibition in children. *Child Develop.*, **58**, 1459–1473.
80. Hayward C., Killen J., Kraemer H., Taylor C. (2000). Predictors of panic attacks in adolescents. *J. Am. Acad. Child Adolesc. Psychiatry*, **39**, 207–214.

CHAPTER

8

Precursors, Early Detection and Prevention of Anxiety Disorders

Dan J. Stein*, Soraya Seedat*, Paul Carey* and Brian Harvey‡

**University of Stellenbosch, Cape Town, South Africa*
‡North West University, Potchefstroom, South Africa

INTRODUCTION

Anxiety disorders are among the most prevalent, disabling and chronic of all the psychiatric disorders [1,2]. The underdiagnosis and undertreatment of these conditions contributes to their enormous personal and economic costs [3,4]. Fortunately, there have been significant advances in understanding their mediating psychobiology and in developing effective interventions [5]. Such advances can be drawn upon to encourage early detection of these disorders and even to consider interventions aimed at prevention. In this chapter we review research relevant to these issues. We begin by considering each of the major anxiety disorders in turn.

GENERALIZED ANXIETY DISORDER

Generalized anxiety disorder (GAD) is characterized by psychic and somatic tension. Although the DSM has focused increasingly on the cognitive aspects of GAD, this disorder often presents with somatic symptoms, and indeed it is the most common anxiety disorder in primary care settings [6]. Although GAD has at times been considered a residual disorder, there is growing evidence that it is in fact an independent disorder, characterized by specific symptomatology, high prevalence and significant disability [7].

Early Detection and Management of Mental Disorders.
Edited by Mario Maj, Juan José López-Ibor, Norman Sartorius, Mitsumoto Sato and Ahmed Okasha.
 ISBN 0-470-01083-5.

GAD is associated with a good deal of psychiatric comorbidity, but no more so than is major depression [8]. The condition has a later onset than most other anxiety disorders, but it tends to precede other comorbid disorders, especially major depression [9]. Other important comorbidities in GAD include somatization disorder, other anxiety disorders, and substance use disorders. The disability that is associated with comorbid GAD and depression is significantly higher than the disability associated with either disorder alone [10].

The psychobiology of GAD is relatively poorly understood. Nevertheless, there is evidence that prefrontal and amygdala circuits are involved, and that serotonergic and GABAergic systems play a particularly important role [11]. Benzodiazepines, 5-HT_{1A} partial agonists, and certain antidepressants – such as tricyclic antidepressants, selective serotonin reuptake inhibitors (SSRIs), and noradrenergic and serotonin selective reuptake inhibitors – have shown efficacy in the treatment of GAD [6].

Given the prevalence of GAD in primary care settings, early detection and management of this condition will require the close participation of primary care providers. GAD patients with somatic symptoms, or with comorbid medical disorders, are at particular risk for failing to receive a psychiatric diagnosis and appropriate treatment. Nevertheless, such patients are also high utilizers of medical care, and are experienced as particularly frustrating by primary care providers [12]. Demonstrating to primary care practitioners that simple screening questions [6] or scales [13] are useful in detecting GAD, and that identified patients respond to treatment, is a crucial step for progress towards early detection and management of this disorder.

To optimize the early detection of GAD, it is also important to ensure that children and adolescents with this disorder are adequately diagnosed and evaluated. There is growing evidence that the SSRIs can be effective in this population [14,15]. Although there is currently little data on the long-term outcome of such patients, it can be speculated that early treatment may prevent the chronicity associated with untreated GAD, and the consequent morbidity.

Early diagnosis and robust treatment of GAD in adults is also an important goal. In patients with comorbid GAD and depression, GAD is most commonly the earliest disorder. Several explanations have been put forward to explain this sequence, but its underlying mechanisms remain poorly understood [16]. There is, however, some evidence that in GAD patients who receive pharmacotherapy, there is decreased likelihood of developing depression [17]. This suggests the plausibility of a neurobiological explanation of the link between earlier GAD and later depression, but additional work is needed to replicate such findings and to delineate the relevant mechanisms.

OBSESSIVE–COMPULSIVE DISORDER

Obsessive–compulsive disorder (OCD) is characterized by intrusive thoughts or images (obsessions) and by repetitive and stereotypic acts (compulsions). In DSM-IV it is made clear that compulsions can be either behaviours or mental acts. Despite the face validity of the clinical distinction between obsessions (which may increase anxiety) and compulsions (which serve to decrease anxiety), factor analyses have increasingly provided evidence for the construct validity of a four-factor model of OCD, including contamination concerns aggressive/checking symptoms, symmetry/ordering concerns and hoarding [18,19].

OCD has a prevalence of around 2%, and some studies have suggested that it is one of the most disabling of all the medical disorders [2]. Studies have demonstrated a remarkably long gap (up to 17 years) between diagnosis and appropriate treatment [20]. Thus, an immediate focus for those interested in preventing the chronicity and morbidity of OCD is the importance of early diagnosis and treatment. Working with consumer advocacy groups and the media may play an important role in increasing awareness, decreasing stigma, and so contributing to earlier and more appropriate intervention [21].

To optimize early detection of OCD, it is particularly important to recognize the group of patients with early onset OCD [22]. Childhood onset OCD patients are more likely to be male and to have comorbid tics. Normal childhood rituals need, however, to be differentiated from pathological OCD symptoms. Fortunately, there is good evidence that many of these patients respond to standard OCD treatments, including pharmacotherapy with the SSRIs [23].

A proportion of childhood-onset cases of OCD can be characterized as having paediatric neuropsychiatric disorders associated with streptococcus (PANDAS). These cases are thought to involve auto-immune responses after infection with this bacterium [24]. This research suggests the possibility that early diagnosis and treatment of streptococcal infection might reduce the incidence of OCD. Nevertheless, the extent to which auto-immune mechanisms account for OCD cases as a whole remains unknown, and such work has not yet been undertaken. An early trial of penicillin prophylaxis in subjects with PANDAS did not prove effective in preventing subsequent OCD symptoms [25]. Penicillin did not, however, effectively prevent streptococcal infection, suggesting that trials with other antibiotics are warranted.

It is theoretically possible that individual and family interventions with high-risk individuals might be useful in enhancing early detection and prevention of OCD. It remains unclear to what extent OCD is caused by genetic versus environmental influences. Nevertheless, it is potentially possible to target individuals at high risk (for example, those with parental OCD), or to target times of higher risk (for example, pregnancy and puerperium [26]). Although it is possible that medication could be used in patients at high risk for OCD, an immediate question is whether cognitive–behavioural therapy (CBT) might not have a role in such cases.

Ultimately, particular neurobiological markers (e.g. abnormal functional brain activity, the presence of particular genetic variants) may prove crucial in targeting individuals at risk for developing OCD. Certainly, there is already evidence that particular variants in the serotonin transporter protein (5-HTTP) gene are associated with high risk for OCD [27]. Nevertheless, at present work on functional imaging and genetic variants in OCD remains primarily within the realm of research.

PANIC DISORDER AND AGORAPHOBIA

Panic disorder is characterized by unexpected panic attacks. These may be followed by panic attacks in response to particular stimuli, and by agoraphobia. Panic disorder with or without agoraphobia is a prevalent and disabling disorder. Panic–depression is a particularly common comorbidity, and contributes to the potentially negative impact of panic disorder [28]. Alcohol and substance abuse and dependence are also frequent comorbidities in panic and other anxiety disorders.

A biological perspective suggests that there are multiple risk factors for the onset of panic disorder [29], including both biological risk factors (e.g. family history) and environmental ones (e.g. separation). Genetic variants may well be important in the pathogenesis of panic, but at present are not clinically useful as risk markers. Long-term studies of anxiety disorders are relatively few, but these provide additional information about resilience and vulnerability factors [30]. Anxiety sensitivity is a trait that predicts frequency and intensity of panic attacks, and that may be responsive to CBT [31].

Patients with panic disorder frequently present to medical practitioners, and may receive a range of unnecessary special investigations. These may include investigation of the cardiovascular, respiratory and gastrointestinal systems. Early detection of panic disorder requires working closely with a range of different practitioners to ensure that panic disorder is entertained in the differential diagnosis of various symptoms.

An influential hypothesis states that panic attacks can be conceptualized in terms of a false suffocation alarm [32]. In this view, conditions characterized by increased PCO_2, such as chronic obstructive pulmonary disorders and asthma, are associated with an increased risk for panic disorder. If correct, then panic disorder could be prevented by optimizing the treatment of such conditions. While this question has received little empirical study to date, there is growing interest in determining the modifiable risk factors for onset and persistence of the comorbidity between respiratory and anxiety disorders [33].

There is also evidence that prior smoking is associated with panic disorder [34]. Thus, it can be hypothesized that decreasing cigarette use in younger populations would help prevent later panic disorder. Prospective studies to assess such questions are difficult, but analysis of long-term epidemiological data could help to address this issue.

Finally, it is possible that early diagnosis and treatment of panic disorder could prevent subsequent agoraphobia, depression and substance use disorders. There is some empirical data to support the assertion that treatment of panic attacks is associated with a lower risk of subsequent depression [35]. Prospective long-term studies are needed to fully understand the course of anxiety disorders such as panic disorder, and to delineate clearly the possible impact of early detection and robust treatment on decreasing symptoms and disability.

POST-TRAUMATIC STRESS DISORDER

By definition, post-traumatic stress disorder (PTSD) occurs in the aftermath of a traumatic event. The characteristic symptoms of the disorder can be divided into intrusive symptoms, avoidance and numbness symptoms, and hyperarousal symptoms. Although initially conceptualized as a normal reaction to an abnormal event, PTSD is increasingly understood as a medical disorder characterized by underlying psychobiological dysfunction [36]. After a traumatic event a range of symptoms is normative; in the majority of cases these gradually diminish, but in PTSD such symptoms persist.

The National Comorbidity Survey in the US found that 60.7% of males and 51.2% of females had experienced a significant traumatic event [37]. The lifetime prevalence of PTSD was 10.4% in females, and 5.0% in males. PTSD is characterized by chronicity of symptoms, significant comorbidity and substantial disability [38]. Early detection and effective treatment is therefore an important goal.

PTSD in combat veterans is well described, and is a routine focus of early detection programmes in the military. It is, however, important to screen for PTSD in populations other than the military. Sexual and physical trauma in children and adolescents is unfortunately a prevalent problem in both the developed and the developing world [39]. Domestic violence is also widespread, and there is a high incidence of PTSD in those exposed to it

[40]. PTSD is associated with high utilization of health care, and screening for exposure to trauma in medical settings is therefore imperative [41]. A range of instruments is available to screen for trauma, interpersonal violence and PTSD [42,43].

There is growing work on risk factors for PTSD [44]. These include demographic factors (e.g. female gender), clinical factors (e.g. dissociation during the trauma, exposure to multiple traumas) and biological variables (e.g. tachycardia, hypocortisolism, decreased dehydroepiandrosterone (DHEA), decreased neuropeptide Y, presence of particular genetic variants) [45]. Symptoms of acute stress disorder after the trauma can be used to determine those at high risk for developing PTSD [46]. Early screening after trauma exposure may also be useful in identifying children at risk for PTSD [47]. There is a need, however, for additional studies to determine how best to screen populations after trauma, in order to optimize the early detection of psychiatric morbidity [48].

Nevertheless, work on psychotherapeutic intervention after exposure to trauma has shown that this is not necessarily helpful. In particular, single-session psychological interventions or "debriefing" does not appear to be an effective intervention [49]. The reason for this failure is unclear, but it may reflect the fact that people process trauma in different ways, and that interventions must be more individualized [50]. More intensive cognitive–behavioural programmes may be effective for those with acute stress disorder [51], or with other risk factors for PTSD such as elevated heart rate [52], although, again, further work is still needed in this area.

There is also a growing interest in using pharmacotherapy to prevent post-traumatic symptoms in the aftermath of trauma. The adrenergic system serves as a general alarm system and its activation may play an important role in facilitating the encoding of emotional memories. Pitman *et al.* [53] have provided evidence that beta-blockers are effective in reducing the psychophysiological reactivity to memory cues of trauma, but had no significant effect on reducing PTSD at 3 months. Subsequent work has, however, provided some indication that PTSD symptoms, as well as PTSD diagnosis, were reduced at 2 months following acute treatment with propranolol [54]. In the immediate aftermath of trauma, severely burned children who received the tricyclic antidepressant imipramine had significantly lower rates of PTSD at 6 months than children who had received chloral hydrate [55]. Benzodiazepines, on the other hand, may exacerbate PTSD symptoms [56]. Additional work with other agents that have different mechanisms of action is needed.

In the future, we can expect approaches to the study of trauma and prevention of its sequelae that integrate biological and psychological approaches. Animal and clinical studies provide an increasingly solid foundation for such work [57]. An interesting recent exemplar of an integrated approach is the work by Fisher *et al.* [58], in which they reported that, in a small sample of maltreated preschool children, a psychosocial intervention undertaken soon after adoption was able to improve behavioural adjustment and to change hypothalamic–pituitary–adrenal (HPA) axis function (as measured by salivary cortisol). The incorporation of genetic and imaging studies into studies of both preventive pharmacotherapy and psychotherapy may be useful in delineating moderators and mediators of such interventions.

SOCIAL ANXIETY DISORDER

Social anxiety disorder (SAD) is characterized by fear of embarrassing oneself in social or performance situations. Subjects with generalized SAD fear several different social situations. SAD is a particularly prevalent and disabling anxiety disorder [59,60]. Thus, subjects with SAD are more likely to be single, are less likely to complete high school or tertiary studies, and are more likely to be unemployed and receive a lower income [6]. It seems reasonable to argue that early intervention for SAD, even in childhood and adolescence, may prevent the negative impact of this disorder. Long-term studies are, however, needed in this area.

SAD has a relatively early onset, and can persist for many years. Comorbid disorders often begin later on [61]. These include major depression, other anxiety disorders and substance use disorders. Simple screening questions [62] or scales, such as the Liebowitz Social Anxiety Scale (LSAS) and the Mini-Social Phobia Inventory (SPIN), are useful for screening for the presence of the disorder [63,64]. However, given that many people with SAD are unaware that they have a treatable medical disorder, and do not present to physicians for care, it is also important to increase awareness of the condition in the community as a whole. Early robust treatment of SAD might conceivably be able to decrease the morbidity of this condition, and prevent secondary comorbidity.

Although anxiety disorders demonstrate relatively high heritability [65], clinical entities are relatively heterogeneous, and there is growing interest in endophenotypes that may be more directly linked to genetic variants. Behavioural inhibition (BI) to the unfamiliar, for example, may be an endophenotype of particular relevance to SAD. Seen in around 20% of young children, it is defined by a stable tendency to be behaviourally restrained in unfamiliar social and non-social situations [66]. A number of similar temperamental styles have been described by other authors [67].

BI has specific biological correlates [68], including an association with the allele of the corticotropin releasing hormone (CRH)-linked locus [69], and increased amygdala response to novel stimuli in adulthood [70]. BI is a risk factor for the subsequent development of anxiety disorders, particularly SAD and panic disorder [71,72]. Withdrawn temperament is a strong predictor of childhood anxiety disorders, a reasonable predictor of adolescent anxiety disorders, and a weak to moderate predictor of adult anxiety disorders [67]. Furthermore, by adolescence early inhibition predicts not only anxiety but also depression, and by adulthood it may predict an even broader range of disorders [67].

An immediate question is whether early identification of children with BI and appropriate interventions are helpful in preventing adult anxiety disorders. There are preliminary data in the affirmative. Inhibited children, aged 3.5 to 4.5 years of age, were recruited to an intervention study via questionnaires distributed to preschools. Interventions were conducted with parents only, with the main aim of providing techniques that help children become more confident and outgoing. Early data from the study of 120 inhibited children suggested that subjects in the intervention group showed a markedly greater reduction in the number of anxiety diagnoses at 12 months relative to controls [67].

A range of other potentially modifiable risks for SAD and anxiety disorders include parental expression of anxiety, parental overprotection and modelling of anxious responses [67]. These factors may further contribute to the development of BI, or may be independent risk factors. Nevertheless, it is notable that most children with BI do not develop anxiety disorders. Therefore it is also important to consider protective factors, such as social support and coping skills. Particular kinds of parental interventions may be able to ensure that BI does not translate into later psychopathology. Ultimately, work delineating the risk and protective factors for anxiety disorders may well lead to novel interventions to prevent the onset of these conditions [73].

SCREENING FOR ANXIETY DISORDERS

In the above discussion of each of the major anxiety disorders, there are overlapping themes. These are highly prevalent, disabling and costly conditions. Despite the availability of effective pharmacotherapy and psychotherapy, they remain underdiagnosed and undertreated [74–77]. Cross-sectional studies of rates of appropriate diagnosis are partly flawed insofar as prevalence of psychiatric disorders is higher in follow-up patients; nevertheless, underdiagnosis is a real problem [78,79]. Thus, there is clearly need for more widespread screening to maximize the chance of early detection and management.

Screening would seem to be particularly relevant in primary care settings [80], although there are also important opportunities for screening in other contexts, including direct screening of the public [81]. A range of screening instruments for anxiety disorders is available for use in primary care [82]. A number have also been studied in more specialized populations, settings and cultures [83–93]. Broad-based questionnaires such as the Primary Care Evaluation of Mental Disorders (PRIME-MD) (for a range of psychiatric disorders) or the Anxiety Screening Questionnaire (for anxiety disorders) may, however, be more useful in the primary care setting than relying on several different measures for individual disorders [94].

Another approach is to rely on a broad but brief measure of distress or negative affectivity, as this construct is perhaps key to a range of different mood and anxiety disorders. Such measures include the General Health Questionnaire (GHQ), the Brief Symptom Inventory-18 (BSI) and the K10/K6 [95,96]. The Hospital Anxiety and Depression Scale (HADS) may be particularly useful in patients with medical disorders, although it also has limitations [91,97]. Patients who score highly on such screening instruments can then be assessed with disorder-specific interviews or scales [98].

It is important to be aware of the costs and possible harms associated with screening [99]. Broad-based questionnaires are time-consuming. Conversely, screens that are too short may fail to identify a range of different disorders. Further work is needed to determine whether the compromise of using measures such as the GHQ or BSI is in fact useful. Computer-administered questionnaires and the Internet provide user-friendly media that may enhance screening strategies [100,101]. Additional work is also necessary to determine the optimal combination of primary care screening, community outreach and screening in more specialized settings.

A systematic review of studies of screening for depression and anxiety disorders has emphasized that screening alone is not sufficient to influence clinicians' behaviour and improve patient outcomes [82]. Screening for depression and anxiety invariably yields false positives, so clinicians may be unwilling to believe screening data. Clinicians who have not been trained in psychiatry may also be uncomfortable managing those who screen positive for these disorders. Screening programmes are enhanced when only positive values are fed back to the clinician, and outcomes are enhanced when screening is integrated with a treatment programme [82,102].

PREVENTION OF ANXIETY DISORDERS

As our understanding of the pathogenesis of anxiety disorders becomes increasingly sophisticated, it may also be possible to develop effective interventions to help prevent their onset [73,103]. In addition, screening strategies discussed above may yield a group of individuals who do not yet have an anxiety disorder, but who are nevertheless at risk should they not receive help. Thus, there is increasing interest in the prevention of childhood anxiety disorders by child-focused methods, parent-focused methods and environmental restructuring methods. Such strategies can be universal, selective or indicated [104]. We discuss each of them in turn.

Universal prevention strategies are provided to entire populations. Lowry-Webster *et al.* [105] assigned 594 children aged 10–13 to CBT conducted by classroom teachers or to assessment only. Barrett and Turner [106] assigned 489 children aged 10–12 years to a psychologist-led programme, a teacher-led programme or to usual care. In both studies, anxiety symptoms were significantly lower in the intervention groups post-treatment, although follow-up data are not yet available. Such efforts require significant resources, such as the close collaboration of schools and teachers, and the cost–benefit ratio must be carefully assessed. In addition, given the relatively stable prevalence of anxiety disorders in epidemiological studies, some scepticism about the extent to which such interventions are valuable may be warranted [107]. Further work is needed to determine the extent to which primary prevention strategies are able to foster protective factors and impact a range of behavioural and emotional problems.

Selective prevention strategies can be targeted at subgroups with a high lifetime or imminent risk of developing a problem after exposure to a biological, psychological or social risk factor. The most commonly studied strategies focus on the occurrence of traumatic or negative life events. Successful programmes have, for example, been developed to help children cope with parental divorce [108], transition to a new school [109], medical [110] and dental [111] procedures, and performances and tests [112]. Interventions for children with anxiety sensitivity [31] or BI [67] also fit under this category. There is relatively less work in adults, despite growing awareness of a range of stressors associated with subsequent anxiety [113]. Although selective prevention strategies require fewer resources than universal strategies, the range of possible harms associated with preventive programmes needs to be borne in mind [114]. More work is also required to develop efficient risk identification procedures and determine the optimal timing of interventions [73].

Indicated prevention strategies are useful when screening has found a pool of individuals at high risk. They may have minimal but detectable symptoms, or biological markers of a disorder. LaFreniere and Capuano [115] randomly assigned 43 anxious–withdrawn preschool children to an intensive intervention programme or non-intervention. Although children in the intervention group did better on a number of outcomes, anxious–withdrawn behaviours decreased in both groups. In another study, Dadds *et al.* [116] screened 1786 children aged 7–14 years, and identified 128 highly anxious children. Children randomized to a 10-week school-based child- and family-focused group intervention had significantly less risk of meeting diagnostic criteria for an anxiety disorder than those assigned to a waiting list at 2-year follow-up. Notably, the benefits of the programme were more apparent in those children with an initial anxiety disorder, and less clear in those with only subclinical anxiety. Some work on secondary prevention strategies has also been done in older subjects: for example, psychological interventions can be useful in college students with high test anxiety [117].

CONCLUSIONS

There have been significant advances in understanding the psychobiology and management of anxiety disorders in recent years [5]. Nevertheless, more attention has been paid to vulnerability to these conditions than to the mechanisms underlying resilience, and there is much room for additional research in this latter area [118]. Furthermore, despite significant progress in this field, there is considerable evidence that the anxiety disorders remain underdiagnosed and undertreated [77,80].

Partnerships with primary care practitioners, consumer advocacy groups and communities may help to raise awareness of these disorders, decrease stigmatization, and encourage early diagnosis and treatment [119]. Further work is needed to fully understand the reasons for pervasive delays in help-seeking in those with anxiety disorders, and to effectively combat this [120,121]. There is a particular need for encouraging treatment-seeking in low referral groups such as children with anxiety disorders, or survivors of domestic violence [122].

Although further prospective long-term studies are needed, timely treatment may well be able to decrease the morbidity and comorbidity associated with the anxiety disorders [17,33]. Increasingly there is also a focus on the prevention of anxiety disorders [103]; there is already promising data in this area, and further effectiveness studies in the community should be undertaken. Future advances in the early detection and prevention of anxiety disorders will depend not only on advances in our understanding of their pathogenesis and molecular biology [123], but also on our ability to work with policy makers and communities to change the perception of psychiatric disorders and to develop innovative methodologies for combating them [21].

ACKNOWLEDGEMENTS

The authors are supported by the Medical Research Council and the National Research Foundation of South Africa.

REFERENCES

1. Kessler R.C., McGonagle K.C., Zhao S., Nelson C.B., Hughes M., Eshleman S., Wittchen H.-U., Kendler K.S. (1994). Lifetime and 12-month prevalence of DSM-III-R psychiatric disorders in the United States: results from the National Comorbidity Survey. *Arch. Gen. Psychiatry*, **51**, 8–19.
2. Murray C.J.L., Lopez A.D. (1996). *Global Burden of Disease: A Comprehensive Assessment of Mortality and Morbidity from Diseases, Injuries and Risk Factors in 1990 and Projected to 2020*, vol. 1. World Health Organization, Harvard, MA.
3. Dupont R.L., Rice D.P., Miller L.S., Shiraki S.S., Rowland C.R., Harwood H.J. (1996). Economic costs of anxiety disorders. *Anxiety*, **2**, 167–172.
4. Greenberg P.E., Sisitsky T., Kessler R.C., Finkelstein S., Berndt E.R., Davidson J.R.T., Ballenger J.C., Fyer A.J. (1999). The economic burden of the anxiety disorders in the 1990s. *J. Clin. Psychiatry*, **60**, 427–435.
5. Stein D.J., Hollander E. (2002). *Textbook of Anxiety Disorders*. American Psychiatric Press, Washington, DC.
6. Ballenger J.C., Davidson J.R., Lecrubier Y., Nutt D.J., Borkovec T.D., Stein D.J., Wittchen H.-U. (2001). Consensus statement on generalized anxiety disorder from the International Consensus Group on Depression and Anxiety. *J. Clin. Psychiatry*, **62** (Suppl. 11), 53–58.
7. Nutt D., Rickels K., Stein D.J. (2002). *Generalized Anxiety Disorder: Symptomatology, Pathogenesis, and Management*. Dunitz, London.
8. Kessler R.C. (2001). The epidemiology of pure and comorbid generalized anxiety disorder. A review and evaluation of recent research. *Acta Psychiatr. Scand.*, **406**, 7–13.
9. Wittchen H.-U., Zhao S., Kessler R.C., Eaton W.W. (1994). DSM-III-R generalized anxiety disorder in the National Comorbidity Survey. *Arch. Gen. Psychiatry*, **51**, 355–364.
10. Stein D.J. (2001). Comorbidity in generalized anxiety disorder: impact and implications. *J. Clin. Psychiatry*, **62** (Suppl. 11), 29–36.
11. Stein D.J., Westenberg H., Liebowitz M.R. (2002). Social anxiety disorder and generalized anxiety disorder: serotonergic and dopaminergic neurocircuitry. *J. Clin. Psychiatry*, **63** (Suppl. 6), 12–19.
12. Roy-Byrne P.P., Katon W. (1997). Generalized anxiety disorder in primary care: the precursor/modifier pathway to increased health care utilization. *J. Clin. Psychiatry*, **58** (Suppl. 3), 34–38.
13. Behar E., Alcaine O., Zuellig A.R., Borkovec T.D. (2003). Screening for generalized anxiety disorder using the Penn State Worry Questionnaire: a receiver operating characteristic analysis. *J. Behav. Ther. Exp. Psychiatry*, **34**, 25–43.
14. Research Unit on Pediatric Psychopharmacology Anxiety Study Group (2001). Fluvoxamine for the treatment of anxiety disorders in children and adolescents. *N. Engl. J. Med.*, **34**, 1279–1285.
15. Rynn M.A., Siqueland L., Rickels K. (2001). Placebo-controlled trial of sertraline in the treatment of children with generalized anxiety disorder. *Am. J. Psychiatry*, **158**, 2008–2014.
16. Stein D. J., Hollander E. (2002). *Anxiety Disorders Comorbid with Depression: Social Anxiety Disorder, Post-Traumatic Stress Disorder, Generalized Anxiety Disorder and Obsessive–Compulsive Disorder*. Dunitz, London.

17. Goodwin R.D., Gorman J.M. (2002). Psychopharmacologic treatment of generalized anxiety disorder and the risk of major depression. *Am. J. Psychiatry*, **159**, 1935–1937.
18. Leckman J.F., Grice D.E., Boardman J., Zhang H., Vitale A., Bondi C., Alsobrook J., Peterson B.S., Cohen D.J., Rasmussen S.A., *et al.* (1997). Symptoms of obsessive–compulsive disorder. *Am. J. Psychiatry*, **54**, 911–917.
19. Lochner C., Stein D.J. (2003). Heterogeneity of obsessive–compulsive disorder: a literature review. *Harv. Rev. Psychiatry*, **11**, 113–132.
20. Hollander E., Stein D.J., Broatch J., Himelein C., Rowland C. (1997). A pharmacoeconomic and quality of life study of obsessive–compulsive disorder. *CNS Spectrums*, **2**, 16–25.
21. Seedat S., Stein D.J., Berk M., Wilson Z. (2002). Barriers to treatment among members of a mental health advocacy group in South Africa. *Soc. Psychiatry Psychiatr. Epidemiol.*, **37**, 483–487.
22. Geller D.A., Biederman J., Faraone S., Agranat A., Cradock K., Hagermose L., Frazier J., Coffey B.J. (2001). Developmental aspects of obsessive–compulsive disorder: findings in children, adolescents, and adults. *J. Nerv. Ment. Dis.*, **189**, 471–477.
23. Geller D.A., Biederman J., Stewart S.E., Mullin B., Martin A., Spencer T. (2003). Which SSRI? A meta-analysis of pharmacotherapy trials in pediatric obsessive–compulsive disorder. *Am. J. Psychiatry*, **160**, 1919–1928.
24. Swedo S.E., Leonard H.L., Garvey M., Mittleman B., Allen A.J., Perlmutter S., Lougee L., Dow S., Zamkoff J., Dubbert B.K., *et al.* (1998). Pediatric autoimmune neuropsychiatric disorders associated with streptococcal infections: clinical description of the first 50 cases. *Am. J. Psychiatry*, **155**, 264–271.
25. Garvey MA., Perlmutter S.J., Allen A.J., Hamburger S., Lougee L., Leonard H.L., Witowski M.E., Dubbert B., Swedo S.E. (1999). A pilot study of penicillin prophylaxis for neuropsychiatric exacerbations triggered by streptococcal infections. *Biol. Psychiatry*, **45**, 1564–1571.
26. Neziroglu F., Anemone R., Yaryura-Tobias J.A. (1992). Onset of obsessive–compulsive disorder in pregnancy. *Am. J. Psychiatry*, **1490**, 947–950.
27. Ozaki N., Goldman D., Kaye W.H., Plotnicov K., Greenberg B.D., Lappalainen J., Rudnick G., Murphy D.L. (2003). Serotonin transporter missense mutation associated with a complex neuropsychiatric phenotype. *Mol. Psychiatry*, **8**, 895, 933–936.
28. Roy-Byrne P.P., Stang P., Wittchen H.-U., Ustun B., Walters E.E., Kessler R.C. (2000). Lifetime panic–depression comorbidity in the National Comorbidity Survey: association with symptoms, impairment, course and help-seeking. *Br. J. Psychiatry*, **176**, 229–235.
29. Gorman J.M., Kent J.M., Sullivan G.M., Coplan J.D. (2000). Neuroanatomical hypothesis of panic disorder, revised. *Am. J. Psychiatry*, **157** 493–505.
30. Yonkers K.A., Bruce S.E., Dyck I.R., Keller M.B. (2003). Chronicity, relapse, and illness – course of panic disorder, social phobia, and generalized anxiety disorder: findings in men and women from 8 years of follow-up. *Depress. Anxiety*, **17**, 173–179.
31. McNally R.J. (2002). Anxiety sensitivity and panic disorder. *Biol. Psychiatry*, **52**, 938–946.
32. Klein D.F. (1993). False suffocation alarms, spontaneous panics, and related conditions: an integrative hypothesis. *Arch. Gen. Psychiatry*, **50**, 306–317.
33. Goodwin R.D. (2003). Asthma and anxiety disorders. *Adv. Psychosom. Med.*, **24**, 51–71.

34. Isensee B., Wittchen H.-U., Stein M.B., Hofler M., Lieb R. (2003). Smoking increases the risk of panic: findings from a prospective community study. *Arch. Gen. Psychiatry*, **60**, 692–700.
35. Goodwin R., Olfson M. (2001). Treatment of panic attack and risk of major depression in the community. *Am. J. Psychiatry*, **158**, 1146–1148.
36. Yehuda R., McFarlane A.C. (1995). Conflict between current knowledge about posttraumatic stress disorder and its original conceptual basis. *Am. J. Psychiatry*, **152**, 1705–1713.
37. Kessler R.C., Sonnega A., Bromet E., Hughes M., Nelson C.B. (1995). Posttraumatic stress disorder in the National Comorbidity Survey. *Arch. Gen. Psychiatry*, **52**, 1048–1060.
38. Kessler R.C. (2002). Posttraumatic stress disorder: the burden to the individual and to society. *J. Clin. Psychiatry*, **61** (Suppl. 5), 4–12.
39. Seedat S., Kaminer D., Lockhat S., Stein D.J. (2000). An overview of posttraumatic stress disorder in children and adolescents. *Primary Care Psychiatry*, **6**, 43–48.
40. Seedat S., Stein D.J. (2000). Trauma and post-traumatic stress disorder in women: a review. *Int. Clin. Psychopharmacol.*, **15** (Suppl. 3), 25–34.
41. Ballenger J.C., Davidson J.R., Lecrubier Y., Nutt D.J., Foa E.B., Kessler R.C., McFarlane A.C., Shalev A.Y. (2000). Consensus statement on posttraumatic stress disorder from the International Consensus Group on Depression and Anxiety. *J. Clin. Psychiatry*, **61** (Suppl. 5), 60–66.
42. Muris P., Merckelbach H., Korver P., Meesters C. (2000). Screening for trauma in children and adolescents: the validity of the Traumatic Stress Disorder Scale for the screen for child anxiety related emotional disorders. *J. Clin. Child Psychol.*, **29**, 406–413.
43. Coker A.L., Pope B.O., Smith P.H., Sanderson M., Hussey J.R. (2001). Assessment of clinical partner violence screening tools. *J. Am. Med. Women's Assoc.*, **56**, 19–23.
44. Brewin C.R., Andrews B., Valentine J.D. (2000). Meta-analysis of risk factors for posttraumatic stress disorder in trauma-exposed adults. *J. Consult. Clin. Psychol.*, **68**, 748–766.
45. Yehuda R. (2004). Risk and resilience in posttraumatic stress disorder. *J. Clin. Psychiatry*, **65** (Suppl. 1), 29–36.
46. Brewin C.R., Rose S., Andrews A., Green J., Tata P., McEvedy C., Turner S., Foa E.B. (2002). Brief screening instrument for post-traumatic stress disorder. *Br. J. Psychiatry*, **181**, 158–162.
47. Stallard P., Velleman R., Baldwin S. (1999). Psychological screening of children for post-traumatic stress disorder. *J. Child Psychol. Psychiatry*, **40**, 1075–1082.
48. Silove D., Blaszczynski A., Manicavasager V., Tyndall K., Petridis A., Hillman K. (2003). Capacity of screening questionnaires to predict psychiatric morbidity 18 months after motor vehicle accidents. *J. Nerv. Ment. Dis.*, **191**, 604–610.
49. Rose S., Bisson J., Wessely S. (2003). A systematic review of single-session psychological interventions (''debriefing'') following trauma. *Psychother. Psychosom.*, **72**, 176–184.
50. Esterling B.A., L'Abate L., Murray E.J., Pennebaker J.W. (1999). Empirical foundations for writing in prevention and psychotherapy: mental and physical health outcomes. *Clin. Psychol. Rev.*, **19**, 79–96.
51. Bryant R., Harvey A., Dang S., Sackville T., Basten C. (1998). Treatment of acute stress disorder: a comparison of cognitive–behavioral therapy and supportive counseling. *J. Consult. Clin. Psychol.*, **66**, 862–866.

52. Gidron Y., Gal R., Freedman S., Twiser I., Lauden A., Snir Y., Benjamin J. (2001). Translating research findings to PTSD prevention: results of a randomized-controlled pilot study. *J. Trauma. Stress*, **14**, 773–780.
53. Pitman R.K., Sanders K.M., Zusman R.M., Healy A.R., Cheema F., Lasko N.B., Cahill L., Orr S.P. (2002). Pilot study of secondary prevention of posttraumatic stress disorder with propranolol. *Biol. Psychiatry*, **51**, 189–192.
54. Vaiva G., Ducrocq F., Jezequel K., Averland B., Lestavel P., Brunet A., Marmar C.R. (2003). Immediate treatment with propranolol decreases posttraumatic stress disorder two months after trauma. *Biol. Psychiatry*, **54**, 947–949.
55. Robert R., Blakeney P.E., Villarreal C., Rosenberg L., Meyer W.J. III (1999). Imipramine treatment in pediatric burn patients with symptoms of acute stress disorder: a pilot study. *J. Am. Acad. Child Adolesc. Psychiatry*, **38**, 873–882.
56. Gelpin E., Bonne E., Peri T., Brandes D., Shalev A.Y. (1996). Treatment of recent trauma survivors with benzodiazepines: a prospective study. *J. Clin. Psychiatry*, **57**, 390–394.
57. Miller Brotman L., Gouley K.K., Klein R.G., Castellanos F.X., Pine D.S. (2003). Children, stress, and context: integrating basic, clinical, and experimental prevention research. *Child Develop.*, **74**, 1053–1057.
58. Fisher P.A., Gunnar M.R., Chamberlain P., Reid J.G. (2000). Preventive intervention for maltreated preschool children: impact on children's behavior, neuroendocrine activity, and foster parent functioning. *Am. Acad. Child Adolesc. Psychiatry*, **39**, 1356–1364.
59. Magee W.J., Eaton W.W., Wittchen H.-U., McGonagle K.A., Kessler R.C. (1996). Agoraphobia, simple phobia, and social phobia in the National Comorbidity Survey. *Arch. Gen. Psychiatry*, **53**, 159–168.
60. Lochner C., Mogotsi M., du Toit P.L., Kaminer D., Niehaus D.J., Stein D.J. (2003). Quality of life in the anxiety disorders: a comparison of obsessive–compulsive disorder, social anxiety disorder, and panic disorder. *Psychopathology*, **36**, 255–262.
61. Kessler R.C., Stang P., Wittchen H.-U., Stein M., Walters E.E. (1999). Lifetime co-morbidities between social phobia and mood disorders in the US National Comorbidity Survey. *Psychol. Med.*, **29**, 555–567.
62. Ballenger J.C., Davidson J.A., Lecrubier Y., Nutt D.J., Bobes J., Beidel D.C., Ono Y., Westenberg H.G. (1998). Consensus statement on social anxiety disorder from the international consensus group on depression and anxiety. *J. Clin. Psychiatry*, **59**, 54–60.
63. Connor K.M., Kobak K.A., Churchill L.E., Katzelnick D., Davidson J.R. (2001). Mini-SPIN: a brief screening assessment for generalized social anxiety disorder. *Depress. Anxiety*, **14**, 137–140.
64. Mennin D.S., Fresco D.M., Heimberg R.G., Schneier F.R., Davies S.O., Liebowitz M.R. (2002). Screening for social anxiety disorder in the clinical setting: using the Liebowitz Social Anxiety Scale. *J. Anxiety Disord.*, **16**, 661–673.
65. Hettema J.M., Neale M.C., Kendler K.S. (2001). A review and meta-analysis of the genetic epidemiology of anxiety disorders. *Am. J. Psychiatry*, **158**, 1568–1578.
66. Kagan J., Reznick J.S., Snidman N. (1987). The physiology and psychology of behavioral inhibition in children. *Child Develop.*, **58**, 1459–1473.
67. Rapee R.M. (2002). The development and modification of temperamental risk for anxiety disorders: prevention of a lifetime of anxiety? *Biol. Psychiatry*, **52**, 947–957.
68. Kagan J., Reznick S., Snidman N. (1988). Biological bases of childhood shyness. *Science*, **240**, 167–171.

69. Smoller J.W., Rosenbaum J.F., Biederman J., Kennedy J., Dai D., Racette S.R., Laird N.M., Kagan J., Snidman N., Hirshfeld-Becker D., *et al.* (2003). Association of a genetic marker at the corticotropin-releasing hormone locus with behavioral inhibition. *Biol. Psychiatry*, **54**, 1376–1381.
70. Schwartz C.E., Wright C.I., Shin L.M., Kagan J., Rauch S.L. (2003). Inhibited and uninhibited infants "grown up": adult amygdalar response to novelty. *Science*, **5627**, 1952–1953.
71. Kagan J., Snidman N. (1999). Early childhood predictors of adult anxiety disorders. *Biol. Psychiatry*, **46**, 1536–1541.
72. Schwartz C.E., Snidman N., Kagan J. (1999). Adolescent social anxiety as an outcome of inhibited temperament in childhood. *J. Am. Acad. Child Adolesc. Psychiatry*, **38**, 1008–1015.
73. Donovan C.L., Spence S.H. (2000). Prevention of childhood anxiety disorders. *Clin. Psychol. Rev.*, **20**, 509–531.
74. Kirmayer L.J., Robbins J.M., Dworkind M., Yaffe M.J. (1993). Somatization and the recognition of depression and anxiety in primary care. *Am. J. Psychiatry*, **150**, 734–741.
75. Sherbourne C.D., Wells K.B., Meredith L.S., Jackson C.A., Camp P. (1996). Comorbid anxiety disorder and the functioning and well-being of chronically ill patients of general medical providers. *Arch. Gen. Psychiatry*, **53**, 889–895.
76. Young A.S., Klap R., Sherbourne C.D., Wells K.B. (2001). The quality of care for depressive and anxiety disorders in the United States. *Arch. Gen. Psychiatry*, **58**, 55–61.
77. Wang P.S., Demler O., Kessler R.C. (2002). Adequacy of treatment for serious mental illness in the United States. *Am. J. Public Health*, **92**, 92–98.
78. Leon A.C., Olfson M., Broadhead W.E., Barrett J.E., Blacklow R.S., Keller M.B., Higgins E.S., Weissman W.W. (1995). Prevalence of mental disorders in primary care. Implications for screening. *Arch. Fam. Med.*, **4**, 857–861.
79. Kessler D., Bennewith O., Lewis G., Sharp D. (2002). Detection of depression and anxiety in primary care: follow-up study. *Br. Med. J.*, **325**, 1016–1017.
80. Lang A.J., Stein M.B. (2002). Screening for anxiety in primary care: why bother? *Gen. Hosp. Psychiatry*, **24**, 365–366.
81. Ritsher J.B., Struening E.L., Hellman F., Guardino M. (2002). Internal validity of an anxiety disorder screening instrument across five ethnic groups. *Psychiatry Res.*, **111**, 199–213.
82. Gilbody S.M., House A.O., Sheldon T.A. (2001). Routinely administered questionnaires for depression and anxiety: systematic review. *Br. Med. J.*, **322**, 406–409.
83. Sinoff G., Ore L., Zlotogorsky D., Tamir A. (1999). Short Anxiety Screening Test – a brief instrument for detecting anxiety in the elderly. *Int. J. Geriatr. Psychiatry*, **14**, 1062–1071.
84. Lee D.T., Wong C.K., Ungvari G.S., Cheung L.P., Haines C.J., Chung T.K. (1997). Screening psychiatric morbidity after miscarriage: application of the 30-item General Health Questionnaire and the Edinburgh Postnatal Depression Scale. *Psychosom. Med.*, **59**, 207–210.
85. Davis T.M., Ross C.J., MacDonald G.F. (2002). Screening and assessing adult asthmatics for anxiety disorders. *Clin. Nurs. Res.*, **11**, 173–189.
86. Dierker L.C., Albano A.M., Clarke G.N., Heimberg R.G., Kendall P.C., Merikangas K.R., Lewinsohn P.M., Offord D.R., Kessler R.C. (2001). Screening for anxiety and depression in early adolescence. *J. Am. Acad. Child Adolesc. Psychiatry*, **40**, 929–936.

87. Weisberg R.B., Paquette J.A. (2002). Screening and treatment of anxiety disorders in pregnant and lactating women. *Women's Health Issues*, **12**, 32–36.
88. Harter M., Reuter K., Gross-Hardt K., Bengel J. (2001). Screening for anxiety, depressive and somatoform disorders in rehabilitation – validity of HADS and GHQ-12 in patients with musculoskeletal disease. *Disabil. Rehabil.*, **23**, 737–744.
89. Franken I.H., Hendriks V.M. (2001). Screening and diagnosis of anxiety and mood disorders in substance abuse patients. *Am. J. Addict.*, **10**, 30–39.
90. El-Rufaie O.E., Absood G.H., Abou-Saleh M.T. (1997). The primary care anxiety and depression (PCAD) scale: a culture-oriented screening scale. *Acta Psychiatr. Scand.*, **95**, 119–124.
91. Le Fevre P., Devereux J., Smith S., Lawrie S.M., Cornbleet M. (1999). Screening for psychiatric illness in the palliative care inpatient setting: a comparison between the Hospital Anxiety and Depression Scale and the General Health Questionnaire-12. *Palliat. Med.*, **13**, 399–407.
92. Muzik M., Klier C.M., Rosenblum K.L., Holzinger A., Umek W., Katschnig H. (2000). Are commonly used self-report inventories suitable for screening postpartum depression and anxiety disorders? *Acta Psychiatr. Scand.*, **102**, 71–73.
93. Payne D.K., Hoffman R.G., Theodoulou M., Dosik M., Massie M.J. (1999). Screening for anxiety and depression in women with breast cancer. Psychiatry and medical oncology gear up for managed care. *Psychosomatics*, **40**, 64–69.
94. Wittchen H.U., Boyer P. (1998). Screening for anxiety disorders. Sensitivity and specificity of the Anxiety Screening Questionnaire (ASQ-15). *Br. J. Psychiatry*, **34S**, 10–17.
95. Goldberg D.P., Rickels K., Downing R., Hesbacher P. (1976). A comparison of two psychiatric screening tests. *Br. J. Psychiatry*, **129**, 61–67.
96. Kessler R.C., Andrews G., Colpe L.J., Hiripi E., Mroczek D.K., Normand S.L., Walters E.E., Zaslavsky A.M. (2002). Short screening scales to monitor population prevalences and trends in non-specific psychological distress. *Psychol. Med.*, **32**, 959–976.
97. Lloyd-Williams M., Friedman T., Rudd N. (2001). An analysis of the validity of the Hospital Anxiety and Depression scale as a screening tool in patients with advanced metastatic cancer. *J. Pain Symptom Manage.*, **22**, 990–996.
98. Goldberg D., Huxley P. (1992). *Common Mental Disorders*. Routledge, London.
99. Wildner M. (2003). Health economic issues of screening programmes. *Eur. J. Pediatr.*, **162** (Suppl. 1), 5–7.
100. Lewis G., Sharp D., Bartholomew J., Pelosi A.J. (1996). Computerized assessment of common mental disorders in primary care: effect on clinical outcome. *Fam. Pract.*, **13**, 120–126.
101. Farvolden P., McBride C., Bagby R.M., Ravitz P. (2003). A web-based screening instrument for depression and anxiety disorders in primary care. *J. Med. Internet Res.* **5**, 23.
102. Stein M.B., Chartier M.J., Hazen A.L., Kozak M.V., Tancher M.E., Lander S., Furer P., Chubaty D., Walker J.R. (1998). A direct-interview family study of generalized social phobia. *Am. J. Psychiatry*, **155**, 90–97.
103. Andrews G., Wilkinson D.D. (2002). The prevention of mental disorders in young people. *Med. J. Australia*, **177S**, 97–100.
104. Mrazek P.J., Haggerty R.J. (1994). *Reducing the Risks for Mental Disorders: Frontiers for Preventive Intervention Research*. National Academy Press, Washington, DC.
105. Lowry-Webster H., Barrett P.M., Dadds M.R. (2001). A universal prevention trial of anxiety and depressive symptomatology in childhood: preliminary data from an Australian study. *Behav. Change*, **18**, 36–50.

106. Barrett P., Turner C. (2001). Prevention of anxiety symptoms in primary school children: preliminary results from a universal school-based trial. *Br. J. Clin. Psychol.*, **40**, 399–410.
107. Leighton A.H., Murphy J.M. (1987). Primary prevention of psychiatric disorders. *Acta Psychiatr. Scand.*, **337S**, 7–22.
108. Short J.L. (1998). Evaluation of a substance abuse prevention and mental health promotion program for children of divorce. *J. Divorce Remarriage*, **28**, 139–155.
109. Felner R.D., Adan A.M. (1988). The School Transition Environment Project: an ecological intervention and evaluation. In: Price R.H., Cowen E.L., Lorion R.P., Ramos-McKay J. (eds) *Fourteen Ounces of Prevention: A Case Book for Practitioners*. American Psychological Association, Washington, DC, pp. 111–122.
110. Klingman A. (1985). Mass inoculation in a community: the effect of primary prevention of stress reactions. *Am. J. Commun. Psychol.*, **13**, 323–332.
111. Weinstein P. (1990). Breaking the worldwide cycle of pain, fear and avoidance: uncovering risk factors and promoting prevention for children. *Ann. Behav. Med.*, **12**, 141–147.
112. Tyron G.S. (1980). The measurement and treatment of test anxiety. *Rev. Educat. Res.*, **50**, 343–372.
113. Hovey J.D., Magana C.G. (2002). Psychosocial predictors of anxiety among immigrant Mexican migrant farmworkers: implications for prevention and treatment. *Cultur. Divers. Ethnic Minor. Psychol.*, **8**, 274–289.
114. Marshall K.G. (1996). Prevention. How much harm? How much benefit? 3. Physical, psychological and social harm. *Can. Med. Ass. J.*, **155**, 169–176.
115. LaFreniere P.J., Capuano F. (1997). Preventive intervention as means of clarifying direction of effects in socialization: anxious–withdrawn preschoolers case. *Develop. Psychopathol.*, **9**, 551–564.
116. Dadds M.R., Holland D.E., Laurens K.R., Mullins M., Barrett P.M., Spence S.H. (1999). Prevention and early intervention for anxiety disorders: a controlled trial. *J. Consult. Clin. Psychol.*, **67**, 145–150.
117. Holahan C.J., Richardson F.C., Puckett S.P., Bell K.F. (2004). Evaluation of two test-anxiety reduction treatments in a secondary prevention program. *Am. J. Commun. Psychol.*, **7**, 679–687.
118. Richardson G.E. (2002). The metatheory of resilience and resiliency. *J. Clin. Psychol.*, **58**, 307–321.
119. Stein D.J., Wessels C., Zungu-Dirwayi N., Berk M., Wilson Z. (2001). Value and effectiveness of consumer advocacy groups: a survey of the anxiety disorders support group in South Africa. *Depress. Anxiety*, **13**, 105–107.
120. Christiana J.M., Gilman S.E., Guardino M., Michelson K., Morselli P.L., Olfson M., Kessler R.C. (2000). Duration between onset and time of obtaining initial treatment among people with anxiety and mood disorders: an international survey of members of mental health patient advocate groups. *Psychol. Med.*, **30**, 693–703.
121. Kessler R.C., Olfson M., Berglund P.A. (1998). Patterns and predictors of treatment contact after first onset of psychiatric disorders. *Am. J. Psychiatry*, **155**, 62–69.
122. Weisz J.R., Weiss B. (1991). Studying the "referability" of child clinical problems. *J. Consult. Clin. Psychol.*, **59**, 266–273.
123. Polyrev T., Weinstock M. (2004). Gender difference in the prevention of hyperanxiety in adult prenatally stressed rats by chronic treatment with amitriptyline. *Psychopharmacology*, **171**, 270–276.

CHAPTER

9

Early Recognition and Management of Depression in Primary Care

Andre Tylee and Paul Walters

Institute of Psychiatry, London, UK

INTRODUCTION

Depression has been designated a major public health problem by the World Health Organization (WHO). To be classified as such, an illness has to satisfy three criteria: it has to be common, increasing in prevalence and treatable. Depression fulfils each of these. The majority of mental health problems are treated in primary care and therefore it is vital that the management of depression in primary care is optimal. In this chapter we shall discuss early recognition and management of depression and explore what interventions can improve the care for patients presenting with depression to their general practitioner.

EPIDEMIOLOGY

Over 90% of patients with mental health problems are treated in primary care alone [1,2]. Shepherd *et al.* [1] estimated that, in the UK, 14% of those registered with their general practitioner (GP) would consult for mental health problems in any one year. The WHO Collaborative Study of Psychiatric Disorders in General Medical Settings found that 26% of GP attendees had at least one psychiatric disorder as defined by ICD-10 criteria [3]. Of these, approximately 17% had current depression. Studies examining consecutive attendees in general practice have estimated between 5% and 15% suffer from major depression [4–6]. In a practice list of 2000 patients, it has been calculated that 60–100 people will suffer from depression [7].

Depressive disorders are also common among children and adolescents, with 2% of school-age children and 4.5% of adolescents suffering from them

Early Detection and Management of Mental Disorders.
Edited by Mario Maj, Juan José López-Ibor, Norman Sartorius, Mitsumoto Sato and Ahmed Okasha.
 ISBN 0-470-01083-5.

[8]. Garralda *et al.* found that 23% of consecutive child attendees aged between 7 and 12 had conspicuous psychiatric morbidity in the form of emotional, conduct or mixed disorders [9]. Among the elderly, up to 16% of those aged over 65 and 10% of those over 75 suffer from depression [10,11].

EARLY RECOGNITION OF DEPRESSION IN PRIMARY CARE

Cross-sectional studies comparing recognition rates of depression by GPs with standardized research interviews have found that between 50% and 70% of patients with depression are missed, though some will be recognized in subsequent consultations [3–6,12–18].

The reasons why depressive disorders appear to have high rates of poor recognition in primary care are complex, and increasingly researchers are beginning to question the validity of these findings. GPs often feel such research does not do them justice and feel unfairly criticized. Cross-sectional studies may not accurately reflect the true proportion of patients with depression that goes unrecognized, as they fail to take into account the longitudinal nature of primary care. Primary care allows a patient to be diagnosed in subsequent visits and so the proportion of missed cases may be lower than that found in cross-sectional studies [19,20]. Kessler *et al.* [21] followed up a cohort of primary care patients over three years and found that only 14% of patients with depression remained unrecognized at the end of this time. Rost *et al.* [22] followed up 98 patients with current major depression who made at least one visit to their GP in the following 6 months and found that 32% remained undetected at 1 year.

Researchers have consistently found that the more severe the depressive illness, the better it is recognized [13,18,23,24]. A categorical definition of depression, as used by most researchers, may not, therefore, be the most appropriate for use in primary care [25]. Depression and anxiety may be better conceptualized as part of the same disorder that represents a continuum, and a dimensional approach to diagnosis may be more epidemiologically valid. Using a dimensional approach, Thompson *et al.* [25] calculated that GPs only missed one "probable case" of depression every 28.6 consultations, and found that only unemployment had an effect on the relationship between severity and recognition, and this increased sensitivity.

Factors Affecting the Early Recognition of Depression in Primary Care

Even if a longitudinal perspective is taken, the early recognition of depression in primary care remains sub-optimal. If a case of probable depression is missed every 29 consultations, this still means that an average GP in the UK will miss one to two cases of probable depression per day. Factors influencing early recognition are therefore important in determining how best to overcome the problem. These can be divided into patient and doctor factors.

Patient Factors Influencing Early Recognition

There are a number of patient factors that determine whether depression is recognized. Particular characteristics of patient groups have been associated with recognition, as has the patient's presentation during the clinical interview. Marks *et al.* [26] found that females are more likely to be assessed as having mental health problems by male GPs (though not by female GPs). However, Gater *et al.* [27], using data from the WHO Study of Psychological Problems in General Health Care, found that sex did not affect the likelihood of depression or anxiety being detected by primary care doctors. It has been recently argued that depression in men is under-diagnosed, and one reason for this may be that men, even though functionally impaired, have fewer symptoms of depression than women [28]. Patients who are middle-aged, unemployed, bereaved or separated and white are more likely to have their mental health problems accurately identified, while younger and older patients and students are more likely to have their mental health problems missed [26]. Patients with comorbid physical illness are also more likely to have their depression missed [4,26,29].

In Germany, Wittchen *et al.* [24] assessed over 20,000 primary care patients and found that recognition of depression by their primary care doctor was increased for those patients with a previous history of depression, older age, and those presenting with psychomotor retardation. Patients presenting with a psychological or social problem are more likely to be recognized, as are patients with more than one psychiatric illness or those who have received a psychiatric diagnosis by their GP in the past year [19]. However, they are also more likely to receive a psychiatric diagnosis when not psychiatrically unwell [19].

Somatization and Early Recognition. Patient presentation in the clinical interview has been shown to affect recognition. This includes not only what the patients present at interview, but also the way in which it is presented. Patients in primary care rarely present with discrete psychological symptoms, and physical symptoms are most often presented at the onset of a depressive illness [13]. The GP is faced with the difficult task of having to disentangle physical and psychological symptomatolgy in order to make a diagnosis. Somatization has been described as the expression of psychological distress through physical symptoms, and is a universal phenomenon [30]. It is common in primary care, and depression often presents with somatized symptoms. Simon and VonKorff [31] analysed data from the National Institute of Mental Health Epidemiological Catchment Area study and found 50% of patients with five or more functional somatic symptoms met criteria for a current psychiatric diagnosis, with strongest associations for depression and anxiety.

Bridges and Goldberg found that depression is more likely to be missed when patients somatized their distress [32]. They defined a patient who somatizes as: (a) not mentioning psychological symptoms, (b) attributing their symptoms to a physical problem when consulting their GP, (c) having symptoms concordant with a psychiatric diagnosis when assessed by research criteria and (d) having somatic symptoms assessed by a researcher as likely to improve with psychiatric treatment [13].

Somatization has also been found to be ubiquitous across cultures [33]. Bridges and Goldberg found that pure somatization accounted for 32% of all DSM-III-R psychiatric illness in primary care [13]. Kirmayer *et al.* assessed 685 patients attending family medical clinics, and found that 76% of those suffering from depression made somatic presentations [34]. They identified three forms of somatic presentation – "initial", "facultative" and "true" somatizers – depending on their willingness to offer or endorse a psychosocial cause for their symptoms. They found that somatizers report lower levels of psychological distress, and are more likely to normalize the cause of their symptoms. They are also less likely to discuss emotional problems with their doctor [35].

Symptom Attribution and Early Recognition. Patients' presentation in primary care is in part determined by how they attribute the cause of their symptoms. Three different patterns of symptom attribution have been described: somatizing, normalizing and psychologizing [36]. The patient's attributional style affects the recognition of depression by GPs [37,38]. Kessler *et al.* found that depressed patients with a normalizing style were less likely to be detected as cases. Patients who tended to psychologize were more likely to be detected, though interestingly patients with a somatizing style were not associated with poor recognition rates. A normalizing attributional style is the most common style in general practice and this may account for low rates of depression recognition [37]. However, somatization in primary care is not necessarily pathological, and Weich *et al.* found more abnormal attachment behaviours in patients who psychologize [39].

Stigma and Early Recognition. Stigma and a lack of awareness of mental health problems are important factors in determining whether patients seek help. A lack of awareness and the stigma surrounding mental health problems is a major problem and contributes to the widespread reluctance to consult and receive appropriate treatment for mental health problems in primary care [40]. Cape and McCulloch examined patients' reasons for not presenting emotional problems to their GP [41]. They interviewed 83 patients with high General Health Questionnaire (GHQ) scores and found 77% had not mentioned emotional problems during the consultation. Of these, 45% did not mention emotional problems because of embarrassment, or not wanting to "trouble" the GP, and 19% were put off by the doctor's behaviour during consultations or feeling the doctor did not have time to discuss the problem.

GP Factors Influencing Early Recognition

GPs vary in their ability to diagnose depression [2,12,26,42,43]. Differences concern knowledge, skills and attitudes. Age and experience in general practice have not been shown to have strong associations with accuracy of diagnosis of depression [26]. However, academically more capable GPs with an appropriate concept of mental illness in primary care are more likely to accurately assess emotionally distressed patients and use more directive interview techniques [12,26,42].

Research on the effect of lengthening the consultation on the ability of GPs to recognize depression conflicts. Marks *et al.* [26] found that doctors with longer consultation times were not better at recognizing depression. In contrast, Howie *et al.* found that longer consultations did improve recognition rates of psychological problems and were met with greater patient satisfaction [44]. Empathy, an interest in psychiatry and asking about family and problems at home are associated with an increased recognition of mental illness [26]. Other reasons why GPs may under-diagnose depression include lack of knowledge about the symptoms and management of depression, being preoccupied with organic illness, underrating the severity and treatability of depression when recognized, and failure to elicit the symptoms of depression during the consultation [45].

The consultation skills of GPs are important in determining their ability to accurately diagnose depression. Most patients present their GP with somatic symptoms, and psychosocial problems are often presented late in the consultation [46,47], even though problems mentioned late in the consultation are as important as those mentioned early on [48]. GPs who make more eye contact, interrupt less, do not appear rushed, use more open questions and are good listeners are more likely to recognize depression [43]. It has also been suggested that the GP's ability to pick up on verbal, vocal and non-verbal cues influences recognition. Davenport *et al.* found that some GPs encouraged these cues, while others actively inhibited them [49].

GPs' attitudes to depression and their clinical behaviour also vary. GPs who are less willing to become actively involved in the treatment of depression and are less willing to explore psychosocial factors have a pessimistic view of depression [50]. Dowrick *et al.* used the Depression Attitude Questionnaire (DAQ) [51] to explore whether there was an association between GPs' attitudes towards depression and their clinical behaviour. They found no correlation between GPs' attitudes as measured by the DAQ and their ability to accurately identify depression, but they did find a positive association between attitudes and ease of management [52].

Improving the Early Recognition of Depression

Approaches to improve the recognition rate of depression in primary care have varied. Generally these approaches have focused on a particular problem area, usually attempting to address one or more of the GP or patient factors found to have an affect on recognition.

Top-Down Approaches

In the UK, the Defeat Depression Campaign, run jointly by the Royal College of Psychiatrists and Royal College of General Practitioners over 5 years (1991–1996), aimed to educate GPs about depression, with the hope of improving recognition and management [53,54]. The outcomes of the campaign were modest, with 40% of GPs having possibly or definitely made changes in their practice according to the questionnaire. The authors recommended that national campaigns need to be supplemented by local practice-based teaching if they are to have an impact on practice and improve care.

The Campaign also aimed to reduce stigma associated with depression, educate the public about depression and its treatment and encourage people to seek help early. Changes in public attitude were small (5–10%) and no changes were found in patients' views of antidepressant treatment. Antidepressant medication was still regarded as addictive and less effective than counselling at the end of the campaign. It seems, therefore, that top-down educational approaches such as this have a limited overall effect, either in changing public awareness or in GP practice.

Can Screening for Depression in Primary Care Improve Early Recognition and Outcome?

High-quality depression care and early treatment rely upon effective recognition and accurate diagnosis. Screening patients in primary care for depression is a possible method of improving early recognition and clinical outcomes of depressed patients.

Mulrow *et al.* [55] reviewed case-finding instruments for depression in the primary care setting and found that instruments used in this respect had reasonable and consistent accuracy. The instruments performed similarly, with good sensitivity (80–90%) but only moderate specificity (70–85%), and there was little to choose between them in terms of their utility in the primary care setting [56]. Whooley *et al.* [57] compared the validity of a two-question case-finding instrument for depression with other validated instruments and found that a positive response to the two-item instrument had a sensitivity of 96% and a specificity of 57%. The two-item instrument involved asking the patient: (a) "Over the past two weeks, have you felt down, depressed or hopeless?" and (b) "Over the past two weeks have you felt little interest or pleasure in doing things?".

Given optimal performance of screening tests, with a prevalence of depression in primary care of 5–10%, the US Preventive Services Task Force (USPSTF) calculated that 25–40% of those screening positive will have major depression [58]. Because of this lower specificity of screening tests, a positive score will necessitate a clinical interview to diagnose a depressive disorder. Pignone *et al.* reviewed the evidence on the effects of depression screening on recognition and clinical outcomes in primary care [59]. They found that feeding back the results of screening to primary care professionals improved recognition of depression. But there was a wide variation in improved recognition between studies (10% to 47%). Immediate feedback of screening results seemed to be more beneficial than delayed feedback. However, Gilbody *et al.* [60] found feeding back screening results only improved recognition rates by clinicians for high scorers, making the routine use of screening instruments costly.

The effect of screening on clinical outcomes of depressed patients in primary care is unclear. Pignone *et al.* found that the results of studies vary, with few reaching statistically significant differences [59]. They concluded that the clinical benefits of screening remain uncertain. In studies in which clinical outcomes were improved by screening, this was part of a comprehensive depression management programme; screening with usual care does not appear to alter clinical outcomes. Dowrick and Buchan examined the effects of feeding back screening results to GPs and found it had no effect on clinical outcome [15]. Gilbody *et al.* concluded that screening might not improve patient outcomes [60].

Valenstein *et al.* [61] have examined the cost-utility of screening for depression in primary care. They found that screening is unlikely to be cost effective until comprehensive structured management programmes for depression are in place; health care organizations would be better off investing in these programmes before investing in screening programmes, and screening in practices that provide "usual depression care" is unlikely to be cost effective.

Many questions about screening and its role in early recognition and management of depression in primary care remain unanswered, such as the frequency of screening, or which age groups are most likely to benefit. A major problem is the efficiency of the screening tools. With a 5% prevalence of major depression in primary care, screening 100 patients would yield 4 true positives and 27 false positives, with 1 false negative [55]. This imposes a considerable burden on busy clinicians, and case-finding restricted to those at high risk of depression may be more efficient than screening [62].

Despite this, the USPSTF concluded that evidence now justifies "screening adults for depression in clinical practices that have systems in place to assure accurate diagnosis, effective treatment and follow-up". Unfortunately, this recommendation does little for those practices that do not have those systems in place and which arguably are the practices most in need of help in identifying cases. What this evidence does show is the importance of a systematic approach to the management of depression in primary care, and whether screening has an important role in this remains to be elucidated.

Using Clinical Guidelines to Improve the Early Detection and Management of Depression in Primary Care

Clinical guidelines have been promoted as a way to improve the quality and consistency of care received by patients in primary care. There is evidence from the general medical setting that guidelines lead to a change in clinical practice and improve patient outcomes [63]. A number of guidelines on the management of depression have been produced [8,64–66]. Littlejohns *et al.* [67] surveyed depression guidelines developed in the UK between 1991 and 1996 and found 45 guidelines that differed considerably in quality. The number is likely to be far larger than this now.

Despite initial optimistic hopes in the ability of clinical guidelines to improve the management of depression in primary care [68], these hopes have not been realized in practice [69]. Though the use of guidelines has been shown to have an impact on the management of some conditions in primary care such as diabetes and possibly asthma [70], their influence on the management of depression in primary care has been less significant.

Studies that have examined the effectiveness of clinical guidelines often combine the implementation of guidelines with educational initiatives. Rutz *et al.* [71] showed that suicide rates decreased and antidepressant prescription increased after an educational programme for GPs consisting of a two-day course delivered by psychiatrists. However, the study was small, with no control group, and the benefits had disappeared after two years [72]. Upton *et al.* [73] evaluated the ICD-10 Primary Health Care mental health guidelines in improving the detection and management of depression in primary care. They found that the guidelines had no impact on the overall detection of mental disorders, accuracy of diagnosis or prescription of antidepressants, and concluded that the success of guidelines in effecting change is uncertain. A study conducted in Groningen by van Os *et al.* [74] found similar disappointing results after implementing a training programme for primary care doctors. No significant improvement in the recognition or accuracy of depression diagnosis was found.

More recently, the Hampshire Depression Project examined the effects of a clinical practice guideline for depression and an educational programme on the detection and outcome of depression in the primary care setting. The guidelines were extensive and included advice on practice organization, roles of non-medical professionals and useful general and local information. The educational initiatives included seminars, video teaching, small group discussions and role-play. Despite this, no differences were found between the intervention and the control group in terms of recognition rates or patient outcomes [75].

There are three problems with existing guidelines on depression management in primary care: the diagnosis is not easy to make in primary care; many primary care professionals doubt the efficacy of antidepressants when there are considerable social difficulties; and patients are reluctant to take medications [76]. Given these problems, Kendrick has suggested that guideline-based interventions are unlikely to have an impact until the evidence base has been improved [76]. Cornwall and Scott [77] examined the content of peer-reviewed depression treatment guidelines and found that only two conformed to the quality standard of a clinical practice guideline. They concluded that the ideal guideline on the management of depression in primary care has yet to be written. However, given that the guidelines used in the Hampshire Depression Project presented the most up to date information, it is unlikely that this is the reason for their apparent failure to change outcomes [78]. Part of the problem may be that guidelines for use in primary care are often derived by specialists, and there is a dissonance which reflects the fact that they treat (and research) different populations.

It has been argued that, to be successful, efforts should be directed towards guideline implementation rather than the production of more and more guidelines [67]. Grol *et al.* found that specific attributes of guidelines determine whether or not they are used in practice [79]. They found that evidence-based recommendations are more likely to be followed than those without a scientific basis, and that precise definitions of recommended performance are needed. Guidelines should be compatible with primary care professionals' value sets, not demand too much change to existing practice and have specific advice on management in specific situations. A small study by Freeman and Sweeney [80] examined the reasons why GPs do not implement evidence-based guidelines. They identified themes that acted as barriers to implementation. These included the doctor–patient relationship, the GPs' feelings about the evidence in relation to their patients, their personal and professional experiences, and the logistics of implementation.

Three levels appear to affect the implementation of depression guidelines in primary care: (a) the quality and attributes of the guidelines; (b) the organizational investment in the guidelines; and (c) the individual characteristics of the primary care professional.

Improving the early recognition and management of depression in primary care through the use of clinical guidelines is therefore a complex process. The guidelines have not only to be of the highest quality, using the most up-to-date evidence available. They also have to conform to specific attributes, and even then may remain unimplemented if there is a failure to take into account organizational obstacles or the context of the doctor–patient relationship and personal experiences of the primary care professional.

A number of studies in the USA have demonstrated improved clinical outcomes using clinical guidelines for depression in primary care, but only as part of enhanced depression management programmes [81–88]. From this work it is clear that clinical guidelines for depression need the associated resources for good dissemination and implementation, and enhanced care processes need to be implemented such as case management, educational initiatives for patients and professionals, and a fluid relationship at the primary–secondary care interface [89]. Without a change in the whole process of care, it is unlikely that clinical guidelines will effect improved clinical outcomes.

Does Recognition Improve Outcome?

Whether increased recognition of depression by GPs improves outcomes has been a contentious issue. Schulberg *et al.* assessed 274 primary care patients and reassessed them six months later [90]. They found that rates of depression at six months were similar for patients in whom depression had been diagnosed and those in whom it had not. They concluded that doctor recognition and treatment did not predict outcome. In contrast, Ormel *et al.* screened nearly 2000 GP attendees in the Netherlands for psychological disorders and found that patients with recognized psychological problems were more likely to receive treatment and had better outcomes (91). Tiemens *et al.* [6] replicated this study, but found that patients in whom psychological disorders were recognized did not have better outcomes. However, those patients that were recognized had more severe depression, and even though the psychological disorder was recognized, this did not mean that those patients were adequately or appropriately treated.

Dowrick *et al.* [15] examined whether detection of depression by GPs affected outcomes and whether disclosure of results from a Beck Depression Inventory had an effect on outcome. They found that diagnosis by GP and disclosure of depression scores failed to have any impact on outcomes. In fact, they found those patients who had been recognized had a worse prognosis than those who remained unrecognized. Simon *et al.* found that recognition improved outcomes at three months, but that at one year there was no difference between those patients with recognized depression and those in whom it was not recognized [92]. GPs are more likely to recognize severe depression and it may be that these patients are less likely to improve because of the severity of their depression and the social difficulties that accompanied it [14]. It appears that, although recognition improves outcome in the short term, it does not improve the long-term prognosis.

Improving the recognition of depression by GPs, therefore, although desirable and important, is by no means the whole solution to improving outcomes for primary care patients with depression, and improving recognition without improving the overall management of depression may not improve long-term outcomes [18,22].

Bottom-up Approaches

To address the problem of low detection of depression in primary care adequately, it is likely that a combination of top-down and bottom-up approaches is needed. Probably a stepped-care approach to depression management will be the most useful in the primary care setting. Initiatives can then be produced aimed at each group of primary care professionals and tailored to meet local needs, with practices and primary care professionals determining the extent of professional responsibilities according to expertise and need at each step. The National Institute for Mental Health in England (NIMHE), as part of the Modernization Agency of the Department of Health, has developed a Primary Care Programme [93,94]. Three of the five programme areas could help improve recognition and management of depression: staff development (through core skills training and "mental health champion" development), commissioning and developing effective partnerships, and empowering primary care user perspectives. Local mental health champion development is achieved through the national "trailblazer" courses. More than 350 participants have already been through the courses and there is increasing international interest from

New Zealand, Australia and the USA in the courses. Courses encourage a bottom-up approach to improving the provision of primary care mental health, eliciting whole-practice learning needs and providing mental health skills training. The courses are modular and participants are paired, one from primary care and one from secondary care, collaborating to define and meet local service development needs and their own learning needs. This fosters close collaborative relationships within pairs and within the group. An adult learner-centred approach is taken in which participants are encouraged to pass on their skills and expertise to others in the group and participants are encouraged to cascade their learning to colleagues in their local service. This process increases the awareness of mental health problems in the whole primary care team and allows innovative services to develop that best meet local needs [95,96]. One of the courses has been independently evaluated with encouraging results [97].

Increasing Public Awareness

An important part of improving early recognition of depression is increasing public awareness. However, as the results from the Defeat Depression Campaign illustrate, modifying public opinion may prove difficult. A recent survey conducted as a baseline measurement of stigmatization of people with mental illnesses for a five-year campaign to reduce the stigma of mental illness ("Changing Minds: Every Family in the Land") found one-quarter of respondents thought people with severe depression were dangerous to others, and one-fifth thought that they could just "pull themselves together" [98]. The evaluation of this five-year campaign is still awaited. However, to complement large national campaigns at a local level, primary care services can play an important part by implementing mental health awareness programmes. These can be developed in conjunction with "expert patients" who can help define the most useful strategies for improving mental health awareness within their community and encouraging people to seek help.

Mental Health Skills Training and Education for Primary Care Professionals

To improve the early recognition and management of depression in primary care, primary care professionals need to have adequate training. In the UK there is a deficit of mental health training for primary care professionals. Few GPs have any higher professional training in mental health [99]. GPs can be successfully trained in mental health management skills, including depression skills, and re-attribution skills for patients who somatize [100–105]. If such teaching is to become widely available in primary care, it is essential that primary care teachers learn how to teach skills to their trainees. A number of studies have shown that it is also possible to train GPs to teach interviewing skills with brief training [104,106].

The World Psychiatric Association has produced a mental health skills training pack for use in primary care [107]. The training pack allows specific mental health skills to be taught through modelling those demonstrated on videos. It encourages the use of role-plays to allow professionals to practise the new skills they have been taught and has information on the planning and running of tutorials in mental health topics.

Practice nurses too have been successfully trained in mental health skills. They have been successfully taught to assess and manage depression [108], can be trained to use problem-solving techniques [109], help monitor compliance and progress [110], and coordinate their patients' care, allowing referral to mental health services where appropriate. Whole practice multi-professional mental health skills training is also successful [111].

EARLY MANAGEMENT OF DEPRESSION IN PRIMARY CARE

Antidepressant Medication

Antidepressant medication is effective in treating major depression in primary care [66]. Mulrow *et al.* have reviewed the efficacy of antidepressant medication in primary care [112]. They found that 63% of depressed patients in primary care improved by at least 50% as measured by rating scales on newer antidepressants, 60% on tricyclics and only 35% on placebo. Newer medications were no more effective that tricyclic antidepressants, but significantly more effective than placebo. Patients in primary care are less likely to drop out of treatment if taking a selective serotonin reuptake inhibitor (SSRI) compared to a tricyclic antidepressant, and SSRIs appear to be better tolerated [113,114]. Because of the prevalence of depression in primary care and the limited availability of psychological treatments in most primary care settings, antidepressant medication remains the mainstay of treatment.

Despite the efficacy of antidepressant medication, there is a wide variation in prescribing practices for depression [115]. Only about 50% of depressed patients receive medication and it is as likely to be a sedative as an antidepressant [3]. If prescribed an antidepressant, few patients receive an adequate dose for an adequate length of time [116], though this appears to have improved with the wider use of SSRIs in primary care [117]. At three-month follow-up, Goldberg *et al.* found that those treated with antidepressant medication have fewer symptoms and are less likely to be suicidal than those treated with sedatives, despite the two groups being identical at outset. The treatment effect is more pronounced for patients suffering from more severe depression. However, by one year all differences had disappeared [115].

More recently, the accusation that tricyclic antidepressants are used by GPs at too low a dose has been contested. Furukawa *et al.* [118] conducted a systematic review of trials comparing low-dose tricyclic antidepressant medication with placebo and concluded that low-dose tricyclics are justified in the treatment of depression. However, further research is needed and it is probably wiser to stick to guideline recommended doses for antidepressant treatment until this research is forthcoming.

Unfortunately, 30–50% of people prescribed antidepressants fail to refill their initial prescriptions and 50–80% of people stop taking antidepressant medication within 6 weeks to 6 months of initiating treatment [119,120], though one study reported compliance rates of 80% at 6 weeks in a primary care sample [121]. Compliance is therefore of the utmost importance. Regular follow-up and monitoring of compliance is a vital part of the primary care team's role. Psychoeducation and drug counselling have been shown to be important in improving compliance rates [110,119]. The reasons for noncompliance with prescribed treatment are complex and may be the most important factors in extrapolating efficacy rates found in research populations to everyday clinical practice [122].

Psychological Therapies and Counselling for Depression in Primary Care

Recent evidence suggests that time-limited psychological treatments are effective in the treatment of mild to moderate depressive disorders in primary care. Cognitive–behaviour therapy (CBT) [123,124], interpersonal therapy (IPT) [125] and problem-solving therapy [126,127] have all been shown to be as effective as antidepressant medication. A recent systematic review of the effectiveness of brief psychological interventions in depression found that patients receiving CBT were significantly more likely than those receiving psychodynamic psychotherapy, interpersonal therapy or supportive therapy to improve [128].

Psychological therapies need skilled people to deliver them and currently access to these treatments is variable. It is possible to train primary care teams to deliver effective psychological interventions. For instance, problem-solving therapy has been successfully taught to nurses, with outcomes similar to those for antidepressant medication [109]. In one recent study comparing general practice-based non-directive counselling, CBT and usual general practice care, patients receiving the psychological treatments recovered quicker then those receiving usual GP care, though by 12 months differences in outcome had disappeared [129].

There are currently several computerized CBT packages that have been developed to treat depression and anxiety [130]. These have the potential to increase access to CBT services and permit increased flexibility of treatment. They may be particularly suitable for a "stepped-care" programme of management. Although to date there have been a number of studies examining the efficacy of computerized CBT, the National Institute for Clinical Excellence in the UK has concluded that as yet there is insufficient evidence to recommend its general introduction [130].

There is a dearth of research evaluating the efficacy of counselling for depression in primary care and what evidence exists is contradictory. Chilvers *et al.* [131] found that generic counselling was as effective as antidepressants for mild to moderate depression, though patients given medication recovered quicker. Counselling can be a useful adjunct to antidepressant medication and it appears to be well liked by patients [132]. Given a choice, patients prefer it to medication [131]. A recent Cochrane review concluded that counselling could lead to modest improvements in the short term but that there were no advantages over care as usual in the long term [133].

When considering psychological treatments in primary care, there are a number of points that should be borne in mind. The therapy should focus on the patient's current problems and the aim should be symptom reduction. Therapists should be trained in the psychotherapeutic modality used and there should be ongoing monitoring of symptoms, with those who fail to respond by 6–8 weeks being reassessed [134].

Self-help and Bibliotherapy

Psychoeducation and self-help have also been shown to be effective in the treatment of depression in primary care [135,136]. What is classed as self-help varies from bibliotherapy, which usually involves learning cognitive–behavioural techniques from written material, to self-help booklets, videos, cassettes and computer programs. Bower *et al.* [137] systematically reviewed the clinical and cost effectiveness of self-help treatments in the primary care setting. They concluded that, though self-help treatments may potentially improve cost effectiveness of treatment in primary care, there was neither the quality nor quantity of research to draw any reliable conclusions. However, a meta-analysis of research into bibliotherapy for depression found that it was as effective as individual and group therapy, though the studies were not limited to primary care populations [138]. At present further research into the effectiveness of self-help and bibliotherapy for depression in primary care is needed.

Enhancing Depression Management in Primary Care

Though individual treatments have been shown to be effective in primary care, there remains the problem that depression may not be recognized, antidepressant medication may not be prescribed at adequate doses, treatment may not be adhered to, and access to psychological treatments is variable [79]. Nutting *et al.* [139] examined the barriers to initiating treatment for depression in accordance with treatment guidelines. They found five main barriers to care: patient noncompliance with visits, patient resistance to treatment, physicians overruling guidelines, patient psychosocial burden and health-care system problems. Doctors felt that the majority of the problems lay with patient-centred factors, their psychosocial circumstances, or attitudes and beliefs about depression and its treatment. Therefore, treatment may best be delivered in packages that are tailored to meet the needs of the individual and address these barriers.

Enhancing the whole process of depression management in primary care using a chronic illness model may be the most effective way of improving outcomes. Katon *et al.* [81,83] demonstrated improved outcomes using a collaborative care model. Collaborative care has been described as a "systematic approach that improves patient education and integrates mental health professionals or other care extenders, such as nurses, into the primary care clinic to help primary care physicians provide treatment in conformity with evidence-based guidelines" [84]. Katon and colleagues developed a collaborative care model that consisted of an extensive educational campaign and training in the implementation of treatment guidelines over a 1-year period, co-management of patients by the primary care doctor and psychiatrist, and reorganized service structures to enhance the role of primary care physicians (including lengthening the initial consultation to 30 minutes, intensive monitoring of the patient to monitor response, allowing more time for patient education, and close collaboration between primary care doctor and the onsite psychiatrist or psychologist). Though this model involved a considerable amount of psychiatrist or psychologist time, they were able to demonstrate an increased adequacy of antidepressant prescribing, improved clinical outcomes, enhanced patient satisfaction, and an increased sense of effectiveness and satisfaction in treating depression among primary care doctors. However, there was no enduring educational effect after the study ended and the multifaceted programme discontinued [82]. This suggests that organizational restructuring and the input of "product champions" is a vital component of enhancing treatment outcomes. The enhanced care approach appeared to be cost effective, despite the increased use of resources, which was offset against improved patient outcomes [140].

A stepped collaborative care approach was also shown to improve outcomes for patients who had not responded to usual primary care treatment. Katon and colleagues found that depressed patients in primary care who had not responded to antidepressant medication at 6–8 weeks were more likely to get adequate treatment, adhere to it and have better clinical outcomes if treated within a collaborative care model than those who continued with treatment as usual by their primary care doctor [84]. This stepped-care model was associated with only modest increases in costs [141].

Other studies have also found that enhanced care involving evidence-based guidelines, patient education, case management and specialist involvement improves outcomes for patients suffering from depression in primary care [85–88]. Rost *et al.* examined the long-term effect of an ongoing enhanced care intervention in primary care [142]. They used a chronic disease management model, which included training for practice staff, screening and practice nurse case-management with active follow-up of patients. Compared with usual care, they found increased remission rates and improved physical and emotional functioning over the 24 months of the study [142]. Koike *et al.* [143] examined the effects of a depression quality improvement programme for depressed patients with comorbid medical illnesses. Again, the quality improvement programme improved rates of treatment and outcome for this population of depressed patients.

Most of the research on enhanced care depression programmes has been conducted in the USA, raising questions about the generalizability of such an approach. More recently, Araya *et al.* compared the effectiveness of a stepped-care programme with usual treatment in low-income women in Santiago, Chile [144]. They found that, despite few resources, at 6-month follow-up 70% of women who had received stepped care had recovered, versus only 30% of those who had received usual care. Further replication studies are required in other countries and with different models of primary care provision to determine whether this model can be successfully generalized. In the UK, a multifaceted approach to detecting and managing primary care depression was effective in only one of the practices in which it was implemented [145]. It appears that only practices familiar with a chronic disease management model may benefit from such approaches, and preliminary work may be necessary in practices that are less well resourced [145].

VonKorff and Goldberg have suggested that efforts to improve the primary care of depression should focus on low-cost case management and close liaison between the GP, case manager and mental health specialist [89]. Within such models, case management (e.g. by a practice nurse) appears to be vital [146]. The case manager is responsible for active follow-up of the patient, assessing the patient's needs, providing education and monitoring the effects of treatments. He or she can also be responsible for consultation with, or referral to, mental health services when needed. Restructuring the delivery of care processes in this way allows interventions, which in isolation may have limited effects to be incorporated into a comprehensive management plan tailored to meet the needs of the individual. These models lend themselves to a whole-team approach and give practice nurses the potential to play a key role in depression management. A three-component model for restructuring depression management in primary care has been suggested as an efficient way of introducing enhanced care programmes [147]. Within this model the practice is "prepared" by educating primary care staff about the process and skills needed to implement guidelines. This educational plan uses predisposing, enabling and reinforcing activities to ensure that collaborative management is implemented and to help address obstacles. Case management and close attention to the mental health interface make up the other components, as suggested by VonKorff and Goldberg [89].

CONCLUSIONS

Depression continues to place a considerable burden on individuals, their families, health-care services and society. Primary care manages the vast majority of patients suffering from depression. Easing the burden of depression will mean that early recognition and diagnosis, followed by appropriate management in the primary care setting, are vital. Evidence suggests that recognition by primary care doctors is sub-optimal. Without improving the early recognition of depression, improvements in treatment cannot occur. Paradoxically, without improving the whole process of depression care, it is unlikely that improvements in recognition will be achieved. Factors which influence recognition of depression in primary care are complex, and even adequate detection does not necessarily equate to improved clinical outcomes. There is growing evidence that organizational restructuring to incorporate a chronic disease model of depression is necessary to improve outcomes. Case management and easy access to mental health specialists are vital in this regard, and a stepped-care approach would appear to be the most feasible way to enhance care. The restructuring of the care model will need the associated additional resources to ensure that practices can implement the changes. Isolated changes in depression care provision seem unlikely to meet with success in the long term.

REFERENCES

1. Shepherd M., Cooper B., Brown A.C., Kalton G. (1966). *Psychiatric Illness in General Practice*. Oxford University Press, London.
2. Goldberg D., Huxley P. (1992). *Common Mental Disorders. A Biosocial Model*. Routledge, London.
3. Ustun T.B., Sartorius N. (1995). *Mental Illness in General Health Care. An International Study*. John Wiley & Sons Ltd, Chichester.
4. Freeling P., Rao B.M., Paykel E.S., Sireling L.I., Burton R.H. (1985). Unrecognised depression in general practice. *Br. Med. J.*, **290**, 1880–1883.
5. Blacker C.V., Clare A.W. (1987). Depressive disorder in primary care. *Br. J. Psychiatry*, **150**, 737–751.
6. Tiemens B.G., Ormel J., Simon G.E. (1996). Occurrence, recognition, and outcome of psychological disorders in primary care. *Am. J. Psychiatry*, **153**, 636–644.
7. Strathdee G., Jenkins R. (1996). Purchasing mental health for primary care. In: Thornicroft G., Strathdee G. (eds) *Commissioning Mental Health Services*. HMSO, London, pp. 77–83.
8. Depression Guideline Panel (1993). *Depression in Primary Care: Detection and Diagnosis 1*. US Department of Health and Human Services, Agency for Health Care Policy and Research, Rockville, MD.
9. Garralda M.E., Bailey D. (1986). Children with psychiatric disorders in primary care. *J. Child Psychol. Psychiatry All. Discipl.*, **27**, 611–624.
10. Livingston G., Hawkins A., Graham N., Blizard B., Mann A. (1990). The Gospel Oak Study: prevalence rates of dementia, depression and activity limitation among elderly residents in inner London. *Psychol. Med.*, **20**, 137–146.
11. Copeland J.R., Davidson I.A., Dewey M.E., Gilmore C., Larkin B.A., McWilliam C., Saunders P.A., Scott A., Sharma V., Sullivan C. (1992). Alzheimer's disease, other dementias, depression and pseudodementia: prevalence, incidence and three-year outcome in Liverpool. *Br. J. Psychiatry*, **161**, 230–239.
12. Goldberg D., Huxley P. (1980). *Mental Illness in the Community. The Pathway to Psychiatric Care*. Tavistock, London.
13. Bridges K., Goldberg D. (1985). Somatic presentation of DSM-III psychiatric disorders in primary care. *J. Psychosom. Res.*, **29**, 563–569.
14. Ronalds C., Creed F., Stone K., Webb S., Tomenson B. (1997). Outcome of anxiety and depressive disorders in primary care. *Br. J. Psychiatry*, **171**, 427–433.
15. Dowrick C., Buchan I. (1995). Twelve month outcome of depression in general practice: does detection or disclosure make a difference? *Br. Med. J.*, **311**, 1274–1276.
16. Wells K.B., Hays R.D., Burnam M.A., Rogers W., Greenfield S., Ware J.E. Jr (1989). Detection of depressive disorder for patients receiving prepaid or fee-for-service care. Results from the Medical Outcomes Study. *JAMA*, **262**, 3298–3302.
17. Simon G.E.M.M., VonKorff M.S. (1995). Recognition, management, and outcomes of depression in primary care. *Arch. Fam. Med.*, **4**, 99–105.
18. Simon G.E., Goldberg D., Tiemens B.G., Ustun T.B. (1999). Outcomes of recognized and unrecognized depression in an international primary care study. *Gen. Hosp. Psychiatry*, **21**, 97–105.
19. Ormel J., Tiemens B. (1995). Recognition and treatment of mental illness in primary care. Towards a better understanding of a multifaceted problem. *Gen. Hosp. Psychiatry*, **17**, 160–164.

20. Freeling P., Tylee A. (1992). Depression in general practice. In: Paykel E.S. (ed.) *Handbook of Affective Disorders*. Churchill Livingstone, Edinburgh, pp. 651–656.
21. Kessler D., Bennewith O., Lewis G., Sharp D. (2002). Detection of depression and anxiety in primary care: follow up study. *Br. Med. J.*, **325**, 1016–1017.
22. Rost K., Zhang M., Fortney J., Smith J., Coyne J., Smith G.R. Jr (1998). Persistently poor outcomes of undetected major depression in primary care. *Gen. Hosp. Psychiatry*, **20**, 12–20.
23. Dowrick C.F. (1995). Case or continuum? Analysing GPs' ability to detect depression in primary care. *Primary Care Psychiatry*, **1**, 255–257.
24. Wittchen H.U., Hofler M., Meister W. (2001). Prevalence and recognition of depressive syndromes in German primary care settings: poorly recognized and treated? *Int. Clin. Psychopharmacol.*, **16**, 121–135.
25. Thompson C., Ostler K., Peveler R.C., Baker N., Kinmonth A. (2001). Dimensional perspective on the recognition of depressive symptoms in primary care: the Hampshire depression project 3. *Br. J. Psychiatry*, **179**, 317–323.
26. Marks J.N., Goldberg D., Hillier V.F. (1979). Determinants of the ability of general practitioners to detect psychiatric illness. *Psychol. Med.*, **9**, 337–353.
27. Gater R., Tansella M., Korten A., Tiemens B.G., Mavreas V.G., Olatawura M.O. (1998). Sex differences in the prevalence and detection of depressive and anxiety disorders in general health care settings: report from the World Health Organization Collaborative Study on Psychological Problems in General Health Care. *Arch. Gen. Psychiatry*, **55**, 405–413.
28. Angst J., Gamma A., Gastpar M., Lepine J.-P., Mendlewicz J., Tylee A. (2002). Gender differences in depression. Epidemiological findings from the European DEPRES I and II studies. *Eur. Arch. Psychiatry Clin. Neurosci.*, **252**, 201–209.
29. Tylee A.T., Freeling P., Kerry S. (1993). Why do general practitioners recognise major depression in one woman patient yet miss it in another? *Br. J. Gen. Pract.*, **43**, 327–330.
30. Reid S., Wessely S. (2001). Somatisation and depression. In: Dawson A., Tylee A. (eds) *Depression: Social and Economic Timebomb*. BMJ Books, London, pp. 55–61.
31. Simon G.E., VonKorff M. (1991). Somatization and psychiatric disorder in the NIMH Epidemiologic Catchment Area study. *Am. J. Psychiatry*, **148**, 1494–1500.
32. Bridges K., Goldberg D. (1987). Somatic presentation of depressive illness in primary care. In: Freeling P., Downey L.J., Malkin J.C. (eds) *The Presentation of Depression: Current Approaches*. Royal College of General Practitioners, London, pp. 9–11.
33. Gureje O., Simon G.E., Ustun T.B., Goldberg D.P. (1997). Somatization in cross-cultural perspective: a World Health Organization study in primary care. *Am. J. Psychiatry*, **154**, 989–995.
34. Kirmayer L.J., Robbins J.M., Dworkind M., Yaffe M.J. (1993). Somatization and the recognition of depression and anxiety in primary care. *Am. J. Psychiatry*, **150**, 734–741.
35. Kirmayer L.J., Robbins J.M. (1996). Patients who somatize in primary care: a longitudinal study of cognitive and social characteristics. *Psychol. Med.*, **26**, 937–951.
36. Robbins J.M., Kirmayer L.J. (1991). Attributions of common somatic symptoms. *Psychol. Med.*, **21**, 1029–1045.
37. Kessler D., Lloyd K., Lewis G., Gray D.P. (1999). Cross sectional study of symptom attribution and recognition of depression and anxiety in primary care. *Br. Med. J.*, **318**, 436–439.

38. Bower P., West R., Tylee A., Hann M. (2000). Symptom attribution and the recognition of psychiatric morbidity. *J. Psychosom. Res.*, **48**, 157–160.
39. Weich S., Lewis G., Mann A. (1996). Effect of early life experiences and personality on the reporting of psychosocial distress in general practice. A preliminary investigation. *Br. J. Psychiatry*, **168**, 116–120.
40. Priest R.G., Vize C., Roberts A., Roberts M., Tylee A. (1996). Lay people's attitudes to treatment of depression: results of opinion poll for Defeat Depression Campaign just before its launch. *Br. Med. J.*, **313**, 858–859.
41. Cape J., McCulloch Y. (1999). Patients' reasons for not presenting emotional problems in general practice consultations. *Br. J. Gen. Pract.*, **49**, 875–879.
42. Millar T., Goldberg D.P. (1991). Link between the ability to detect and manage emotional disorders: a study of general practitioner trainees. *Br. J. Gen. Pract.*, **41**, 357–359.
43. Goldberg D.P., Jenkins L., Millar T., Faragher E.B. (1993). The ability of trainee general practitioners to identify psychological distress among their patients. *Psychol. Med.*, **23**, 185–193.
44. Howie J.G.R., Porter A.M.D., Heaney D.J., Hopton J.L. (1991). Long to short consultation ratio: a proxy measure of quality in general practice. *Br. J. Gen. Pract.*, **41**, 48–52.
45. Schulberg H.C., McClelland M. (1987). A conceptual model for educating primary care providers in the diagnosis and treatment of depression. *Gen. Hosp. Psychiatry*, **9**, 1–10.
46. Burack R.C., Carpenter R.R. (1983). The predictive value of the presenting complaint. *J. Fam. Pract.*, **16**, 749–754.
47. Tylee A., Freeling P., Kerry S., Burns T. (1995). How does the content of consultations affect the recognition by general practitioners of major depression in women? *Br. J. Gen. Pract.*, **45**, 578.
48. Beckman H.B., Frankel R.M. (1984). The effect of physician behavior on the collection of data. *Ann. Intern. Med.*, **101**, 692–696.
49. Davenport S., Goldberg D., Millar T. (1987). How psychiatric disorders are missed during medical consultations. *Lancet*, **2**, 439–441.
50. Ross S., Moffat K., McConnachie A., Gordon J., Wilson P. (1999). Sex and attitude: a randomized vignette study of the management of depression by general practitioners. *Br. J. Gen. Pract.*, **49**, 17–21.
51. Botega N., Mann A., Blizard R., Wilkinson G. (1992). General practitioners and depression – first use of the Depression Attitude Questionnaire. *Int. J. Methods Psychiatr. Res.*, **2**, 169–180.
52. Dowrick C., Gask L., Perry R., Dixon C., Usherwood T. (2000). Do general practitioners' attitudes towards depression predict their clinical behaviour? *Psychol. Med.*, **30**, 413–419.
53. Paykel E.S., Hart D., Priest R.G. (1998). Changes in public attitudes to depression during the Defeat Depression Campaign. *Br. J. Psychiatry*, **173**, 519–522.
54. Rix S., Paykel E.S., Lelliott P., Tylee A., Freeling P., Gask L., Hart D. (1999). Impact of a national campaign on GP education: an evaluation of the Defeat Depression Campaign. *Br. J. Gen. Pract.*, **49**, 99–102.
55. Mulrow C.D., Williams J.W.J., Gerety M.B., Ramirez G., Montiel O.M., Kerber C. (1995). Case-finding instruments for depression in primary care settings. *Ann. Intern. Med.*, **122**, 913–921.
56. Williams J.W.J., Noel P.H.P., Cordes J.A.M., Ramirez G.D., Pignone M.M. (2002). Is this patient clinically depressed? *JAMA*, **287**, 1160–1170.

57. Whooley M.A.M., Avins A.L.M., Miranda J.P., Browner W.S.M.M. (1997). Case-finding instruments for depression: two questions are as good as many. *J. Gen. Intern. Med.*, **12**, 439–445.
58. US Preventive Services Task Force (2002). Screening for depression: recommendations and rationale. *Ann. Intern. Med.*, **136**, 760–764.
59. Pignone M.P.M., Gaynes B.N.M., Rushton J.L.M., Burchell C.M.M., Orleans C.T.P., Mulrow C.D.M., Lohr K.N.P. (2002). Screening for depression in adults: a summary of the evidence for the US Preventive Services Task Force. *Ann. Intern. Med.*, **136**, 765–776.
60. Gilbody S.M., House A.O., Sheldon T.A. (2001). Routinely administered questionnaires for depression and anxiety: systematic review. *Br. Med. J.*, **322**, 406–409.
61. Valenstein M.M., Vijan S.M., Zeber J.E.M., Boehm K.M., Buttar A.M. (2001). The cost-utility of screening for depression in primary care. *Ann. Intern. Med.*, **134**, 345–360.
62. Kroenke K.M. (2001). Depression screening is not enough. *Ann. Intern. Med.*, **134**, 418–420.
63. Grimshaw J.M., Russell I.T. (1993). Effect of clinical guidelines on medical practice: a systematic review of rigorous evaluations. *Lancet*, **342**, 1317–1322.
64. Paykel E.S., Priest R.G. (1992). Recognition and management of depression in general practice: concensus statement. *Br. Med. J.*, **305**, 1198–1202.
65. Depression Guideline Panel (1993). *Depression in Primary Care: Treatment of Major Depression* 2. US Department of Health and Human Services, Agency for Health Care Policy and Research, Rockville, MD.
66. Anderson I.M., Nutt D.J., Deakin J.F. (2000). Evidence-based guidelines for treating depressive disorders with antidepressants: a revision of the 1993 British Association for Psychopharmacology guidelines. British Association for Psychopharmacology. *J. Psychopharmacol.*, **14**, 3–20.
67. Littlejohns P., Cluzeau F., Bale R., Grimshaw J., Feder G., Moran S. (1999). The quantity and quality of clinical practice guidelines for the management of depression in primary care in the UK. *Br. J. Gen. Pract.*, **49**, 205–210.
68. NHS Centre for Reviews and Dissemination (1993) The treatment of depression in primary care. *Eff. Health Care Bull.*, **1** (5).
69. NHS Centre for Reviews and Dissemination (2002). Improving the recognition and management of depression in primary care. *Eff. Health Care Bull.*, **7** (5).
70 Feder G., Griffiths C., Highton C., Eldridge S., Spence M., Southgate L. (1995). Do clinical guidelines introduced with practice-based education improve care of asthmatic and diabetic patients? A randomised controlled trial in general practices in east London. *Br. Med. J.*, **311**, 1473–1478.
71. Rutz W., von Knorring L., Walinder J. (1989). Frequency of suicide on Gotland after systematic postgraduate education of general practitioners. *Acta Psychiatr. Scand.*, **80**, 151–154.
72. Rutz W., von Knorring L., Walinder J. (1992). Long-term effects of an educational program for general practitioners given by the Swedish Committee for the Prevention and Treatment of Depression. *Acta Psychiatr. Scand.*, **85**, 83–88.
73. Upton M.W., Evans M., Goldberg D.P., Sharp D.J. (1999). Evaluation of ICD-10 PHC mental health guidelines in detecting and managing depression within primary care. *Br. J. Psychiatry*, **175**, 476–482.
74. van Os T.W., Ormel J., van den Brink R.H., Jenner J.A., Van Der M.K., Tiemens B.G., van der D.W., Smit A., van den B.W. (1999). Training primary care

physicians improves the management of depression. *Gen. Hosp. Psychiatry*, **21**, 168–176.
75. Thompson C., Kinmonth A.L., Stevens L., Peveler R.C., Stevens A., Ostler K.J., Pickering R.M., Baker N.G., Henson A., Preece J., *et al.* (2000). Effects of clinical-practice guideline and practice-based education on detection and outcome of depression in primary care: Hampshire Depression project randomised controlled trial. *Lancet*, **355**, 185–191.
76. Kendrick T. (2000). Why can't GPs follow guidelines on depression? We must question the basis of the guidelines themselves. *Br. Med. J.*, **320**, 200–201.
77. Cornwall P.L., Scott J. (2000). Which clinical practice guidelines for depression? An overview for busy practitioners. *Br. J. Gen. Pract.*, **50**, 908–911.
78. Peveler R., Kendrick T. (2001). Treatment delivery and guidelines in primary care. *Br. Med. Bull.*, **57**, 193–206.
79. Grol R., Dalhuijsen J., Thomas S., Veld C., Rutten G., Mokkink H. (1998). Attributes of clinical guidelines that influence use of guidelines in general practice: observational study. *Br. Med. J.*, **317**, 858–861.
80. Freeman A.C., Sweeney K. (2001). Why general practitioners do not implement evidence: qualitative study. *Br. Med. J.*, **323**, 1100–1102.
81. Katon W., Von Korff M., Lin E., Walker E., Simon G.E., Bush T., Robinson P., Russo J. (1995). Collaborative management to achieve treatment guidelines. Impact on depression in primary care. *JAMA*, **273**, 1026–1031.
82. Lin E.H., Katon W.J., Simon G.E., VonKorff M., Bush T.M., Rutter C.M., Saunders K.W., Walker E.A. (1997). Achieving guidelines for the treatment of depression in primary care: is physician education enough? *Med. Care*, **35**, 831–842.
83. Katon W., Robinson P., Von Korff M., Lin E., Bush T., Ludman E., Simon G., Walker E. (1996). A multifaceted intervention to improve treatment of depression in primary care. *Arch. Gen. Psychiatry*, **53**, 924–932.
84. Katon W., VonKorff M., Lin E., Simon G., Walker E., Unutzer J., Bush T., Russo J., Ludman E. (1999). Stepped collaborative care for primary care patients with persistent symptoms of depression: a randomized trial. *Arch. Gen. Psychiatry*, **56**, 1109–1115.
85. Katzelnick D.J., Simon G.E., Pearson S.D., Manning W.G., Helstad C.P., Henk H.J., Cole S.M., Lin E.H., Taylor L.H., Kobak K.A. (2000). Randomized trial of a depression management program in high utilizers of medical care. *Arch. Fam. Med.*, **9**, 345–351.
86. Hunkeler E.M., Meresman J.F., Hargreaves W.A., Fireman B., Berman W.H., Kirsch A.J., Groebe J., Hurt S.W., Braden P., Getzell M., *et al.* (2000). Efficacy of nurse telehealth care and peer support in augmenting treatment of depression in primary care. *Arch. Fam. Med.*, **9**, 700–708.
87. Rost K., Nutting P., Smith J., Werner J., Duan N. (2001). Improving depression outcomes in community primary care practice: a randomized trial of the quEST intervention. Quality Enhancement by Strategic Teaming. *J. Gen. Intern. Med.*, **16**, 143–149.
88. Wells K.B., Sherbourne C., Schoenbaum M., Duan N., Meredith L., Unutzer J., Miranda J., Carney M.F., Rubenstein L.V. (2000). Impact of disseminating quality improvement programs for depression in managed primary care: a randomized controlled trial. *JAMA*, **283**, 212–220.
89. VonKorff M., Goldberg D. (2001). Improving outcomes in depression. *Br. Med. J.*, **323**, 948–949.

90. Schulberg H.C., McClelland M., Gooding W. (1987). Six-month outcomes for medical patients with major depressive disorders. *J. Gen. Intern. Med.*, **2**, 312–317.
91. Ormel J., van den B.W., Koeter M.W., Giel R., Van Der M.K., Van De W.G., Wilmink F.W. (1990). Recognition, management and outcome of psychological disorders in primary care: a naturalistic follow-up study. *Psychol. Med.*, **20**, 909–923.
92. Simon G.E., Goldberg D., Tiemens B.G., Ustun T.B. (1999). Outcomes of recognized and unrecognized depression in an international primary care study. *Gen. Hosp. Psychiatry*, **21**, 97–105.
93. Department of Health (2002). *First Year Strategy for NIMHE*. NIMHE/Department of Health, Leeds.
94. Tylee A. (2003). The Primary Care Programme of the National Institute for Mental Health in England (NIMHE). *Primary Care Mental Health*, **1**, 1–3.
95. Dwyer M. (2002). Trailblazers. *J. Primary Care Mental Health*, **6**, 17.
96. Walters P. (2003). Trailblazers – an update. *J. Primary Care Mental Health*, **7**.
97. Brown C., Bullock A., Wakefield S. (2002). *Evaluation of the Trailblazers Mental Health Teaching the Teachers Course in the West Midlands*. University of Birmingham, Birmingham.
98. Crisp A.H., Gelder M.G., Rix S., Meltzer H.I., Rowlands O.J. (2000). Stigmatisation of people with mental illnesses. *Br. J. Psychiatry*, **177**, 4–7.
99. Tylee A. (2001). Management of depression in primary care. In: Dawson A., Tylee A. (eds) *Depression: Social and Economic Timebomb*. BMJ Books, London, pp. 85–92.
100. Morriss R.K., Gask L. (2002). Treatment of patients with somatized mental disorder: effects of reattribution training on outcomes under the direct control of the family doctor. *Psychosomatics*, **43**, 394–399.
101. Evans A., Gask L., Singleton C., Bahrami J. (2001). Teaching consultation skills: a survey of general practice trainers. *Med. Educ.*, **35**, 222–224.
102. Gask L. (1998). Small group interactive techniques utilizing videofeedback. *Int. J. Psychiatry Med.*, **28**, 97–113.
103. Bowman F.M., Goldberg D.P., Millar T., Gask L., McGrath G. (1992). Improving the skills of established general practitioners: the long-term benefits of group teaching. *Med. Educ.*, **26**, 63–68.
104. Gask L., Goldberg D., Boardman J., Craig T., Goddard C., Jones O., Kiseley S., McGrath G., Millar T. (1991). Training general practitioners to teach psychiatric interviewing skills: an evaluation of group training. *Med. Educ.*, **25**, 444–451.
105. Gask L., Goldberg D., Porter R., Creed F. (1989). The treatment of somatization: evaluation of a teaching package with general practice trainees. *J. Psychosom. Res.*, **33**, 697–703.
106. Naji S.A., Maguire G.P., Fairbairn S.A., Goldberg D.P., Faragher E.B. (1986). Training clinical teachers in psychiatry to teach interviewing skills to medical students. *Med. Educ.*, **20**, 140–147.
107. Goldberg D., Gask L., Sartorius N. (2001). *Training Physicians in Mental Health Skills*. World Psychiatric Association, New York.
108. Mann A., Blizard R., Murray J. (1998). An evaluation of practice nurses working with general practitioners to treat people with depression. *Br. J. Gen. Pract.*, **48**, 875–879.
109. Mynors-Wallis L. (1996). *The Training of Community Nurses in Problem Solving Treatment*. Intelligence NHS Mental Health R&D Programme.

110. Peveler R., George C., Kinmonth A.L., Campbell M., Thompson C. (1999). Effect of antidepressant drug counselling and information leaflets on adherence to drug treatment in primary care: randomised controlled trial. *Br. Med. J.*, **319**, 612–615.
111. Tylee A. (1999). Training the whole primary care team in common mental disorders. In: Tansella M., Thornicroft G. (eds) *Mental Disorders in Primary Care*. Routledge, London, pp. 194–207.
112. Mulrow C.D.M., Williams J.W.J., Chiquette E.P., Aguilar C.M., Hitchcock-Noel P.P., Lee S.M., Cornell J.P., Stamm K.B. (2000). Efficacy of newer medications for treating depression in primary care patients. *Am. J. Med.*, **108**, 54–64.
113. Martin R.M., Hilton S.R., Kerry S.M., Richards N.M. (1997). General practitioners' perceptions of the tolerability of antidepressant drugs: a comparison of selective serotonin reuptake inhibitors and tricyclic antidepressants. *Br. Med. J.*, **314**, 646–651.
114. MacGillivray S., Arroll B., Hatcher S., Ogston S., Reid I., Sullivan F., Williams B., Crombie I. (2003). Efficacy and tolerability of selective serotonin reuptake inhibitors compared with tricyclic antidepressants in depression treated in primary care: systematic review and meta-analysis. *Br. Med. J.*, **326**, 1014.
115. Goldberg D., Privett M., Ustun B., Simon G., Linden M. (1998). The effects of detection and treatment on the outcome of major depression in primary care: a naturalistic study in 15 cities. *Br. J. Gen. Pract.*, **48**, 1840–1844.
116. Donoghue J.M.M.R., Tylee A.D. (1996). The treatment of depression: prescribing patterns of antidepressants in primary care in the UK. *Br. J. Psychiatry*, **168**, 164–168.
117. Dunn R.L., Donoghue J.M., Ozminkowski R.J., Stephenson D., Hylan T.R. (1999). Longitudinal patterns of antidepressant prescribing in primary care in the UK: comparison with treatment guidelines. *J. Psychopharmacol.*, **13**, 136–143.
118. Furukawa T.A., McGuire H., Barbui C. (2002). Meta-analysis of effects and side effects of low dosage tricyclic antidepressants in depression: systematic review. *Br. Med. J.*, **325**, 991.
119. Lin E.H., VonKorff M., Katon W., Bush T., Simon G.E., Walker E., Robinson P. (1995). The role of the primary care physician in patients' adherence to antidepressant therapy. *Med. Care*, **33**, 67–74.
120. Lawrenson R.A., Tyrer F., Newson R.B., Farmer R.D. (2000). The treatment of depression in UK general practice: selective serotonin reuptake inhibitors and tricyclic antidepressants compared. *J. Affect. Disord.*, **59**, 149–157.
121. George C.F., Peveler R.C., Heiliger S., Thompson C. (2000). Compliance with tricyclic antidepressants: the value of four different methods of assessment. *Br. J. Clin. Pharmacol.*, **50**, 166–171.
122. Mendlewicz J. (2001). Optimising antidepressant use in clinical practice: towards criteria for antidepressant selection. *Br. J. Psychiatry*, **179** (Suppl. 42), S1–S3.
123. Scott C., Tacchi M.J., Jones R., Scott J. (1997). Acute and one-year outcome of a randomised controlled trial of brief cognitive therapy for major depressive disorder in primary care. *Br. J. Psychiatry*, **171**, 131–134.
124. Appleby L., Warner R., Whitton A., Faragher B. (1997). A controlled study of fluoxetine and cognitive–behavioural counselling in the treatment of postnatal depression. *Br. Med. J.*, **314**, 932–936.

125. Schulberg H.C., Block M.R., Madonia M.J., Scott C.P., Rodriguez E., Imber S.D., Perel J., Lave J., Houck P.R., Coulehan J.L. (1996). Treating major depression in primary care practice. Eight-month clinical outcomes. *Arch. Gen. Psychiatry*, **53**, 913–919.
126. Mynors-Wallis L., Gath D. (1997). Predictors of treatment outcome for major depression in primary care. *Psychol. Med.*, **27**, 731–736.
127. Mynors-Wallis L.M., Gath D.H., Day A., Baker F. (2000). Randomised controlled trial of problem solving treatment, antidepressant medication, and combined treatment for major depression in primary care. *Br. Med. J.*, **320**, 26–30.
128. Churchill R., Hunot V., Corney R., Knapp M., McGuire H., Tylee A., Wessely S. (2001). A systematic review of controlled trials of the effectiveness and cost-effectiveness of brief psychological treatments for depression. *Health Technol. Assess.*, **5** (35).
129. Ward E., King M., Lloyd M., Bower P., Sibbald B., Farrelly S., Gabbay M., Tarrier N., Addington-Hall J. (2000). Randomised controlled trial of non-directive counselling, cognitive–behaviour therapy, and usual general practitioner care for patients with depression. I: Clinical effectiveness. *Br. Med. J.*, **321**, 1383–1388.
130. Kaltenthaler E., Shackley P., Stevens K., Beverley C., Parry G., Chilcott J. (2002). A systematic review and economic evaluation of computerised cognitive behaviour therapy for depression and anxiety. *Health Technol. Assess.*, **6**, 1–89.
131. Chilvers C., Dewey M., Fielding K., Gretton V., Miller P., Palmer B., Weller D., Churchill R., Williams I., Bedi N., *et al.* (2001). Antidepressant drugs and generic counselling for treatment of major depression in primary care: randomised trial with patient preference arms. *Br. Med. J.*, **322**, 772–775.
132. Friedli K., King M.B., Lloyd M., Horder J. (1997). Randomised controlled assessment of non-directive psychotherapy versus routine general-practitioner care. *Lancet*, **350**, 1662–1665.
133. Bower P., Rowland N., Mellor C., Heywood P., Godfrey C., Hardy R. (2002). Effectiveness and cost effectiveness of counselling in primary care. *Cochrane Database of Systematic Reviews*, CD001025.
134. Schulberg H.C., Katon W.J., Simon G.E., Rush A.J. (1999). Best clinical practice: guidelines for managing major depression in primary medical care. *J. Clin. Psychiatry*, **60** (Suppl. 7), 19–26.
135. Dowrick C., Dunn G., Ayuso-Mateos J.L., Dalgard O.S., Page H., Lehtinen V., Casey P., Wilkinson C., Vazquez-Barquero J.L., Wilkinson G. (2000). Problem solving treatment and group psychoeducation for depression: multicentre randomised controlled trial. Outcomes of Depression International Network (ODIN) group. *Br. Med. J.*, **321**, 1450–1454.
136. Williams C. (2001). Use of written cognitive–behavioural therapy self-help materials to treat depression. *Adv. Psychiatr. Treat.*, **7**, 233–240.
137. Bower P., Richards D., Lovell K. (2001). The clinical and cost-effectiveness of self-help treatments for anxiety and depressive disorders in primary care: a systematic review. *Br. J. Gen. Pract.*, **51**, 838–845.
138. Cuijpers P. (1997). Bibliotherapy in unipolar depression: a meta-analysis. *J. Behav. Ther. Exper. Psychiatry*, **28**, 139–147.
139. Nutting P.A., Rost K., Dickinson M., Werner J.J., Dickinson P., Smith J.L., Gallovic B. (2002). Barriers to initiating depression treatment in primary care practice. *J. Gen. Intern. Med.*, **17**, 103–111.

140. VonKorff M., Katon W., Bush T., Lin E.H., Simon G.E., Saunders K., Ludman E., Walker E., Unutzer J. (1998). Treatment costs, cost offset, and cost-effectiveness of collaborative management of depression. *Psychosom. Med.*, **60**, 143–149.
141. Simon G.E., Katon W.J., VonKorff M., Unutzer J., Lin E.H., Walker E.A., Bush T., Rutter C., Ludman E. (2001). Cost-effectiveness of a collaborative care program for primary care patients with persistent depression. *Am. J. Psychiatry*, **158**, 1638–1644.
142. Rost K., Nutting P., Smith J.L., Elliott C.E., Dickinson M. (2002). Managing depression as a chronic disease: a randomised trial of ongoing treatment in primary care. *Br. Med. J.*, **325**, 934.
143. Koike A.K., Unutzer J., Wells K.B. (2002). Improving the care for depression in patients with comorbid medical illness. *Am. J. Psychiatry*, **159**, 1738–1745.
144. Araya R., Rojas G., Fritsch R., Gaete J., Rojas M., Simon G., Peters T.J. (2003). Treating depression in primary care in low-income women in Santiago, Chile: a randomised controlled trial. *Lancet*, **361**, 995–1000.
145. Scott J., Thorne A., Horn P. (2002). Quality improvement report: effect of a multifaceted approach to detecting and managing depression in primary care. *Br. Med. J.*, **325**, 951–954.
146. Simon G.E., VonKorff M., Rutter C., Wagner E. (2000). Randomised trial of monitoring, feedback, and management of care by telephone to improve treatment of depression in primary care. *Br. Med. J.*, **320**, 550–554.
147. Oxman T.E., Dietrich A.J., Williams Jr J.W., Kroenke K. (2002). A three-component model for reengineering systems for the treatment of depression in primary care. *Psychosomatics*, **43**, 441–450.

CHAPTER

10

The Prodromes and Early Detection of Alzheimer's Disease

Michael Zaudig

Windach Hospital and Institute for Neurobehavioral Research and Therapy, Windach, Germany

INTRODUCTION

Over the past two decades, an increased scientific effort has been devoted to gaining an understanding not only of the epidemiology, genetics and biochemical pathogenesis of Alzheimer's disease (AD), but also of how to detect in individuals with subclinical or preclinical forms of the disorder [1]. Identification of such individuals will become a clinical and public health imperative once effective therapeutic measures are developed. Mild cognitive impairment (MCI) defines a transitional stage between normal ageing and dementia and reflects the clinical situation where a person has memory complaints but no evidence of dementia [2].

TERMINOLOGY, CLASSIFICATION AND DEFINITION OF MCI

In this chapter, the term MCI is used to describe subjects with cognitive impairment that is not severe enough to meet the criteria for dementia (DSM-IV, ICD-10, National Institute of Neurological and Communicative Disorders and Stroke – Alzheimer's Disease and Related Disorders Association (NINCDS-ADRDA) criteria) and in whom the cognitive impairment is not related to vascular disorders, Parkinson's disease, brain neoplasm, head trauma, drugs, alcohol or thyroid dysfunction. The term MCI as used in this chapter means objective (measured by neuropsychological tests) mild cognitive impairment with insidious onset and slow deterioration in older people. MCI currently is seen as a harbinger of AD.

Early Detection and Management of Mental Disorders.
Edited by Mario Maj, Juan José López-Ibor, Norman Sartorius, Mitsumoto Sato and Ahmed Okasha.
 ISBN 0-470-01083-5.

The term "preclinical AD" refers to subjects who have objective mild cognitive impairment and who then develop AD. Consequently the diagnosis of preclinical AD can only be made retrospectively.

According to Feinstein [3], classification must perform three principal functions: (a) denomination (i.e. assigning a common name to a group of phenomena); (b) qualification (i.e. enriching the informativeness of the name or category by adding relevant descriptive features such as typical symptoms, age at onset and severity); and (c) prediction (i.e. a probabilistic statement about the expected course and outcome of the named entity as well as a statement about its likely response to treatment). Because of the diversity of origins and presentation, the term MCI does not represent a unitary or uniform phenomenon. Rather, it represents a broad category, often multifactorial, multiform and dynamic. There is still no commonly accepted definition of MCI. Classification systems like the DSM-IV and ICD-10 provide concepts which are only tangentially related to the above-mentioned notion of MCI (mild neurocognitive disorder in the DSM-IV; mild cognitive disorder in the ICD-10). There is an urgent need to establish a valid MCI category in future editions of these systems.

Reviewing the literature on MCI, it is evident that some confusion exists concerning the specific boundaries of the condition. There are several possible contributing factors to this inconsistency in the literature, such as the different sources of study participants, the differences in reference points for normal ageing (no cognitive impairment, NCI) as well as reference points for dementia, and the use of different rating scales. Typically, MCI is thought to have a degenerative basis and to progress gradually to dementia and likely to AD. To define MCI, a description of the onset and course of the disorder is necessary. Typically MCI evolves gradually; there is no acute onset. The course is chronic, usually insidious at onset, and develops slowly but steadily over a period of many years. This period can be as short as two or three years, but may also be considerably longer. Progression rate depends on the severity of MCI.

Basic criteria to identify those likely to decline to dementia (AD) over time might be:

- Presence of a mild cognitive impairment which is objectified by neuropsychological tests or screening tests like the Structured Interview for the Assessment of Dementia (SIDAM [4]) or the Cambridge Examination for Mental Disorders of the Elderly (CAMDEX [5]).
- Evidence of a progression of cognitive impairment over time (at least 6 months).
- Subjective cognitive impairment.
- Cognitive impairment which is verified by an informant.

- Insidious onset with slow deterioration. While the onset usually seems difficult to pinpoint in time, realization by others that the cognitive problems exist may come more or less suddenly.
- Exclusion of systemic or brain disease (e.g. hypothyroidism, hypercalcaemia, vitamin B12 deficiency, neurosyphilis, normal-pressure hydrocephalus or subdural haematoma), absence of a sudden apoplectic onset or of neurological signs of focal damage such as hemiparesis, sensory loss or visual field defects.
- Exclusion of dementia.
- Exclusion of clinically relevant depressions, states of subnormal cognitive functioning attributable to a severely impoverished social environment and limited education, and mild or moderate mental retardation.
- There are no or at least very mild problems in activities of daily living (ADL), measured by means of a sensitive scale. ADL performance may also be declining.

EPIDEMIOLOGY

Ritchie *et al.* [6] reported the prevalence of MCI and age-associated cognitive decline (AACD) in a representative population to be 3.2% and 19.3%, respectively. Lopez *et al.* [7] found that 22% of subjects aged 75 years or older had MCI. In more detail, the prevalence increased with age from 19% in people younger than 75 years, to 29% in those older than 85 years. These authors found that the prevalence of MCI, amnestic-type was 6% and that of MCI, multiple cognitive deficit-type was 16%. The prevalence rates for MCI and related conditions reflect differences in cohort characteristics and in the criteria used to define MCI.

DIFFERENTIAL DIAGNOSIS

In diagnosing MCI, physicians need to be aware of the salient features of normal brain ageing and the boundaries between normal brain ageing and dementia. MCI currently is seen as a harbinger of AD. If so, a list of conditions that can produce dementia apart from AD have to be excluded. They include metabolic disorders, endocrine disorders, nutritional disorders, toxic conditions, infectious processes, neoplastic disorders, normal-pressure hydrocephalus, cerebrovascular events and other conditions of known and unknown aetiology (e.g. prion diseases, Pick's disease, frontal lobe dementias, Lewy body dementia, parkinsonian dementia and human immunodeficiency virus (HIV) infection).

Several studies involving elderly subjects from the general population have indicated that depression is a risk factor for AD [8–11]. However, it is not clear from the literature whether depression can predict AD in subjects with MCI. Some studies reported that most depressed subjects with cognitive impairment develop AD, but these studies lacked a control group of non-depressed subjects with MCI [12,13]. Other studies indicated that depression itself can cause cognitive impairment that mimics the cognitive impairment seen in AD and that the cognitive impairment in depressed subjects was reversible after the improvement of the depression [14]. One important question still is, therefore, how subjects with preclinical AD or MCI can be differentiated from subjects with depression-related cognitive impairment.

DIAGNOSTIC BORDERS

MCI refers to a transitional state between normal ageing and dementia [1]. To describe the borders of MCI in the elderly, a strict delineation from both healthy and demented individuals is necessary, since the threshold for dementia diagnosis (or healthy status) may vary considerably among clinicians and criteria. How comparable are the DSM-IV, ICD-10 and NINCDS-ADRDA criteria for dementia? Only very limited data are available on this issue. Kukull *et al.* [15] found that the DSM-III-R criteria were more specific in diagnosing dementia, whereas the NINCDS-ADRDA criteria were more sensitive. Waite *et al.* [16] and Erkinjuntti *et al.* [17] found that the DSM-III-R criteria for dementia seemed to be more inclusive than the DSM-IV criteria. There is a need to compare ICD-10 and DSM-IV thresholds for dementia, otherwise heterogeneous diagnoses and prevalence data on MCI and dementia will result, affecting disease estimates.

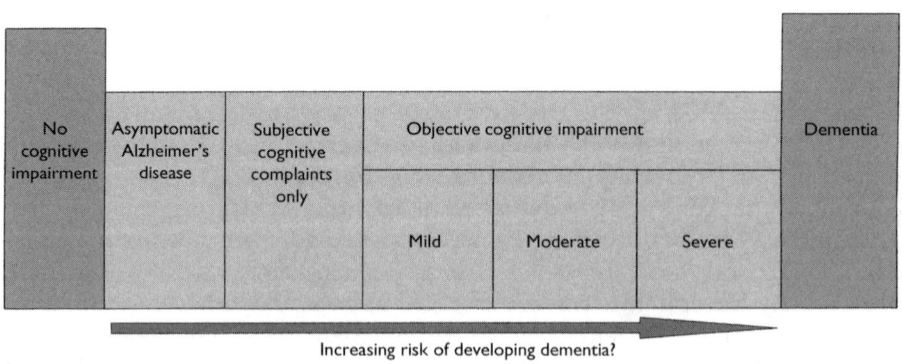

Figure 10.1 Spectrum of cognitive disorders in the elderly

The same is true for healthy individuals. Morris *et al.* [18] were using strict criteria in delineating MCI from healthy subjects by defining even very mild impairment (not only memory failure) as abnormal (MCI). More MCI cases and fewer healthy subjects will result with this approach (Figure 10.1).

FOLLOW-UP STUDIES OF MCI AND RATES OF CONVERSION TO AD

Several follow-up studies have reported annualized rates of conversion from MCI to dementia, with a range from 3.7% to 25% (Table 10.1). Most studies have rates of between 10% and 15%. Where additional domains to memory loss are affected, rates of conversion are much higher (25% per year) [29].

Palmer *et al.* [31] found the relative risks of progressing to dementia in non-demented subjects with mild, moderate or severe cognitive impairment to be 3.6, 5.4 and 7.0 respectively. The more impaired, the higher the risk of conversion to dementia [18,31].

ASSESSMENT

At present, there is a great variety of assessment instruments in geriatric psychiatry; the older tendency to proliferation of classifications has been replaced by a tendency to proliferation of instruments. There are now many rating scales, interviews and questionnaires that measure cognitive symptoms of dementia and of MCI. Some measures encompass a large range of problems (e.g. the SIDAM or the CAMDEX); others focus on one or more specific areas. Some require little or no training to administer (e.g. the Mini Mental State Examination, MMSE [32]); others require administration by trained clinicians. Some instruments, like the SIDAM or CAMDEX, have a broader range of purposes: for example diagnosis (DSM-IV or ICD-10), measurement of cognitive symptoms, assessment of ADL and screening (Table 10.2). In general, there are cognitive screening tests, observer/informant-based instruments and ADL/instrumental ADL (IADL) scales. The only instrument comprising a cognitive screening test, observer- and informant-based information, an ADL scale, and ICD-10 and DSM-IV criteria for dementia is the SIDAM [4,33].

One of the biases inherent in the assessment of MCI [38] is that the same scales developed to document AD are used to estimate rates of conversion to AD, creating a self-fulfilling prophecy. Memory complaints are the core

Table 10.1 Recent follow-up studies of mild cognitive impairment (MCI)

Authors	Subjects	Follow-up	Percentage developing dementia	Annual rates of conversion (%)
Flicker *et al.* [19]	MCI	2 years	50	25
Tierney *et al.* [20]	Memory impairment	2 years	28	14
Bowen *et al.* [21]	Isolated memory loss	4 years	48	12
Devanand *et al.* [22]	Questionable dementia	2.7 years	41	15
Wolf *et al.* [23]	MCI	3 years	20	6.7
Krasucki *et al.* [24]	MCI	4.5 years	100	22
Petersen *et al.* [25]	MCI	1 year	10–15	10
Black [26]	MCI	3 years	30	10
McKelvey *et al.* [27]	MCI	3 years	53	17.7
Daly *et al.* [28]	MCI	3 years	18	6
Ritchie *et al.* [6]	MCI	3 years	11.1	3.7
Ritchie *et al.* [6]	Age-associated cognitive decline	3 years	28.6	9.5
Bozoki *et al.* [29]	MCI (multiple domains)	2 years	50	25
Morris *et al.* [18]	MCI	5 years	20–60 (depending on a clinical rating)	4–12
Waite *et al.* [16]	MCI	3 years	21	7
	(with extrapyramidal signs)	(mean)	34	11.3
	(with vascular features)		38	12.7
Tabert [30]	MCI	2 years (average)	25	12.5
Palmer *et al.* [31]	Cognitive impairment, non-demented	3 years	35	11.7

feature of MCI, but the measurement of cognitive functions in addition to memory is important, not least to show that they are normal.

Beside neuropsychological batteries and single tests, there are only two clinical screening instruments which allow a broad assessment of MCI: the Cambridge Cognitive Examination (CAMCOG), part of the CAMDEX [5], and the SIDAM Score (SISCO), part of the SIDAM [4]. Both instruments allow the exclusion of dementia, but only the SIDAM is derived from

TABLE 10.2 Instruments for the identification of mild cognitive impairment (MCI) and dementia

	General cognitive screening test	Observer/ informant-based instrument	ADL/ IADL	Dementia criteria		
				Any	ICD-10	DSM-IV
MMSE [32]	+	–	–	–	–	–
ADAS [34]	+	–	–	–	–	–
GDS [37]	–	+	(+)	+	–	–
CDR [35]	–	+	(+)	+	–	–
CAMDEX [5]	+	+	+	+	–	–
SIDAM [4]	+	+	+	–	+	+
CIE [36]	+	+	+	–	+	–

ADAS, Alzheimer's Disease Assessment Scale; ADL, activities of daily living; CAMDEX, Cambridge Examination for Mental Disorders of the Elderly; CDR, Clinical Dementia Rating; CIE, Canberra Interview of the Elderly; GDS, Global Deterioration Scale; IADL, instrumental activities of daily living; MMSE, Mini Mental State Examination; SIDAM, Structured Interview for the Assessment of Dementia.

ICD-10 and DSM-IV algorithms. Both have included the MMSE. The MMSE is valid only in the assessment of dementia, therefore instruments like the CAMDEX or SIDAM should be preferred. Also very useful are batteries like the Consortium to Establish a Registry for Alzheimer's Disease (CERAD) measures [39], including a sensitive test like the Word List Delayed Recall (WLDR), which has predictive power concerning the development of MCI and dementia.

Useful staging instruments are the Global Deterioration Scale (GDS [37]) and the Clinical Dementia Rating (CDR [35]). The CDR describes a continuum from normal ageing (CDR 0) through questionable dementia (CDR 0.5), to mild (CDR 1), moderate (CDR 2) and severe dementia (CDR 3). Although some authors believe that CDR 0.5 is equivalent to MCI, others contend that CDR 0.5 actually describes a broader population, including mild AD [40]. The GDS stages subjects from GDS 1 (normal) to GDS 2 (subjective memory impairment), GDS 3 (mild cognitive decline and mild dementia), and GDS 4 through 8 (more severe stages of dementia).

An ideal assessment of all domains of MCI is presented in Table 10.3.

ACTIVITIES OF DAILY LIVING (ADL)

The assessment of daily functioning based on reports is particularly important: the core criteria for the diagnosis of dementia include proven impairment in

Table 10.3 Domains to be assessed for a diagnosis of MCI, with examples of the relevant instruments

- Memory complaints: Informant Questionnaire on Cognitive Decline in the Elderly (IQCODE [41])
- Objective memory impairment: Word List Delay Recall (WLDR [2])
- General cognitive functions: Cambridge Examination for Mental Disorders of the Elderly (CAMDEX [5]) or Structured Interview for the Assessment of Dementia (SIDAM [4])
- Dementia: CAMDEX or SIDAM
- Staging: Global Deterioration Scale (GDS [37]) or Clinical Dementia Rating (CDR [35])
- Activities of daily living: ADL International Scale (ADL-IS [42])

professional and social activities. New ADL scales to assess subtle changes in social activities in MCI patients have been developed (e.g. the ADL International Scale, ADS-IS [42]). Preliminary data demonstrated high correlations between ADL scores and GDS 2 and 3 stages. The higher significance of informant-reported than self-reported functional deficits has been emphasized [30]: informant-reported disabilities are more predictive of the future development of AD, particularly if there is a discrepancy between informants' reports and self-reports.

ADL deficits are integral components of dementia and ADL measures are most important in the diagnosis of dementia, but there are no guidelines as to what constitutes ADL restriction in MCI [1]. ADL deficits are commonly observed in incipient AD up to 2 years before diagnosis [6,43]. It has been hypothesized that ADL changes may be seen in MCI if lower thresholds are used to define restriction. Ritchie *et al.* [6] could find a difference between MCI and AACD criteria concerning ADL performance.

ASYMPTOMATIC AD

Preclinical AD

Objective and measurable cognitive loss is the hallmark in those people who develop AD, but there is good evidence that even earlier stages of the disease can be defined. It is possible to postulate a very early asymptomatic stage, where subtle cognitive changes occur over time, indistinguishable from normal ageing, and where there is no evidence of cognitive impairment but the neuropathological changes typical for AD are already present.

Several clinicopathologic studies of older adults with mild cognitive decline before death demonstrated large numbers of neurofibrillarly tangles and amyloid plaques sufficient for the diagnosis of AD. These pathological lesions develop over time. Therefore, the process that underlies AD must begin in a preclinical stage that precedes clinically detectable cognitive change probably by years.

Preclinical AD cases [18,44] resemble very mild AD cases pathologically. AD lesions must be present for a sufficiently long time to produce neuronal or synaptic loss before cognitive symptoms (MCI) appear. Preclinical AD indicates a stage in which there is no cognitive impairment [18,44–46].

Goldman *et al.* [45] reported longitudinal psychometric data from 24 cases analysed in the study of Price *et al.* [44]. None of the preclinical AD cases declined in psychometric performance with time; their mean performance was close to that of the healthy non-demented group. These and previous results support a model in which AD has a subtle transition from healthy ageing before identifiable cognitive loss.

Cognitive "Decliners" within Normal Neuropsychological Limits

In their prospective study, Collie *et al.* [47] used the WLDR, among other tests, on five occasions during a 2-year period in a cohort of 101 healthy older subjects. The results suggest that, during follow-up, subtle episodic memory decline can be detected among healthy older people before an objective memory deficit is evident using standard clinical criteria. Episodic memory decline as measured by performance on the WLDR remained within the normal limits. These data suggest that subtle cognitive decline can be detected in non-demented and higher performing older people by using serial administration of reliable and valid neuropsychological tests over an extended period before these people meet conventional clinical criteria for MCI [47].

Combination of Presymptomatic AD and APOE-ε4 Allele

Bookheimer *et al.* [48] found that among older people who had the APOE-ε4 allele and a normal memory for their age, both the magnitude and the extent of brain activation (as measured by functional magnetic resonance imaging, fMRI) during verbal memory challenge were greater than those among similar subjects who had the APOE-ε3 allele. These patterns of brain activation correlated with the degree of memory decline among subjects who were retested two years later. The authors concluded that older persons with APOE-ε4 have alterations in brain function without obvious cognitive impairment. A challenging task requiring memory (e.g. delayed-recall test) resulted in increased MRI signal intensity in presymptomatic subjects at genetic risk for AD. Brain activation might therefore be used to predict subsequent decline in memory.

SUBJECTIVE COGNITIVE IMPAIRMENT

Subjective Memory Complaints

There is emerging evidence from most community longitudinal studies that memory complaints do predict dementia or subsequent decline on cognitive tests [40,49,50]. Other studies found a stronger association between complaints and measures of depression and anxiety [51,52]. Hogan and Ebly [53] found that informant-based report of memory loss predicted progression to dementia in cognitively impaired non-demented (CIND) subjects. Schofield *et al.* [54] reported that memory complaints were associated with cognitive decline but only in cognitively impaired individuals. Palmer *et al.* [31] found, in a 6-year prospective population-based study of 212 CIND subjects, that absence of subjective memory complaints predicted improvement (odds ratio = 5.4).

In a prospective longitudinal community study ($n = 331$ aged over 75 years), Jorm *et al.* [52] showed that memory complaints do reflect perceptions of past memory performance and are also an early manifestation of memory impairment. This longitudinal analysis over 7–8 years demonstrates that memory complaints serve as a precursor of memory impairment in older people.

Ritchie *et al.* [6] further confirmed that memory complaints verified by neuropsychological assessment are not benign and should not be dismissed as a normal feature of ageing. Within a separate cognitive complaint cohort followed over 3 years, the conversion rate to AD (18% incidence over 3 years) was much higher than that observed in the general population.

Combination of Subjective Memory Complaints and APOE-ε4

Dik *et al.* [55] investigated to what extent subjective memory complaints and APOE-ε4 allele carriage predict future cognitive decline in cognitively intact elderly persons, by evaluating both their separate and combined effects. 1168 subjects from a prospective population-based study, aged 62–85 years, were evaluated for APOE-ε4, and memory complaints were assessed at baseline, and after 3 and 6 years. Furthermore, in all participants it was determined whether they met criteria for AACD at the 6-year follow-up. These authors reported that both memory complaints and APOE-ε4 allele carriage predicted cognitive decline at an early stage. Memory complaints were associated with a greater rate of decline in almost all cognitive measures. APOE-ε4 allele carriers also had a greater rate of cognitive decline after 6 years. The effects of memory complaints and APOE-ε4 allele carriage were additive: subjects with both factors had a two times higher cognitive decline than did subjects without both factors. Almost 50% of the APOE-ε4 allele carriers with memory complaints had AACD within 6 years.

This finding highlights the importance of subjective memory complaints even at an early stage when objective tests are still unable to detect cognitive deficits. They are especially important for elderly carriers of the APOE-ε4 allele, because they have an increased risk for AD [1]. Objective cognitive impairment became significant after 3 years and even more after 6 years [55].

Subjective Cognitive Complaints (Not Only Memory)

In the Rotterdam Scan Study, a prospective general population study, 1049 elderly non-demented individuals were assessed to investigate the relationship between cerebral white matter lesions (WML) and subjective cognitive dysfunction [56]. The concept of subjective cognitive failure is more comprehensive and broadly defined than memory complaints and may be a prelude to objective cognitive impairment. The authors found periventricular and subcortical WML to be associated with subjective cognitive failures and in particular with progression of these failures even in the absence of objective cognitive impairment. Subjects who reported retrospectively a 5-year progression of subjective cognitive failure had the most severe periventricular WML. These data suggest that the progression of subjective cognitive failures might be an early warning sign related to progression of WML [56].

BIOLOGICAL MARKERS

Biomarkers may be helpful in identifying subtypes of MCI, increasing the accuracy of clinical diagnosis, identifying those at risk, exploring the biology and monitoring progression of disease and effect of treatment. However, there are no definitive data on the usefulness of biomarkers in classifying MCI. There are some biomarkers in the cerebrospinal fluid (CSF) which have been used as indicators of Alzheimer's disease. Abnormal hyperphosphorylation of the microtubule-associated protein tau and its incorporation into neurofibrillary tangles are major hallmarks of the pathogenesis of AD. Hampel *et al.* [57] found that the p-tau proteins in CSF come closest to fulfilling the criteria of a biological marker of AD. There was even a tendency for p-tau proteins to perform differently in the discrimination of primary dementia disorders from AD. According to Sunderland *et al.* [58], all subjects with MCI who convert to AD have high CSF tau values, in contrast to non-progressive MCI. Since CSF tau levels do not increase during the course of AD, measurement of CSF tau might be used effectively for identifying incipient AD among those patients diagnosed as having MCI [59]. In a prospective 2-year follow-up, Okamura *et al.* [60] found that the CSF-cerebral blood flow (CBF) index (based on CSF tau levels divided by regional CBF in the posterior cingulate cortex) was useful in predicting AD in subjects with MCI.

NEUROPATHOLOGY AND NEUROIMAGING

Neuroimaging evidence of hippocampal shrinkage has been demonstrated in people with MCI, and atrophy in that region predicts the development of AD in those at high risk. Kantarci *et al.* [61] looked at the diagnostic accuracy of magnetic resonance hippocampal volumetry and spectroscopy in patients with MCI, in normal older people and in patients with AD. Hippocampal volumes and *N*-acetylaspartate/creatine spectroscopy were the most sensitive assessments discriminating MCI from AD. Changes in metabolic brain imaging may be an earlier and more sensitive predictor of later impairment both in cross-sectional [62] and in longitudinal studies of those at risk of developing dementia [63].

A recent study [44] could demonstrate that very mild AD cases (CDR 0.5) consistently have extensive diffuse and neuritic amyloid plaques throughout the neocortex and neurofibrillary tangles in and around the hippocampus, and meet pathological criteria for AD. These data indicate that the onset of objective cognitive decline and the diagnosis of very mild AD (CDR 0.5) correlate closely with the onset of neuronal loss in the hippocampus and entorhinal cortex (ERC), two areas that are particularly critical for memory processing. Similar findings were reported by Kordower *et al.* [64], with a marked cell loss in the layer II entorhinal cortex in cases with MCI. Data of this study indicate that atrophy and loss of layer II neurons occur in MCI prior to the onset of dementia and suggest that these changes are not exacerbated in early AD. Du *et al.* [65] found that volume reductions in the ERC and hippocampus may be early signs of AD pathology that can be measured using MRI. ERC and hippocampal volume were significantly reduced in MCI compared with NCI subjects. The same was true comparing AD with MCI. Further evidence for hippocampal volume reduction in

MCI/CDR 0.5 is reported by Wolf *et al.* [23]. Left-sided and posterior hippocampal MRI measures were most accurate in classifying CDR 0 and CDR 0.5. DeSanti *et al.* [62] could demonstrate that cross-sectional positron emission tomography (PET) measures of hippocampal metabolism and volume were superior in classifying healthy and MCI subjects. These data show that in MCI hippocampal changes exist without significant neocortical changes.

MANAGEMENT OF MCI

The aims of the management of subjects with MCI are: (a) to reduce symptoms or at least prevent them becoming worse and (b) to delay the decline to dementia. At present, three approaches can be distinguished: (a) counselling and support for the patient and relatives, (b) non-pharmacological treatment and (c) pharmacological treatment.

It is only recently that clinicians have recognized the need to support cognitively impaired patients and their care-giving families. The patient needs to be reassured about the decline of his/her cognitive capacities, learn to live with his/her errors and not feel ashamed of them. The intervention should concentrate on improving the patient's self-esteem.

Non-pharmacological therapy for elderly subjects with MCI has not been frequently implemented. Most interventions have been directed at the healthy elderly with subjective memory complaints, with or without objective memory impairment. The main goal has been the improvement of memory functions by memory training programmes. There is still a need for developing intervention programmes to improve coping styles and the quality of life of patients with MCI.

At present no studies of agents like nootropics, antioxidants, anti-inflammatory drugs and oestrogens in MCI patients have been reported. A number of agents like donepezil, rivastigmine, galantamine and memantine are currently being evaluated in MCI patients. Treatments which stabilize or reverse deposition of amyloid plaques or abnormal phosphorylation of tau protein will have a more significant role in impeding the progression of the disease than neurotransmitter-replacement therapies [2].

To date there is still no evidence that MCI, once diagnosed, can be successfully treated, but some treatment studies are now in publication.

CONCLUSIONS

An optimal diagnostic validation [66] of MCI should include: a careful clinical description, the delineation of a potential diagnostic category, a reliable method to assess symptoms, epidemiological studies, outcome/follow-up studies, laboratory and genetic studies. The above-mentioned elements are only partially available. The major problem is the heterogeneity of the MCI concept as a harbinger of AD. There are too many definitions of MCI, which do not allow comparison of epidemiological, outcome, laboratory and genetic studies. Research should focus on one reliable and valid diagnosis of MCI, and there is hope that at least some of what is now designated as MCI will be accepted in the future.

On the basis of the results of the studies reviewed above, it may be concluded that the following may predict progression to AD [1]: impairment of episodic memory, impairment in other cognitive domains, presence of APOE-ε4 allele, reduced temporo-parietal glucose metabolism and blood flow, neuronal loss in the entorhinal cortex and layer II and CA I of the hippocampus, brain activation of the hippocampus during cognitive stress tests, purely subjective cognitive impairment and the degree of functional impairment. Hybrid prediction models may provide the more accurate identification of individuals who are at risk for AD.

REFERENCES

1. Zaudig M. (2002). Mild cognitive impairment in the elderly. *Curr. Opin. Psychiatry*, **15**, 387–393.
2. Burns A., Zaudig M. (2002). Mild cognitive impairment in older people. *Lancet*, **360**, 1963–1965.
3. Feinstein A.R. (1972). Clinical biostatistics: 13. On homogeneity, taxonomy, and nosography. *Clin. Pharmacol. Ther.*, **13**, 114–129.
4. Zaudig M., Mittelhammer J., Hiller W., Pauls A., Thora C., Morinigo A., Mombour W. (1991). SIDAM – a structured interview for the diagnosis of dementia of the Alzheimer type, multi-infarct dementia and dementias of other etiology according to ICD-10 and DSM-III-R. *Psychol. Med.*, **21**, 225–236.
5. Roth M., Thym E., Mountjoy C.Q., Huppert F.A, Hendrie H., Verma S., Goddard R. (1986). CAMDEX. A standardized instrument for the diagnosis of mental disorders in the elderly with special reference to the early detection of dementia. *Br. J. Psychiatry*, **149**, 698–709.
6. Ritchie K., Artero S., Touchon J. (2001). Classification criteria for mild cognitive impairment. A population-based validation study. *Neurology*, **56**, 37–42.
7. Lopez O.L., Jagust W.J., DeKosky S.T., Becker J.T., Fitzpatrick A., Breitner J., Lyketsos C., Jones B., Kawas C., Carlson M., *et al.* (2003). Prevalence and classification of mild cognitive impairment in the Cardiovascular Health Study Cognition Study. Part 1. *Arch. Neurol.*, **60**, 1385–1389.
8. Visser P.J. (2000). *Predictors of Alzheimer Type Dementia in Subjects with Mild Cognitive Impairments*. Maastricht University Press, Maastricht, pp. 134–139.
9. Devanand D., Sano M., Tang M., Taylor S., Gurland B., Wilder D., Stern Y., Mayeux R. (1996). Depressed mood and the incidence of Alzheimer's disease in the elderly living in the community. *Arch. Gen. Psychiatry*, **53**, 175–182.

10. Jorm A., van Duijn C., Chandra V., Fratiglioni L., Graves A., Heyman A. (1991). Psychiatric history and related disorders as risk factors for Alzheimer's disease: a collaborative re-analysis of case-control studies. *Int. J. Epidemiol.*, **20**, 43–47.
11. Yaffe K., Blackwell T., Gore R., Sands L., Reus V., Browner W. (1999). Depressive symptoms and cognitive decline in nondemented elderly women. *Arch. Gen. Psychiatry*, **56**, 425–430.
12. Alexopoulous G.S., Meyers B.S., Young J.C., Mattis S., Kakuma T. (1993). The course of geriatric depression with "reversible dementia": a controlled study. *Am. J. Psychiatry*, **150**, 1693–1699.
13. Kral V., Emery O. (1989). Long-term follow-up of depressive pseudodementia. *Can. J. Psychiatry*, **34**, 445–466.
14. Hill C.D., Stoudemire A., Morris R., Martino-Salzman D., Markwalter H.R. (1992). Similarities and differences in memory deficits in patients with primary dementia and depression-related cognitive dysfunction. *J. Neuropsychiatr. Clin. Neurosci.*, **5**, 277–282.
15. Kukull W.A., Larson E.P., Reifler B.V., Lampe T.H., Jerby M.S., Hughes J.P. (1990). The validity of 3 clinical diagnostic criteria for Alzheimer's disease. *Neurology*, **40**, 1364–1369.
16. Waite L.M., Broe G.A., Grayson D.A., Creasey H. (2001). Preclinical syndromes predict dementia: the Sydney older persons study. *J. Neurol. Neurosurg. Psychiatry*, **71**, 296–302.
17. Erkinjuntti T., Ostbye T., Steenhuis R., Palo J. (1997). The effect of different diagnostic criteria on the prevalence of dementia. *N. Engl. J. Med.*, **337**, 1667–1674.
18. Morris J.C., Storandt M., Miller J.P., McKeel D.W., Price J.L., Rubin E.H., Berg L. (2001). Mild cognitive impairment represents early-stage Alzheimer's disease. *Arch. Neurol.*, **58**, 397–405.
19. Flicker C., Ferris S.H., Reisberg B. (1991). Mild cognitive impairment in the elderly: predictors of dementia. *Neurology*, **41**, 1006–1009.
20. Tierney M.C., Szalai J.P., Snow W.G., Fisher R.H., Nores A., Nadon G., Dann E., St. George-Hylop P.H. (1996). Prediction of probable Alzheimer's disease in memory-impaired patient: a prospective longitudinal study. *Neurology*, **46**, 661–665.
21. Bowen J., Teri L., Kukull W., McCormick W., McCurry S.M., Larson E.B. (1997). Progression to dementia in patients with isolated memory loss. *Lancet*, **349**, 763–765.
22. Devanand D.P., Folz M., Gorlyn M., Moeller J.R., Stern Y. (1997). Questionable dementia: clinical course and predictors of outcome. *J. Am. Geriatr. Soc.*, **45**, 321–328.
23. Wolf H., Grunwald M., Ecke G.M., Bettin S., Zedlick D., Dannenberg C., Dietrich J., Eschrich K., Arendt T., Gertz H.J. (1998). The prognosis of mild cognitive impairment in the elderly. *J. Neural Transm.*, **54**, 31–50.
24. Krasucki J.S., Alexander G.E., Horwitz B., Daly E.M., Murphy D.G., Rapoport S.J., Schapiro M.B. (1998). Volumes of medial temporal lobe structures in patients with Alzheimer's disease and mild cognitive impairment (and in healthy controls). *Biol. Psychiatry*, **43**, 60–68.
25. Petersen R.C., Smith G.E., Waring S.C., Irnik R.J., Tangalos E.G., Kokmen E. (1999). Mild cognitive impairment. Clinical characterization and outcome. *Arch. Neurol.*, **56**, 303–308.
26. Black S.E. (1999). Can SPECT predict the future for mild cognitive impairment? *Can. J. Neurol. Sci.*, **26**, 4–6.

27. McKelvey R., Bergman H., Stern J. (1999). Lack of prognostic significance of SPECT abnormalities in elderly subjects with a mild memory loss. *Can. J. Neurol. Sci.*, **26**, 23–28.
28. Daly E., Zaitchik D., Copeland M., Schmahmann J., Gunther J., Albert M. (2000). Predicting conversion to Alzheimer disease using standardized clinical information. *Arch. Neurol.*, **57**, 675–680.
29. Bozoki A., Giordani B., Heidebrink J.L., Berent S., Foster N.L. (2001). Mild cognitive impairments predict dementia in nondemented elderly patients with memory loss. *Arch. Neurol.*, **58**, 401–416.
30. Tabert M.H., Albert S.M. (2002). Functional deficits in patients with mild cognitive impairment. Prediction of AD. *Neurology*, **58**, 758–764.
31. Palmer K., Wang H., Bäckman L., Winblad B., Fratiglioni L. (2002). Differential evolution of cognitive impairment in nondemented older persons: results from the Kungsholmen Project. *Am. J. Psychiatry*, **159**, 436–442.
32. Folstein M.F., Folstein S.E., McHugh P.R. (1975). Mini-Mental-State: a practical method for grading the cognitive state of patients for the clinician. *J. Psychiatr. Res.*, **12**, 189–198.
33. Zaudig M., Hiller W. (1996). *SIDAM-Handbuch. Strukturiertes Interview für die Diagnose einer Demenz vom Alzheimer Typ, der vaskulären Demenz und Demenzen anderer Ätiologien nach DSM-III-R, DSM-IV und ICD-10*. Hans Huber, Bern.
34. Mohs R.C., Rosen W.G., Davis K.L. (1983). The Alzheimer's disease assessment scale: an instrument for assessing treatment efficacy. *Psychopharmacol. Bull.*, **19**, 448–450.
35. Hughes C.P., Berg L., Danziger W.L., Coben L.A., Martin R.L. (1982). A new clinical scale for the staging of dementia. *Br. J. Psychiatry*, **140**, 566–572.
36. Henderson A.S. (1992). The Canberra Interview for the Elderly: a new field instrument for the diagnoses of dementia and depression by ICD-10 and DSM-III-R. *Acta Psychiatr. Scand.*, **85**, 105–113.
37. Reisberg B., Ferris S.H., Leon M.J., Crook T. (1982). The Global Deterioration Scale (GDS): an instrument for the assessment of primary degenerative dementia (PDD). *Am. J. Psychiatry*, **139**, 1135–1139.
38. Ritchie K., Touchon J. (2000). Mild cognitive impairment: conceptual basis and current nosological status. *Lancet*, **355**, 225–228.
39. Welsh K.A., Butters N., Hughes J.P., Mohs R.C., Heyman A. (1992). Detection on staging of dementia in Alzheimer's disease. Use of the Neuropsychological Measures developed for the Consortium to Establish a Registry for Alzheimer's Disease. *Arch. Neurol.*, **49**, 448–452.
40. Petersen R.C., Doody R., Kurz A., Mohs R., Morris J.C., Rabins P.V., Ritchie K., Russor M., Thal L., Winblad B. (2001). Current concepts in mild cognitive impairment. *Neurology*, **58**, 1985–1992.
41. Jorm A.F., Jacomb P.A. (1989). The Informant Questionnaire on Cognitive Decline in the Elderly (IQCODE): socio-demographic correlates, reliability, validity and some norms. *Psychol. Med.*, **19**, 1015–1022.
42. Reisberg B., Finkel S., Overall J., Schmidt-Gollas N., Kanowski S., Hulla F., Selan S., Wilms H.-U., Lehfeld H., Heininger K., *et al.* (2001). The Alzheimer's Disease Activities of Daily Living International Scale (ADL-IS). *Int. Psychogeriatr.*, **13**, 163–181.
43. Touchon J., Ritchie K. (1999). Prodromal cognitive disorder in Alzheimer's disease. *Int. J. Geriatr. Psychiatry*, **14**, 556–563.

44. Price J.L., Ko A.I., Wade M.J., Tsou S.K., McKell D.W., Morris J.C. (2001). Neuron number in the entorhinal cortex and CA I in preclinical Alzheimer disease. *Arch. Neurol.*, **58**, 1395–1402.
45. Goldman W.P., Price J.L., Storandt M., Grant E.A., McKeel D.W., Rubin E.H., Morris J.C. (2001). Absence of cognitive impairment or decline in preclinical Alzheimer's disease. *Neurology*, **56**, 361–367.
46. Price J.L., Morris J.C. (1999). Tangles and plaques in non-demented aging and preclinical Alzheimer's disease. *Ann. Neurol.*, **45**, 358–368.
47. Collie A., Maruff P., Shafiq-Antonacci R., Smith M., Hallup M., Schofield R.P., Maslers C.C., Currie J. (2001). Memory decline in healthy older people. Implication for identifying mild cognitive impairment. *Neurology*, **56**, 1533–1538.
48. Bookheimer S.Y., Strojwas M.H., Cohen M.S., Saunders A.M., Pericak-Vance M.A., Mazziota J.C., Small G.W. (2000). Patterns of brain activation in people at risk for Alzheimer's disease. *N. Engl. J. Med.*, **343**, 450–456.
49. Schmand B., Jonker C., Geerlings M.I., Lindeboom J. (1997). Subjective memory complaints in the elderly: depressive symptoms and future dementia. *Br. J. Psychiatry*, **171**, 373–376.
50. Geerlings M.E., Jonker C., Bouter L.M., Ader J.J., Schmand B. (1999). Association between memory complaints and incident Alzheimer's disease in elderly people with normal baseline cognition. *Am. J. Psychiatry*, **156**, 531–537.
51. Jorm A.F., Chistensen H., Korten A.E., Henderson A.S., Jacomb P.A., Mackinnon A. (1997). Do cognitive complaints either predict future cognitive decline or reflect past cognitive decline? A longitudinal study of an elderly community sample. *Psychol. Med.*, **27**, 91–98.
52. Jorm A.F., Christensen H., Korten A.E., Jacomb P.A., Henderson A.S. (2001). Memory complaints as a precursor of memory impairment in older people: a longitudinal analysis over 7–8 years. *Psychol. Med.*, **31**, 441–449.
53. Hogan D.B., Ebly E.M. (2000). Predicting who will develop dementia in a cohort of Canadian seniors. *Can. J. Neurol. Sci.*, **27**, 18–24.
54. Schofield P.W., Marder K., Dooneief G., Jacobs D.M., Sano M., Stern Y. (1997). Association of subjective memory complaints with subsequent cognitive decline in community-dwelling elderly individuals with baseline cognitive impairment. *Am. J. Psychiatry*, **154**, 609–615.
55. Dik M.G., Jonker C., Comijs H.C., Bouter L.M., Twisk J.W.R., van Kamp G.J., Deeg D.J.H. (2001). Memory complaints and APOE-ε4 accelerate cognitive decline in cognitively normal elderly. *Neurology*, **57**, 217–222.
56. DeGroot J.C., deLeuw F.E., Oudkerk M., Hofman A., Jolles J., Breteler M.M.B. (2001). Cerebral white matter lesions and subjective cognitive dysfunction. The Rotterdam Scan Study. *Neurology*, **56**, 1539–1545.
57. Hampel H., Buerger K., Zinkowski R., Teipel S.J., Goernitz A., Andreasen N., Sjoegren M., DeBernardis J., Kerkman D., Ichiguro K., *et al.* (2004). Measurement of phosphorylated tau epitopes in the differential diagnoses of Alzheimer's disease. A comparative cerebrospinal fluid study. *Arch. Gen. Psychiatry*, **61**, 95–102.
58. Sunderland T., Wolozin B., Galasko D. (1999). Longitudinal stability of CSF tau levels in Alzheimer patients. *Biol. Psychiatry*, **46**, 750–755.
59. Galasko D. (1999). Cerebrospinal fluid opens a window on Alzheimer's disease. *Arch. Neurol.*, **56**, 655–656.
60. Okamura N., Arai H., Maroyama M., Iguchi M., Mazui T., Tanji H., Seki T., Hirai H., Chiba H., Itoh M., *et al.* (2002). Combined analysis of CSF tau levels and [(123)I] iodoamphetamine SPECT in mild cognitive impairment: implications for a novel predictor of Alzheimer's disease. *Am. J. Psychiatry*, **159**, 474–476.

61. Kantarci K., Xu Y., Shiung M.M. (2002). Comparative diagnostic utility of different MR modalities in mild cognitive impairment and Alzheimer's disease. *J. Dem. Geriatr. Cogn. Dis.*, **14**, 198–207.
62. DeSanti S., DeLion M.J., Rusinek H., Convit A., Tarshik C.Y., Roche A., Tsui W.H., Kandil E., Boppana M., Daisly K., *et al.* (2001). Hippocampal formation glucose metabolism and volume losses in MCI and AD. *Neurobiol. Aging*, **22**, 529–539.
63. Kennedy A.M., Frackowiak R.S., Newman S.K. (1995). Deficits in cerebral glucose metabolism demonstrated by positron emission tomography in individuals at risk of familial Alzheimer's disease. *Neurosci. Lett.*, **186**, 17–20.
64. Kordower J.H., Chu Y., Stebbins G.T., Dekosky S.T., Cochran E.J., Bennet D., Mufson E.J. (2001). Loss and atrophy of layer II entorhinal cortex neurons in elderly people with mild cognitive impairment. *Neurology*, **49**, 202–213.
65. Du A.T., Schuff N., Amend D., Laakso M.P., Hsu Y.Y., Jagust W.J., Yaffe K., Kramer J.H., Reed B., Norman D., *et al.* (2001). Magnetic resonance imaging of the entorhinal cortex and hippocampus in mild cognitive impairment and Alzheimer's disease. *J. Neurol. Neurosurg. Psychiatry*, **71**, 441–447.
66. Robins E., Guze S. (1970). Establishment of diagnostic validity in psychiatric illnesses: its application to schizophrenia. *Am. J. Psychiatry*, **126**, 983–987.

Index

Early Detection and Management of Mental Disorders.
Edited by Mario Maj, Juan José López-Ibor, Norman Sartorius, Mitsumoto Sato and Ahmed Okasha.
 ISBN 0-470-01083-5.